Advanced Dental Materials: From Design to Application

Advanced Dental Materials: From Design to Application

Guest Editors

**Josip Kranjčić
Tina Poklepovic Pericic**

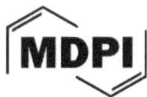

Basel • Beijing • Wuhan • Barcelona • Belgrade • Novi Sad • Cluj • Manchester

Guest Editors

Josip Kranjčić
School of Dental Medicine
University of Zagreb
Zagreb
Croatia

Tina Poklepovic Pericic
School of Medicine
University of Split
Split
Croatia

Editorial Office
MDPI AG
Grosspeteranlage 5
4052 Basel, Switzerland

This is a reprint of the Special Issue, published open access by the journal *Materials* (ISSN 1996-1944), freely accessible at: www.mdpi.com/journal/materials/special_issues/7532343325.

For citation purposes, cite each article independently as indicated on the article page online and using the guide below:

Lastname, A.A.; Lastname, B.B. Article Title. *Journal Name* **Year**, *Volume Number*, Page Range.

ISBN 978-3-7258-3202-6 (Hbk)
ISBN 978-3-7258-3201-9 (PDF)
https://doi.org/10.3390/books978-3-7258-3201-9

© 2025 by the authors. Articles in this book are Open Access and distributed under the Creative Commons Attribution (CC BY) license. The book as a whole is distributed by MDPI under the terms and conditions of the Creative Commons Attribution-NonCommercial-NoDerivs (CC BY-NC-ND) license (https://creativecommons.org/licenses/by-nc-nd/4.0/).

Contents

About the Editors . . . . **vii**

Preface . . . . **ix**

Josip Kranjcic and Tina Poklepovic Pericic
Advanced Dental Materials: From Design to Application
Reprinted from: *Materials* **2024**, *17*, 3667, https://doi.org/10.3390/ma17153667 . . . . **1**

Nazli Aydin, Selin Celik Oge, Ogulcan Guney, Onur Okbaz and Yasar Sertdemir
A Comparison of the Shear Bond Strength between a Luting Composite Resin and Both Machinable and Printable Ceramic–Glass Polymer Materials
Reprinted from: *Materials* **2024**, *17*, 4697, https://doi.org/10.3390/ma17194697 . . . . **3**

Wolfgang Bömicke, Franz Sebastian Schwindling, Peter Rammelsberg and Stefan Rues
Bond Strength of Milled and Printed Zirconia to 10-Methacryloyloxydecyl Dihydrogen Phosphate (10-MDP) Resin Cement as a Function of Ceramic Conditioning, Disinfection and Ageing
Reprinted from: *Materials* **2024**, *17*, 2159, https://doi.org/10.3390/ma17092159 . . . . **15**

Lara Berger, Ragai-Edward Matta, Christian Markus Weiß, Werner Adler, Manfred Wichmann and José Ignacio Zorzin
Effect of Luting Materials on the Accuracy of Fit of Zirconia Copings: A Non-Destructive Digital Analysis Method
Reprinted from: *Materials* **2024**, *17*, 2130, https://doi.org/10.3390/ma17092130 . . . . **29**

Josip Vuksic, Ana Pilipovic, Tina Poklepovic Pericic and Josip Kranjcic
The Influence of Contemporary Denture Base Fabrication Methods on Residual Monomer Content, Flexural Strength and Microhardness
Reprinted from: *Materials* **2024**, *17*, 1052, https://doi.org/10.3390/ma17051052 . . . . **43**

Josip Vuksic, Ana Pilipovic, Tina Poklepovic Pericic and Josip Kranjcic
Tensile Bond Strength between Different Denture Base Materials and Soft Denture Liners
Reprinted from: *Materials* **2023**, *16*, 4615, https://doi.org/10.3390/ma16134615 . . . . **58**

Zbigniew Raszewski, Katarzyna Chojnacka, Marcin Mikulewicz and Abdulaziz Alhotan
Bioactive Glass-Enhanced Resins: A New Denture Base Material
Reprinted from: *Materials* **2023**, *16*, 4363, https://doi.org/10.3390/ma16124363 . . . . **71**

Koudai Nagata, Keitaro Inaba, Katsuhiko Kimoto and Hiromasa Kawana
Accuracy of Dental Models Fabricated Using Recycled Poly-Lactic Acid
Reprinted from: *Materials* **2023**, *16*, 2620, https://doi.org/10.3390/ma16072620 . . . . **84**

Nicolae Daniel Olteanu, Ionut Taraboanta, Tinela Panaite, Carina Balcos, Sorana Nicoleta Rosu and Raluca Maria Vieriu et al.
Color Stability of Various Orthodontic Clear Aligner Systems after Submersion in Different Staining Beverages
Reprinted from: *Materials* **2024**, *17*, 4009, https://doi.org/10.3390/ma17164009 . . . . **95**

Ragai Edward Matta, Lara Berger, Moritz Loehlein, Linus Leven, Juergen Taxis and Manfred Wichmann et al.
Stress Distribution within the Peri-Implant Bone for Different Implant Materials Obtained by Digital Image Correlation
Reprinted from: *Materials* **2024**, *17*, 2161, https://doi.org/10.3390/ma17092161 . . . . **107**

Kana Wakamori, Koudai Nagata, Toshifumi Nakashizu, Hayato Tsuruoka, Mihoko Atsumi and Hiromasa Kawana
Comparative Verification of the Accuracy of Implant Models Made of PLA, Resin, and Silicone
Reprinted from: *Materials* **2023**, *16*, 3307, https://doi.org/10.3390/ma16093307 117

Xin Zhang, Yuxuan Zhang, Ying Li, Xiaoming Wang and Xueqin Zhang
Restorative Dental Resin Functionalized with Calcium Methacrylate with a Hydroxyapatite Remineralization Capacity
Reprinted from: *Materials* **2023**, *16*, 6497, https://doi.org/10.3390/ma16196497 128

Anna A. Forysenkova, Inna V. Fadeeva, Dina V. Deyneko, Alevtina N. Gosteva, Georgy V. Mamin and Darya V. Shurtakova et al.
Polyvinylpyrrolidone—Alginate—Carbonate Hydroxyapatite Porous Composites for Dental Applications
Reprinted from: *Materials* **2023**, *16*, 4478, https://doi.org/10.3390/ma16124478 145

Aniruddha Pal, Ayako Oyane, Tomoya Inose, Maki Nakamura, Erika Nishida and Hirofumi Miyaji
Fabrication of Ciprofloxacin-Immobilized Calcium Phosphate Particles for Dental Drug Delivery
Reprinted from: *Materials* **2024**, *17*, 2035, https://doi.org/10.3390/ma17092035 161

Franz-Josef Schröter and Nicoleta Ilie
Pushout Bond Strength in Coronal Dentin: A Standardization Approach in Comparison to Shear Bond Strength
Reprinted from: *Materials* **2023**, *16*, 5667, https://doi.org/10.3390/ma16165667 176

About the Editors

Josip Kranjčić

Josip Kranjčić is a prosthodontist and an Associate Professor at the University of Zagreb School of Dental Medicine.

As a student, he was the best in his year, earning five consecutive Dean's Awards. Since 2011, he has been employed as an Assistant at the Department of Fixed Prosthodontics at the School of Dental Medicine in Zagreb. In 2014, he spent time at the Smithsonian Institution in Washington, D.C., USA, where he researched the characteristics of the temporomandibular joint in North American historical populations as part of his doctoral dissertation. That same year, he also participated in the "Young Prosthodontic Educators Workshop", organized by the International College of Prosthodontists in Germany. He successfully defended his doctoral dissertation, titled "Research on Anthropometric Measures of Temporomandibular Joint's Articular Eminence on Historical Samples" in 2016. He also completed his specialization in prosthetic dentistry in 2016. In 2017, he was promoted to Assistant Professor, and in 2022, he was appointed Associate Professor at the Department of Fixed Prosthodontics, University of Zagreb School of Dental Medicine.

As a specialist in prosthetic dentistry, he works at the University Hospital "Dubrava" in Zagreb. He has participated in scientific projects funded by the Croatian Science Foundation. He has published several scientific and professional papers in domestic and international journals and has actively participated in numerous international conferences. He is also a Guest Editor for the scientific journal *Materials*.

Tina Poklepovic Pericic

Tina Poklepović Peričić is a prosthodontist and an Assistant Professor at the University of Split School of Medicine, where she teaches research methodology and prosthodontics.

Since 2009, she has been actively involved in the voluntary work of Cochrane Croatia, first as a dental medicine coordinator and from 2015 to 2022 as a co-director of the Centre.

Her interests include systematic reviews, the dissemination of evidence, and education. Since 2019, she has been a member of the international GRADE working group, which assesses the certainty of research evidence and develops clinical practice guidelines.

She has authored various papers on evidence synthesis, clinical practice guidelines, and scientific methodology.

She has also been a reviewer for several scientific journals and an Editorial Board Member for *BMC Medical Research Methodology*, *Systematic Reviews*, and *Frontiers in Medicine*.

In addition to leading an ongoing EU project on fact-checking, she led the international Erasmus + project "Evidence Implementation in Clinical Practice" and has been coordinating the global initiative "Informed Health Choices" in Croatia, which deals with teaching children and the public about critical thinking regarding health issues. She collaborated with the WHO in collecting and analyzing the available evidence for selecting and using the essential medicines list and is now involved in a WHO project on ageing. Also, Tina Poklepović Peričić recently joined the European WHO Network for Clinical Practice Guidelines. She was a clinical advisor to the Cochrane Clinical Answers and participated in the EVBRES (Evidence-Based Research) COST Action CA-17117 project on evidence-based research.

Preface

The field of dental materials has seen remarkable advancements in recent years, with innovative designs and applications transforming modern dental practice. This reprint, *Advanced Dental Materials: From Design to Application*, aims to provide a comprehensive overview of the latest developments in dental material science, exploring underlying principles, cutting-edge technologies, and real-world applications. It is intended for dental professionals, researchers, and students who seek a deeper understanding of the materials shaping the future of dentistry. We hope that this work will inspire further exploration and innovation, bridging the gap between material design and clinical use.

Josip Kranjčić and Tina Poklepovic Pericic
Guest Editors

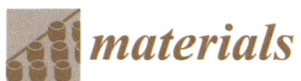 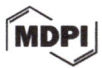

Editorial

Advanced Dental Materials: From Design to Application

Josip Kranjcic [1,2,*] and Tina Poklepovic Pericic [3,*]

1. Department of Prosthodontics, University Hospital Dubrava, Av. Gojka Šuška 6, 10000 Zagreb, Croatia
2. Department of Fixed Prosthodontics, University of Zagreb School of Dental Medicine, Gunduliceva 5, 10000 Zagreb, Croatia
3. School of Medicine, University of Split, Šoltanska 2, 21000 Split, Croatia
* Correspondence: kranjcic@sfzg.unizg.hr (J.K.); tinapoklepovic@gmail.com (T.P.P.)

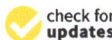

Citation: Kranjcic, J.; Poklepovic Pericic, T. Advanced Dental Materials: From Design to Application. *Materials* **2024**, *17*, 3667. https://doi.org/10.3390/ma17153667

Received: 12 July 2024
Accepted: 20 July 2024
Published: 25 July 2024

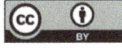

Copyright: © 2024 by the authors. Licensee MDPI, Basel, Switzerland. This article is an open access article distributed under the terms and conditions of the Creative Commons Attribution (CC BY) license (https://creativecommons.org/licenses/by/4.0/).

The title of this Special Issue is "Advanced Dental Materials: From Design to Application". This is a very specific topic related to the rapid development of dentistry and, therefore, also of dental materials. The expectations of patients and the requirements of dentists are also increasing daily. Significant efforts are being invested in developing and improving the properties of the dental materials used in daily practice. The aesthetic properties of the materials are very important, but so are their mechanical and physical properties, i.e., their ability to withstand the stresses of a very dynamic environment—the oral cavity.

This Special Issue provides readers with up-to-date information on the properties of various materials: ceramics, acrylic resin, and composite materials, as well as dental alloys and their application in the field of prosthodontics using analog and digital technologies—additive and subtractive manufacturing technologies.

Twelve high-quality research papers were published in this Special Issue, covering a period of almost one and a half years. More than 60 authors from many institutions worldwide have contributed to the published articles.

Matta RE et al. (1) contributed a paper entitled "Stress Distribution within the Peri-Implant Bone for Different Implant Materials Obtained by Digital Image Correlation"; Bömicke W et al. (2) contributed a paper entitled "Bond Strength of Milled and Printed Zirconia to 10-Methacryloyloxydecyl Dihydrogen Phosphate (10-MDP) Resin Cement as a Function of Ceramic Conditioning, Disinfection and Ageing"; Berger L et al. (3) contributed a paper entitled "Effect of Luting Materials on the Accuracy of Fit of Zirconia Copings: A Non-Destructive Digital Analysis Method"; Pal A et al. (4) contributed a paper entitled "Fabrication of Ciprofloxacin-Immobilized Calcium Phosphate Particles for Dental Drug Delivery"; Vuksic J et al. (5,6) contributed papers entitled "The Influence of Contemporary Denture Base Fabrication Methods on Residual Monomer Content, Flexural Strength and Microhardness" and "Tensile Bond Strength between Different Denture Base Materials and Soft Denture Liners"; Zhang X et al. (7) contributed a paper entitled "Restorative Dental Resin Functionalized with Calcium Methacrylate with a Hydroxyapatite Remineralization Capacity"; Schröter FJ et al. (8) contributed a paper entitled "Pushout Bond Strength in Coronal Dentin: A Standardization Approach in Comparison to Shear Bond Strength"; Forysenkova AA et al. (9) contributed a paper entitled "Polyvinylpyrrolidone–Alginate–Carbonate Hydroxyapatite Porous Composites for Dental Applications"; Raszewski Z et al. (10) contributed a paper entitled "Bioactive Glass-Enhanced Resins: A New Denture Base Material"; Wakamori K et al. (11) contributed a paper entitled "Comparative Verification of the Accuracy of Implant Models Made of PLA, Resin, and Silicone", and Nagata K et al. (12) contributed a paper entitled "Accuracy of Dental Models Fabricated Using Recycled Poly-Lactic Acid".

This Special Issue provides readers with many scientific facts, but also serves as a link between science and clinical practice. We would also like to express our sincere thanks to all the authors who have contributed to this Special Issue. Their valuable research has made this Special Issue possible and we greatly appreciate their efforts.

Author Contributions: Both authors equally contributed to this research. All authors have read and agreed to the published version of the manuscript.

Conflicts of Interest: The authors declare no conflicts of interest.

List of Contributions:

1. Matta, R.E.; Berger, L.; Loehlein, M.; Leven, L.; Taxis, J.; Wichmann, M.; Motel, C. Stress Distribution within the Peri-Implant Bone for Different Implant Materials Obtained by Digital Image Correlation. *Materials* **2024**, *17*, 2161. https://doi.org/10.3390/ma17092161.
2. Bömicke, W.; Schwindling, F.S.; Rammelsberg, P.; Rues, S. Bond Strength of Milled and Printed Zirconia to 10-Methacryloyloxydecyl Dihydrogen Phosphate (10-MDP) Resin Cement as a Function of Ceramic Conditioning, Disinfection and Ageing. *Materials* **2024**, *17*, 2159. https://doi.org/10.3390/ma17092159.
3. Berger, L.; Matta, R.-E.; Weiß, C.M.; Adler, W.; Wichmann, M.; Zorzin, J.I. Effect of Luting Materials on the Accuracy of Fit of Zirconia Copings: A Non-Destructive Digital Analysis Method. *Materials* **2024**, *17*, 2130. https://doi.org/10.3390/ma17092130.
4. Pal, A.; Oyane, A.; Inose, T.; Nakamura, M.; Nishida, E.; Miyaji, H. Fabrication of Ciprofloxacin-Immobilized Calcium Phosphate Particles for Dental Drug Delivery. *Materials* **2024**, *17*, 2035. https://doi.org/10.3390/ma17092035.
5. Vuksic, J.; Pilipovic, A.; Poklepovic Pericic, T.; Kranjcic, J. The Influence of Contemporary Denture Base Fabrication Methods on Residual Monomer Content, Flexural Strength and Microhardness. *Materials* **2024**, *17*, 1052. https://doi.org/10.3390/ma17051052.
6. Vuksic, J.; Pilipovic, A.; Poklepovic Pericic, T.; Kranjcic, J. Tensile Bond Strength between Different Denture Base Materials and Soft Denture Liners. *Materials* **2023**, *16*, 4615. https://doi.org/10.3390/ma16134615.
7. Zhang, X.; Zhang, Y.; Li, Y.; Wang, X.; Zhang, X. Restorative Dental Resin Functionalized with Calcium Methacrylate with a Hydroxyapatite Remineralization Capacity. *Materials* **2023**, *16*, 6497. https://doi.org/10.3390/ma16196497.
8. Schröter, F.-J.; Ilie, N. Pushout Bond Strength in Coronal Dentin: A Standardization Approach in Comparison to Shear Bond Strength. *Materials* **2023**, *16*, 5667. https://doi.org/10.3390/ma16165667.
9. Forysenkova, A.A.; Fadeeva, I.V.; Deyneko, D.V.; Gosteva, A.N.; Mamin, G.V.; Shurtakova, D.V.; Davydova, G.A.; Yankova, V.G.; Antoniac, I.V.; Rau, J.V. Polyvinylpyrrolidone—Alginate—Carbonate Hydroxyapatite Porous Composites for Dental Applications. *Materials* **2023**, *16*, 4478. https://doi.org/10.3390/ma16124478.
10. Raszewski, Z.; Chojnacka, K.; Mikulewicz, M.; Alhotan, A. Bioactive Glass-Enhanced Resins: A New Denture Base Material. *Materials* **2023**, *16*, 4363. https://doi.org/10.3390/ma16124363.
11. Wakamori, K.; Nagata, K.; Nakashizu, T.; Tsuruoka, H.; Atsumi, M.; Kawana, H. Comparative Verification of the Accuracy of Implant Models Made of PLA, Resin, and Silicone. *Materials* **2023**, *16*, 3307. https://doi.org/10.3390/ma16093307.
12. Nagata, K.; Inaba, K.; Kimoto, K.; Kawana, H. Accuracy of Dental Models Fabricated Using Recycled Poly-Lactic Acid. *Materials* **2023**, *16*, 2620. https://doi.org/10.3390/ma16072620.

Disclaimer/Publisher's Note: The statements, opinions and data contained in all publications are solely those of the individual author(s) and contributor(s) and not of MDPI and/or the editor(s). MDPI and/or the editor(s) disclaim responsibility for any injury to people or property resulting from any ideas, methods, instructions or products referred to in the content.

Article

A Comparison of the Shear Bond Strength between a Luting Composite Resin and Both Machinable and Printable Ceramic–Glass Polymer Materials

Nazli Aydin [1,2,*], Selin Celik Oge [1], Ogulcan Guney [3], Onur Okbaz [3] and Yasar Sertdemir [4]

1. Department of Prosthodontics, Faculty of Dentistry, Cukurova University, Adana 01250, Turkey; selincelik@cu.edu.tr
2. The Abdi Sutcu Vocational School of Health Services, Cukurova University, Adana 01790, Turkey
3. Faculty of Dentistry, Cukurova University, Adana 01250, Turkey; ogulcanguney04@gmail.com (O.G.); onurokbaz98@gmail.com (O.O.)
4. Department of Biostatistics and Medical Informatics, Faculty of Medicine, Cukurova University, Adana 01790, Turkey; yasarser@cu.edu.tr
* Correspondence: nazli.yesilyurt.aydin@gmail.com

Abstract: This study aims to compare the shear bond strength (SBS) and Weibull characteristics between a luting composite resin and both printable and two different machinable ceramic–glass polymer materials. A total of 36 substrates were prepared, with 12 in each group. Printable substrates (12 mm × 12 mm × 2 mm) were printed by using permanent crown resin (3D-PR). Machinable substrates were obtained from Cerasmart 270 (CS) and Vita Enamic (VE) blocks (2 mm in thickness). The bonding surfaces of substrates were polished and airborne abraded (50 μm Al_2O_3). A self-adhesive luting composite resin (RelyX U200, 3M ESPE, St. Paul, MN, USA, SLC) was applied on substrates with the help of a cylindrical (Ø3 × 3 mm) mold. The SBS test was conducted using a universal test machine. The SBSs of three materials were compared using a one-way analysis of variance (ANOVA) ($\alpha = 0.05$). The Weibull modulus was calculated for each material. The Kruskal–Wallis and chi-square tests were carried out for the failure mode analysis. There was no significant difference between the SBSs of the three materials ($p = 0.129$). The Weibull modulus was 3.76 for the 3D-PR, 4.22 for the CS, and 6.52 for the VE group. Statistical analysis showed no significant difference between the failure modes of the groups ($p = 0.986$). Mixed-failure fractures were predominantly observed in all three groups. The results show that the SBS of the SLC to printable 3D-PR is comparable to that of CS and VE material. Failure modes of printable 3D-PR show similar results with two different machinable ceramic–glass polymers.

Keywords: three-dimensional printing; 3D printed permanent resin; printable permanent resin; ceramic glass polymer materials; shear bond strength; self-adhesive luting composite

1. Introduction

Chairside computer-aided design and computer-aided manufacturing (CAD/CAM) technology and CAD/CAM dental materials have been evolving and diversifying [1–5]. Currently, ceramics and composites are available esthetic materials in this field, and they have many advantages and disadvantages [1,3,5]. Therefore, ceramic–glass polymer materials were developed to combine the benefits of ceramics and composites, such as lower abrasive effects, durability, ease of fabrication, polishability, and intraoral reparability because of their resin content [2,6]. Polymer-infiltrated-ceramic network materials (VITA Enamic) (VE) and force-absorbing hybrid ceramics (Cerasmart 270) (CS) are commercially available machinable ceramic–glass polymer materials [5,7–11]. These materials are highly attractive for dental practice, as they are industrially polymerized blocks with no need for any post-milling processes such as firing or curing [5,7].

Additive manufacturing (AM) is also a part of CAD/CAM technology, along with subtractive manufacturing (SM) [12–15]. AM saves material as it only uses the amount of the definitive product and can produce more complex geometries, unlike the SM [16,17]. Furthermore, the manufacturers recommend that the built object require a post-processing step (such as cleaning with alcohol and post-polymerization) in order to stabilize the mechanical and biological properties [12,14,18]. One of the printable ceramic–glass polymer materials, VarseoSmile Crown Plus (3D-PR), has recently been developed for permanent restorations that can be printed in one session [15,19–21].

The strength and durability of the bond between the restoration and luting agent are one of the most crucial factors for the restoration's success [3,8,9,18,22–24]. Ideally, luting composite resins are suggested for long-term successful restorations [3,4,8,25,26]. Self-adhesive luting composite resins (SLCs) have commonly been used as modern luting agents that eliminate the preprocessing of teeth tissue [4,22,26,27]. The adhesion of SLC to tooth structure has been clarified and documented in great detail in previous studies [22,26,28]. However, the factors affecting the restoration side are also important. The susceptibility of the bonding surface to physical or chemical modification is determined by the type of material and fabrication technique, such as casting, pressing, sintering, and machining [3,29].

In the literature, the mechanical and optical properties of 3D-PR have been compared with machinable ceramic–glass polymer materials, but no studies have compared the bond strengths with an SLC [15,20]. There are many laboratory studies evaluating the bond strengths of SLC to machinable ceramic–glass polymer materials [4,6,9,23,30]. The in vitro comparison of a printable ceramic–glass polymer material with machinable ones can be a useful method for pre-estimating the clinical performance of bond strength. Prior to clinical dental applications, Weibull statistics are important for evaluating the reliability of bond strength tests and understanding specimens' structural reliability and strength properties [26,31–33]. Whereas limited data are available on the bond strength of 3D printed temporary resin to luting composite resins, the authors are unaware of previous research on 3D-PR [18,34].

The purpose of this study is to compare the shear bond strengths (SBSs) of an SLC to printable 3D-PR and two different machinable ceramic–glass polymers, VE and CS; and then evaluate the Weibull distribution of tested materials. The null hypothesis stated that there would be no difference in terms of the SBS of the SLC to the printable 3D-PR, and machinable VE or CS.

2. Materials and Methods

According to our power analysis, to detect a difference of MPa ≥ 2 with 80% power and a 0.05 significance level at a standard deviation of 2.5, a total of 36 samples, 12 per group, were calculated. Table 1 describes the information about the materials used in this study. Randomization was performed using a web-based, free tool (research randomizer Version 4.0, access date: 8 January 2021, http://www.randomizer.org) to eliminate bias across groups in specimen selection. This in vitro study required no ethical approval.

Table 1. Manufacturers and contents of the materials used in the study.

	Material	Manufacturer	Composition	Lot Number
Machinable Blocks	(CS) Cerasmart 270	GC Dental Products, Leuven, Belgium	Organic part: Bis-MEPP, UDMA, DMA Inorganic part: 71 wt% silica (0.02 µm) and barium glass (0.3 µm) nanoparticles	2102176
	(VE) VITA Enamic	VITA Zahnfabrik, Bad Säckingen, Germany	Organic part: UDMA, TEGDMA Inorganic part: 86 wt% glass ceramic (SiO_2, Al_2O_3, Na_2O, K_2O, and other oxides)	73340

Table 1. Cont.

Material		Manufacturer	Composition	Lot Number
Printable Resin	(3D-PR) VarseoSmile Crown Plus is distributed by Formlabs as Permanent Crown	Bego, Bremen, Germany	4′-isopropylidiphenol, ethoxylated and 2-methylprop-2enoic acid. Silanized dental glass, methyl benzoylformate, diphenyl (2,4,6-trimethylbenzoyl) phosphine oxide, 30–50 wt% inorganic fillers (particle size 0.7 μm)	600163
Self-adhesive luting composite	(SLC) RelyX™ U200	3M ESPE, St. Paul, MN, USA	Base paste: Silane-treated glass filler, 2-propenoic acid, 2-methyl 1,1′-[1-(hydroxymethyl)-1,2-ethanediyl] ester, triethylene dimethacrylate, sodium persulfate andper—3,5,5-trimethylhexanoate t-butyl. Catalyst paste: Silanated filler, dimethacrylate, silane-treated filler, sodium p-toluenesulfonate,1-benzyl-5-phenyl-baric acid, calcium salts, 1,12-dodecane dimethacrylate, calcium hydroxide and titanium dioxide (~70 wt% filler)	7784355

2.1. Preparation of Substrates

Using CAD software (free version, access date: 4 December 2021, https://www.blender.org; Blender Foundation, The Netherlands, Amsterdam), 3D-PR substrates with dimensions of 12 mm × 12 mm × 2 mm were designed and exported as a standard tessellation language (STL) file. According to the STL data, twelve 3D-PR substrates were printed by using a 3D printer (Form 3B; Formlabs, Somerville, MA, USA) (90 degrees printing orientation, LED, λ = 405 nm, the layer thickness of 50 μm). After the printing was complete, the substrates were immersed in isopropyl alcohol (IPA $\geq$ 99%) for 3 min in a washer (Form Wash; Formlabs, Somerville, MA, USA). Then, they were polymerized in a unit (Form Cure; Formlabs, Somerville, MA, USA) at 60 °C for 20 min. After the supports had been eliminated, the second polymerization was carried out for 20 min.

Next, 2 mm thickness machinable VE and CS substrates were cut from each block using a water-cooled cutting instrument (Accutom-10; Struers, OH, USA). Subsequently, all substrates were embedded in autopolymerized acrylic resin (Imicryl SC; Imicryl Dental Materials, Konya, Turkey) with a silicone mold (3 cm × 2.5 cm × 2 cm) (Presigum; President Dental GmbH, Germany). The bonding surfaces were polished with silicon carbide abrasive papers (800- and 1200-grit) to standardize them. Then, each substrate underwent 50 μm Al_2O_3 airborne particle abrasion (Korox 50; Bego, Bremen, Germany) for 15 s at a pressure of 0.1 MPa at a distance of 10 mm. After ultrasonically cleaning with distilled water, they were air-dried.

2.2. Application of Luting Composite Resin

After machinable and printable substrates were prepared, the SLC was mixed and filled to the top of the cylindrical silicone mold (Ø3 × 3 mm) (Presigum; President Dental GmbH, Germany). The light power intensity of the light polymerization unit (Rainbow LED Curing Light, Liang Ya Dental Equipment Co., Ltd., Guangzhou, China) was measured to 950 mW/cm^2 (Demetron LED Radiometer, SDS Kerr, Middleton, WI, USA). The top surfaces of the specimens were polymerized for 20 s. After removing the silicone mold, the specimens were polymerized on the four proximal sides and the top for 20 s each in order to polymerize them completely. Before testing for SBS, every specimen was submerged in distilled water to 37 $\pm$ 2 °C for 24 $\pm$ 2 h.

2.3. Shear Bond Strength (SBS) Test

A universal test machine (Testometric M500-25AT; Testometric Co., Ltd., Rochdale, UK) was used to perform the macro-SBS test at the crosshead speed of 1 mm/min until the specimens failed (Figure 1). A notch-shaped rod was used to apply the testing load. The bonding interface was parallel to the loading direction. Failure loads were recorded, and SBS values of the specimens were calculated using the formula: SBS = $\frac{L}{A}$, where L is the load at failure (Newton), and A is the specimen's bonding area (mm^2). The mean SBS was calculated for each study group.

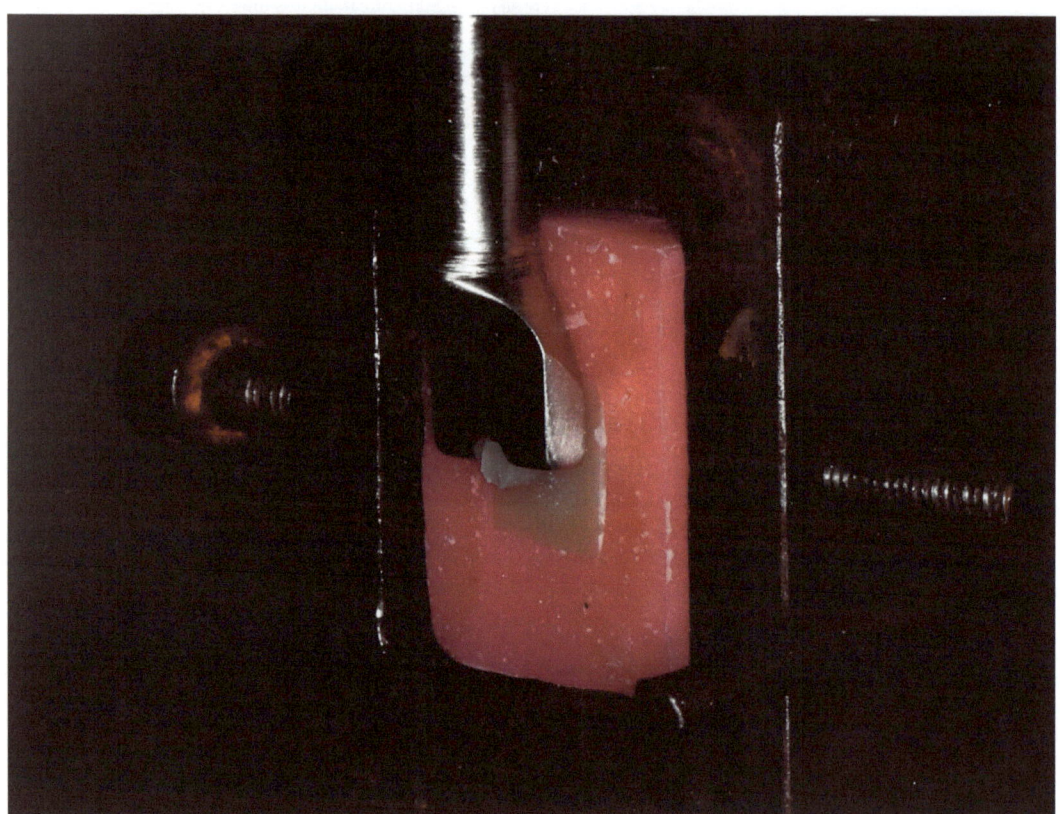

Figure 1. Shear bond strength test design.

2.4. Microscopic Characterization of Failure Modes

The failure modes were analyzed by using an optical microscope (×40 Zeiss Primostar; Carl Zeiss, Germany) after the SBS test was completed. Failure modes were categorized as (1) adhesive, failure at the bonding line, no remnants from SLC; (2) mixed, failure line comprises both restorative material and luting composite (partially restorative material, partially SLC visible); (3) cohesive failure in luting composite, fracture surface consists of only SLC; (4) cohesive failure in restorative material, fracture surface consists of only restorative material. The scanning electron microscope (SEM) (FEI; Quanta 650 FEG, Salem, OR, USA.) was used to acquire representative photographs of failure modes at a magnification of ×80 (Figure 2a–c).

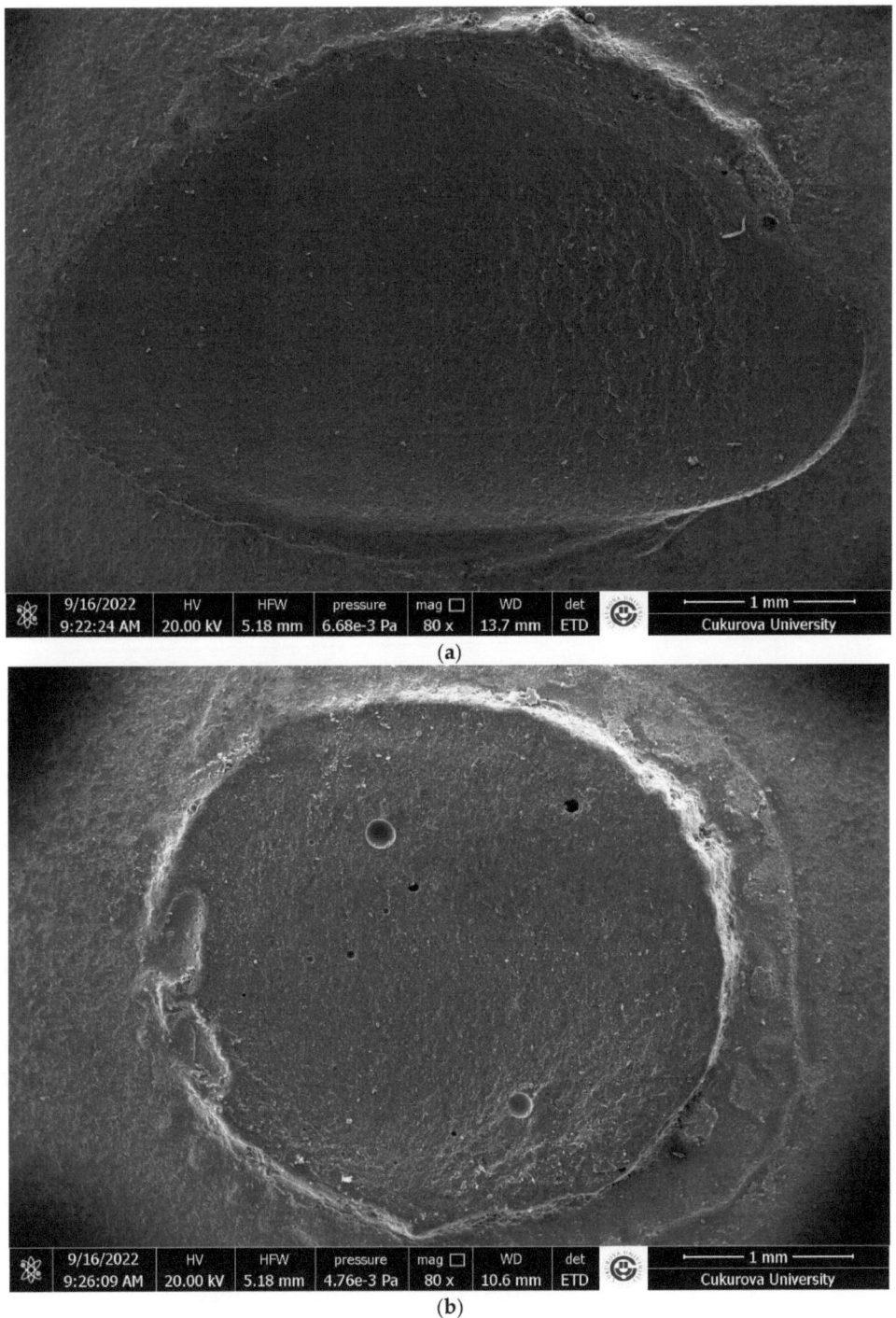

Figure 2. *Cont.*

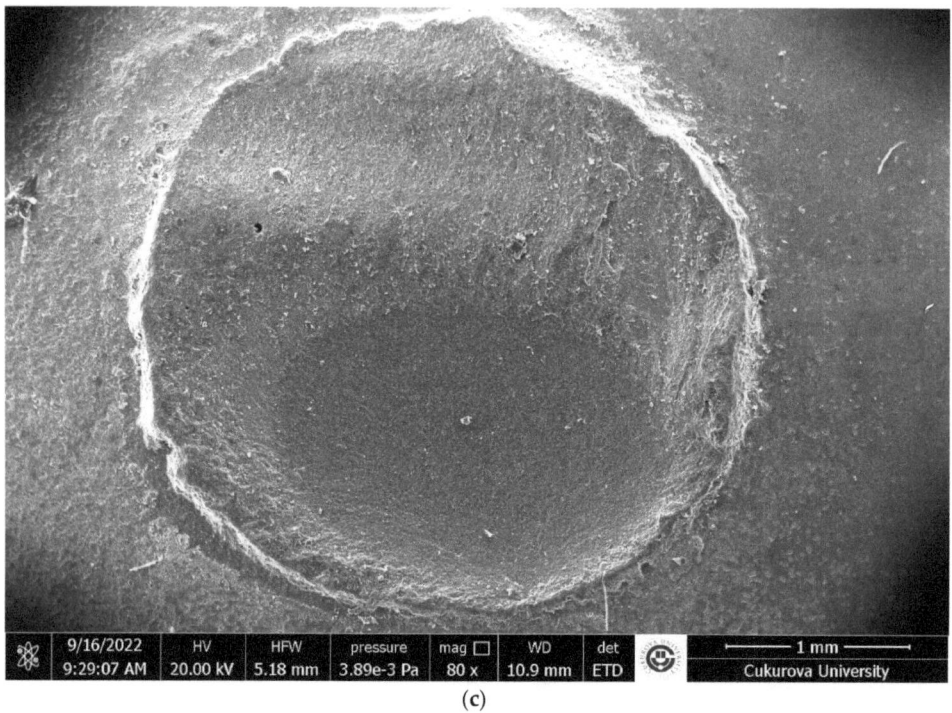

(c)

Figure 2. (a) Cohesive failure in restorative material, scanning electron microscope image (×80 magnification). (b) Cohesive failure in luting composite, scanning electron microscope image (×80 magnification). (c) Mixed failure, scanning electron microscope image (×80 magnification).

2.5. Statistical Analysis

A statistical software program (IBM SPSS v20.0; IBM Corp., Armonk, NY, USA) was used for the statistical analysis of the collected data. The Levene test showed that the data were normally distributed. In addition to the descriptive analysis, a 1-way analysis of variance (ANOVA) was used for evaluating the SBS measurements ($\alpha = 0.05$). The Kruskal–Wallis test and chi-square test were used for the failure mode analysis. In addition, a Weibull analysis was conducted and Weibull modulus' were calculated [31].

3. Results

3.1. Shear Bond Strength (SBS) and Weibull Modulus

Table 2 represents the mean SBSs and standard deviations for all tested groups. The highest mean SBS value (12.03 ± 2.11 MPa) was observed in the VE, and the lowest mean SBS value (9.74 ± 2.88 MPa) was observed in the 3D-PR, among the tested groups. Statistically, the variance was homogeneous among groups ($p = 0.529$). There was no significant difference among the three groups (ANOVA, $p = 0.129$). In accordance with the Weibull analysis (Figure 3), the highest Weibull modulus was observed for VE ($m = 6.52$) followed by CS ($m = 4.22$), and the data for the machinable ceramic–glass polymer materials were distributed uniformly. Although the lowest Weibull modulus was seen for the 3D-PR ($m = 3.76$), a printable ceramic–glass polymer was also observed to have a homogeneous distribution.

Table 2. Mean and standard deviation (SD) of the shear bond strength (MPa) with confidence intervals (95% CI) values of tested groups.

Material	N	Mean ± SD (MPa)	95% CI	p
3D-PR (Permanent Crown)	12	9.74 ± 2.88	[7.91; 11.58]	
VE (VITA Enamic)	12	12.03 ± 2.11	[10.68; 13.37]	0.129
CS (Cerasmart 270)	12	11.02 ± 2.96	[9.13; 12.90]	

ANOVA.

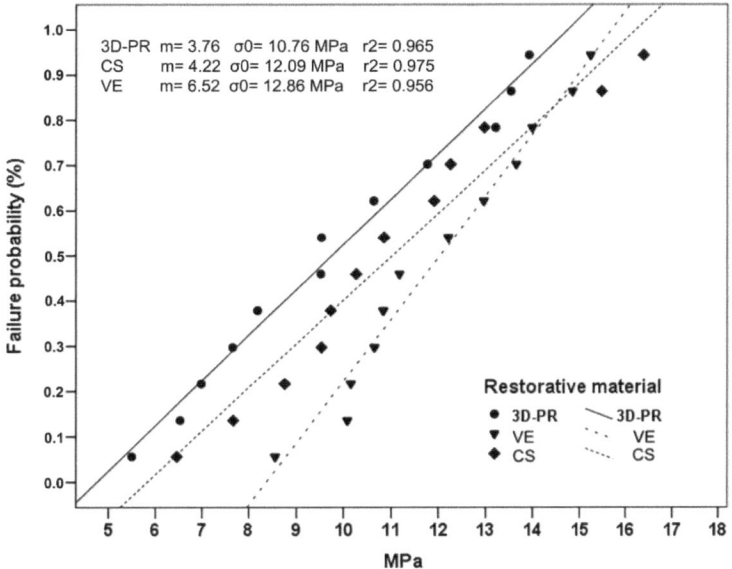

Figure 3. Weibull plots of tested ceramic–glass polymer materials.

3.2. Distribution of the Failure Modes

Distribution of the failure modes was also examined, and there was no significant difference between the three groups (Table 3). Mixed-failure fractures were predominantly observed in all groups. Adhesive failure mode was not observed in any groups. When the relationship between failure modes and SBS is examined, it was seen that the mean SBS of the specimens showing a cohesive failure in luting composite was significantly lower (Table 4).

Table 3. Distribution of failure modes.

	Adhesive n (%)	Mixed n (%)	Cohesive-Material n (%)	Cohesive-Luting Composite n (%)	p
3D-PR (Permanent Crown)	0 (0)	7 (58.3)	2 (16.7)	3 (25)	
VE (VITA Enamic)	0 (0)	8 (66.7)	2 (16.7)	2 (16.7)	0.986
CS (Cerasmart 270)	0 (0)	7 (58.3)	2 (16.7)	3 (25)	

Chi-Square test; $p < 0.05$.

Table 4. Comparing the mean shear bond strength (MPa) of failure modes.

Failure Mode	Mean ± SD (n)	p
Adhesive	- (0)	
Cohesive-Material	11.1 ± 3 (6)	0.033
Cohesive-luting composite	8.9 ± 1.6 (8)	
Mixed	11.6 ± 2.7 (22)	

Kruskal–Wallis; $p < 0.05$.

4. Discussion

The number of ways that novel 3D-printable resins can be used in dentistry is growing quickly [12–14,19]. But to use it as a fixed dental prosthesis, you need a luting composite resin to make a bond that is stable and lasts a long time [18]. Printable ceramic–glass polymer materials are clinically promising because of the material savings and the ability to create more complex geometries compared to machinable ones. Different manufacturing methods may be effective in the bond strength of ceramic–glass polymers to the luting composite resin. The research showed that no significant difference was found between SBS of SLC to printable 3D-PR material, and to machinable ceramic–glass polymer materials (CS and VE). Therefore, the null hypothesis was not rejected.

There are many research studies to improve the bond quality of ceramic–glass polymer materials with different luting composite resins [3–5,8,9,30,35]. In this study, SLC was preferred because it is widespread and easy to use [9,22]. The present research focused on the effect of different manufacturing methods on the bond strength; improving the bond quality of ceramic–glass polymer materials was beyond the scope of this study, but future research should evaluate these.

Machinable ceramic–glass polymer materials are polymerized at higher rates (up to 96%) under high pressure and temperature, leaving few free monomers for copolymerization with luting composite monomers [36–39]. The lower degrees of conversion (76.11%) reported in the literature for 3D-PR might indicate better adhesion, but the results did not show this [40]. It should be taken into account that when a parameter is changed in the manufacturing or post-processing, the degree of conversion will be affected and also probably affect the bonding performance [41]. According to the literature [10,35,37,39], it has been suggested that micro-retentive surfaces be generated prior to luting by either airborne particle abrasion or hydrofluoric acid etching for VE and CS. According to the literature, 50 μm Al_2O_3 airborne particle abrasion resulted in better bond strength values [3,37,42]; 0.1–0.2 MPa is the recommended airborne particle abrasion pressure for machinable ceramic–glass polymers and is lower than the pressure prescribed for metal and ceramic restorations. Thus, 0.1 MPa was chosen because of concerns that airborne particle-abraded machinable ceramic–glass polymers at higher pressures would cause subsurface fractures [38]. Because previous researchers have shown that airborne particle abrasion for more than 30 s reduces bond strength for machinable ceramic–glass polymers, 15 s was used [24]. Therefore, the pretreatment with 0.4 MPa 50 μm Al_2O_3 airborne particle abrasion was reported to have the highest bond strengths for temporary printable resin [18]. It is generally believed that silane application increases bond strength following the formation of micro-retentive areas. However, there have been no consistent reports on the effectiveness of silane for bonding of ceramic–glass polymer materials, so silane application has not been used [36,43,44].

The shear test and micro-tensile test are the most common methods used to measure bond strength in the dental literature. Both advantages and disadvantages have been extensively discussed and explained in the past [27,32]. The SBS test has been reported to be the fastest and most convenient method of obtaining accurate results, and there is a good correlation between in vitro SBS data and clinical bond performance [27]. Although it is believed that the stress is more uniformly distributed during a micro-tensile test, specimen preparation is extremely challenging, and bond strength tends to increase with smaller bonding areas [45]. After a direct comparison of the various test results, the use of Weibull statistics has been proposed to provide more information because bond strength tests have low reliability [31,32].

According to Barutcugil et al. [9], the SBS of the SLC to VE specimens was reported to be 9.139 ± 2.428 MPa. In another study, the SBS of the SLC to the specimens was reported to be 12.69 ± 2.32 MPa for VE and 10.76 ± 2.23 MPa for CS [30]. The results of the current study are similar to other studies in the literature (the SBS of VE was 12.03 ± 2.11 MPa and CS was 11.02 ± 2.96 MPa). The SBS value of the newly introduced 3D-PR (9.74 ± 2.88 MPa) is slightly lower than the others. This may be because, unlike the pre-polymerized machinable blocks compared in the study, post-polymerization was required for printable 3D-PR. Mostafavi et al. [46] reported that post-processing procedures in AM affect the accuracy of the material being tested. Considering that the quality of post-processing depends on the operator, pre-polymerized machinable blocks are the more standard method. Although this study indicated that there was no significant difference in the ability to bond to SLC between machinable and printable ceramic–glass polymer materials, different post-processing procedures may alter the results. Future studies may be considered to compare the effect of different post-processing procedures on bond strength. However, SBSs of all tested materials in this study had enough to ensure good clinical performance, as a limit of 10–13 MPa is considered the minimum for acceptable clinical bond strength [47,48].

According to failure mode analysis, machinable and printable ceramic–glass polymers exhibited comparable failure modes in the present study. The predominant failure mode was a mixed failure, and there was no adhesive failure in all three groups. These findings were compatible with SBS values. Cohesive and mixed modes are preferable to adhesive failure mode because adhesive failure mode is typically related to low bond strength values [2,8,35]. In the study conducted by Sresthadatta et al. [30], adhesive failure was observed in all control specimens that had no surface treatment. Then, adhesive failure modes decreased and mixed-failure modes increased in surface treatment groups [30]. However, cohesive failure in the material is not a sign of a strong bond; rather, it may also be explained by the mechanics of the test and the brittleness of the components involved [45]. Barutcugil et al. [9] observed 50% adhesive, 40% mixed, and 10% cohesive failure in airborne particle-abraded VE specimens with macro-shear test (approximately 3 mm^2). The increased mixed failure rates of the VE group (66.7%) may depend on an expanded bonded area (7.06 mm^2) and the use of a notch-shaped rod in the present study. A notch-shaped rod was used instead of a knife-edge rod for testing in order to avoid inhomogeneous stress concentrations [45]. Nagasawa et al. [4] reported that the airborne particle-abraded CS group failed only cohesively within the ceramic using the macro-shear test (28.26 mm^2). Concerns have been reported that the macro SBS test procedure results in cohesive failure of the substrate due to inhomogeneous stress distribution dependent on the expanded bonded area [9,27,31,32].

There is no single value to specify the strength of brittle materials such as resin composites, ceramics, and tooth structures due to the variability in the existence of strength-controlling defects in these [32]. Weibull statistics are suggested to both specify the strength of brittle materials and to improve the reliability and interpretation of bond strength tests [26,31–33]. According to Figure 3, both printable and machinable materials showed homogeneous distribution, and VE showed higher Weibull modulus compared to CS and 3D-PR, respectively. Unexpectedly, CS and 3D-PR showed similar slopes. This shows that the same types of defects are active in both sets of specimens. Unlike industrially polymerized CS and VE, 3D-PR resin has to undergo post-processing (such as cleaning with alcohol and post-curing) and appears to have been able to be achieved consistently, although complete polymerization is dependent on the operator. It is seen that the SBSs are parallel to the filler ratios of the substrates, respectively. 3D-PR was the less compliant material since it consists of 30–50 wt% of fillers, explaining its lower Weibull modulus with SLC (70 wt%). It appears that structural reliability increases when the luting agent and substrate are well-matched [31,49]. Nagasawa et al. [4] reported that the 70 μm Al$_2$O$_3$ airborne particle-abraded CS with another SLC (G-CEM one; GC) had a 4.8 ± 0.5 Weibull modulus. This Weibull modulus was similar with the present study's result for CS (m = 4.22). Another study [26] examined the strength of the same SLC (RelyX U200; 3M) with dentin and enamel and found the Weibull modulus to be 5.2 and 6.7, respectively. With this information, it is possible to say that SLC has similar reliability on both sides of the adhesive sandwich containing the tooth and restoration. In addition, another issue to consider with SLCs is which light curing unit is preferred for polymerization, because the compatibility of the wavelength range of the light curing unit with photoinitiators is reported to affect bond strength [50].

The present study investigated the effect of different manufacturing methods on the SBS between ceramic–glass polymer materials and SLC using a simplified surface treatment with airborne particle abrasion. This study's design has several limitations. The fact that the materials compared have different filler ratios makes it difficult to establish a direct relationship when comparing production methods, but the study is important in terms of comparing accessible production methods. As far as the authors are aware, no permanent 3D printing ceramic–glass polymer resin currently has a filler ratio above 50%. In the future, if 3D permanent resins with higher filler content are introduced to the market, the results must be updated. When the bond between the SLC and the restorative material was evaluated, no seating pressure was provided, and air bubbles as a function of thickness may have led to the failure (Figure 2b). In addition, the SBS of cohesive failure in luting composite was found to be significantly lower (Table 4). It is difficult to compare results to clinical situations because it does not replicate the oral environment. Nevertheless, in vitro studies still can serve for ranking the materials within the same conditions. Different test techniques can be used to determine the bond strength of materials. This study's findings can be used for screening purposes, but they must be confirmed by additional research employing the micro-tensile and fracture toughness test. More studies are needed to evaluate the long-term durability of the new 3D-PR, including the aging process and thermal cycle, different adhesive systems, and different surface treatment strategies.

5. Conclusions

The following conclusions were reached within the limits of this study:

1. There is no difference in the SBS of the SLC to both printable 3D-PR and machinable ceramic–glass polymers, VE or CS. SBSs of all tested materials had enough to ensure good clinical performance.
2. The lowest Weibull modulus was seen for the printable 3D-PR, but both printable and machinable materials in the present study have shown a homogenous distribution.
3. In the failure modes of both printable and machinable materials in the present study, there is no difference, and the predominant failure mode was mixed mode for 3D-PR, VE, and CS.

Author Contributions: Conceptualization, N.A., S.C.O., O.G. and O.O.; methodology, N.A., S.C.O., O.G. and O.O.; investigation, N.A., O.G. and O.O.; data curation, N.A. and Y.S.; formal analysis, Y.S.; validation, N.A., S.C.O. and Y.S.; resources, N.A., O.G. and O.O.; writing—original draft preparation, N.A.; writing—review and editing, N.A., S.C.O., O.G., O.O. and Y.S.; visualization, N.A.; project administration, N.A.; funding acquisition, N.A. All authors have read and agreed to the published version of the manuscript.

Funding: This study was supported by the Scientific Research Projects Coordination Unit of Cukurova University, project number TSA-2021-14200.

Institutional Review Board Statement: Not applicable.

Informed Consent Statement: Not applicable.

Data Availability Statement: The raw data supporting the conclusions of this article will be made available by the authors on request.

Acknowledgments: Presented as an oral presentation at the International Dental Congress on Additive Manufacturing (IDCAM) (Cukurova University, Faculty of Dentistry), Adana, Turkey, 18–19 March 2022. The authors would like to thank Yurdanur Ucar for her contributions in assembling the research team.

Conflicts of Interest: The authors declare no conflicts of interest.

References

1. Awada, A.; Nathanson, D. Mechanical Properties of Resin-Ceramic CAD/CAM Restorative Materials. *J. Prosthet. Dent.* **2015**, *114*, 587–593. [CrossRef] [PubMed]
2. Alp, G.; Subaşı, M.G.; Johnston, W.M.; Yilmaz, B. Effect of Different Resin Cements and Surface Treatments on the Shear Bond Strength of Ceramic-Glass Polymer Materials. *J. Prosthet. Dent.* **2018**, *120*, 454–461. [CrossRef] [PubMed]
3. Sarahneh, O.; Günal-Abduljalil, B. The Effect of Silane and Universal Adhesives on the Micro-Shear Bond Strength of Current Resin-Matrix Ceramics. *J. Adv. Prosthodont.* **2021**, *13*, 292–303. [CrossRef]
4. Nagasawa, Y.; Eda, Y.; Shigeta, H.; Ferrari, M.; Nakajima, H.; Hibino, Y. Effect of Sandblasting and/or Priming Treatment on the Shear Bond Strength of Self-Adhesive Resin Cement to CAD/CAM Blocks. *Odontology* **2022**, *110*, 70–80. [CrossRef]
5. Çelik, E.; Sahin, S.C.; Dede, D.Ö. Shear Bond Strength of Nanohybrid Composite to the Resin Matrix Ceramics after Different Surface Treatments. *Photomed. Laser Surg.* **2018**, *36*, 424–430. [CrossRef]
6. Cekic-Nagas, I.; Ergun, G.; Egilmez, F.; Vallittu, P.K.; Lassila, L.V.J. Micro-Shear Bond Strength of Different Resin Cements to Ceramic/Glass-Polymer CAD-CAM Block Materials. *J. Prosthodont. Res.* **2016**, *60*, 265–273. [CrossRef] [PubMed]
7. Castro, E.F.; Azevedo, V.L.B.; Nima, G.; de Andrade, O.S.; Dias, C.T.S.; Giannini, M. Adhesion, Mechanical Properties, and Microstructure of Resin-Matrix CAD-CAM Ceramics. *J. Adhes. Dent.* **2020**, *22*, 421–431. [CrossRef]
8. Secilmis, A.; Ustun, O.; Kecik Buyukhatipoglu, I. Evaluation of the Shear Bond Strength of Two Resin Cements on Different CAD/CAM Materials. *J. Adhes. Sci. Technol.* **2016**, *30*, 983–993. [CrossRef]
9. Barutcigil, K.; Barutcigil, Ç.; Kul, E.; Özarslan, M.M.; Buyukkaplan, U.S. Effect of Different Surface Treatments on Bond Strength of Resin Cement to a CAD/CAM Restorative Material. *J. Prosthodont.* **2019**, *28*, 71–78. [CrossRef]
10. Mine, A.; Kabetani, T.; Kawaguchi-Uemura, A.; Higashi, M.; Tajiri, Y.; Hagino, R.; Imai, D.; Yumitate, M.; Ban, S.; Matsumoto, M.; et al. Effectiveness of Current Adhesive Systems When Bonding to CAD/CAM Indirect Resin Materials: A Review of 32 Publications. *Jpn. Dent. Sci. Rev.* **2019**, *55*, 41–50. [CrossRef]
11. Papathanasiou, I.; Kamposiora, P.; Dimitriadis, K.; Papavasiliou, G.; Zinelis, S. In Vitro Evaluation of CAD/CAM Composite Materials. *J. Dent.* **2023**, *136*, 104623. [CrossRef]
12. Dawood, A.; Marti, B.M.; Sauret-Jackson, V.; Darwood, A. 3D Printing in Dentistry. *Br. Dent. J.* **2015**, *219*, 521–529. [CrossRef]
13. Alharbi, N.; Wismeijer, D.; Osman, R.B. Additive Manufacturing Techniques in Prosthodontics: Where Do We Currently Stand? A Critical Review. *Int. J. Prosthodont.* **2017**, *30*, 474–484. [CrossRef]
14. Jockusch, J.; Özcan, M. Additive Manufacturing of Dental Polymers: An Overview on Processes, Materials and Applications. *Dent. Mater. J.* **2020**, *39*, 345–354. [CrossRef]
15. Grzebieluch, W.; Kowalewski, P.; Grygier, D.; Rutkowska-Gorczyca, M.; Kozakiewicz, M.; Jurczyszyn, K. Printable and Machinable Dental Restorative Composites for Cad/Cam Application—Comparison of Mechanical Properties, Fractographic, Texture and Fractal Dimension Analysis. *Materials* **2021**, *14*, 4919. [CrossRef]
16. Lim, N.K.; Shin, S.Y. Bonding of Conventional Provisional Resin to 3D Printed Resin: The Role of Surface Treatments and Type of Repair Resins. *J. Adv. Prosthodont.* **2020**, *12*, 322–328. [CrossRef]
17. Tahayeri, A.; Morgan, M.C.; Fugolin, A.P.; Bompolaki, D.; Athirasala, A.; Pfeifer, C.S.; Ferracane, J.L.; Bertassoni, L.E. 3D Printed versus Conventionally Cured Provisional Crown and Bridge Dental Materials. *Dent. Mater.* **2018**, *34*, 192–200. [CrossRef]
18. Lankes, V.; Reymus, M.; Liebermann, A.; Stawarczyk, B. Bond Strength between Temporary 3D Printable Resin and Conventional Resin Composite: Influence of Cleaning Methods and Air-Abrasion Parameters. *Clin. Oral Investig.* **2023**, *27*, 31–43. [CrossRef]
19. Schweiger, J.; Edelhoff, D.; Güth, J.F. 3d Printing in Digital Prosthetic Dentistry: An Overview of Recent Developments in Additive Manufacturing. *J. Clin. Med.* **2021**, *10*, 2010. [CrossRef]
20. Çakmak, G.; Oosterveen-Rüegsegger, A.L.; Akay, C.; Schimmel, M.; Yilmaz, B.; Donmez, M.B. Influence of Polishing Technique and Coffee Thermal Cycling on the Surface Roughness and Color Stability of Additively and Subtractively Manufactured Resins Used for Definitive Restorations. *J. Prosthodont.* **2024**, *33*, 467–474. [CrossRef]
21. Demirel, M.; Diken Türksayar, A.A.; Donmez, M.B. Fabrication Trueness and Internal Fit of Hybrid Abutment Crowns Fabricated by Using Additively and Subtractively Manufactured Resins. *J. Dent.* **2023**, *136*, 104621. [CrossRef]
22. Hitz, T.; Stawarczyk, B.; Fischer, J.; Hämmerle, C.H.F.; Sailer, I. Are Self-Adhesive Resin Cements a Valid Alternative to Conventional Resin Cements? A Laboratory Study of the Long-Term Bond Strength. *Dent. Mater.* **2012**, *28*, 1183–1190. [CrossRef]
23. Bayazıt, E.Ö. Microtensile Bond Strength of Self-Adhesive Resin Cements to CAD/CAM Resin-Matrix Ceramics Prepared with Different Surface Treatments. *Int. J. Prosthodont.* **2019**, *32*, 433–438. [CrossRef]
24. Tekçe, N.; Tuncer, S.; Demirci, M. The Effect of Sandblasting Duration on the Bond Durability of Dual-Cure Adhesive Cement to CAD/CAM Resin Restoratives. *J. Adv. Prosthodont.* **2018**, *10*, 211–217. [CrossRef]

25. Malament, K.A.; Socransky, S.S. Survival of Dicor Glass-Ceramic Dental Restorations over 16 Years. Part III: Effect of Luting Agent and Tooth or Tooth-Substitute Core Structure. *J. Prosthet. Dent.* **2001**, *86*, 511–519. [CrossRef]
26. Fehrenbach, J.; Münchow, E.A.; Isolan, C.P.; Brondani, L.P.; Bergoli, C.D. Structural Reliability and Bonding Performance of Resin Luting Agents to Dentin and Enamel. *Int. J. Adhes. Adhes.* **2021**, *107*, 102863. [CrossRef]
27. Van Meerbeek, B.; Peumans, M.; Poitevin, A.; Mine, A.; Van Ende, A.; Neves, A.; De Munck, J. Relationship between Bond-Strength Tests and Clinical Outcomes. *Dent. Mater.* **2010**, *26*, e100–e121. [CrossRef]
28. Manso, A.P.; Carvalho, R.M. Dental Cements for Luting and Bonding Restorations: Self-Adhesive Resin Cements. *Dent. Clin. N. Am.* **2017**, *61*, 821–834. [CrossRef]
29. Mair, L.; Padipatvuthikul, P. Variables Related to Materials and Preparing for Bond Strength Testing Irrespective of the Test Protocol. *Dent. Mater.* **2010**, *26*, e17–e23. [CrossRef]
30. Sresthadatta, P.; Sriamporn, T.; Klaisiri, A.; Thamrongananskul, N. Effect of Surface Treatments on Shear Bond Strength of Resin Cement to Hybrid Ceramic Materials. *J. Int. Dent. Med. Res.* **2021**, *14*, 125–135.
31. Quinn, J.B.; Quinn, G.D. A Practical and Systematic Review of Weibull Statistics for Reporting Strengths of Dental Materials. *Dent. Mater.* **2010**, *26*, 135–147. [CrossRef]
32. Scherrer, S.S.; Cesar, P.F.; Swain, M.V. Direct Comparison of the Bond Strength Results of the Different Test Methods: A Critical Literature Review. *Dent. Mater.* **2010**, *26*, e78–e93. [CrossRef]
33. Beyabanaki, E.; Ashtiani, R.E.; Moradi, M.; Namdari, M.; Mostafavi, D.; Zandinejad, A. Biaxial Flexural Strength and Weibull Characteristics of a Resin Ceramic Material after Thermal-Cycling. *J. Prosthodont.* **2023**, *32*, 721–727. [CrossRef]
34. Holmer, L.; Othman, A.; Lührs, A.K.; von See, C. Comparison of the Shear Bond Strength of 3D Printed Temporary Bridges Materials, on Different Types of Resin Cements and Surface Treatment. *J. Clin. Exp. Dent.* **2019**, *11*, e367–e372. [CrossRef]
35. Elsaka, S.E. Bond Strength of Novel CAD/CAM Restorative Materials to Self-Adhesive Resin Cement: The Effect of Surface Treatments. *J. Adhes. Dent.* **2014**, *16*, 531–540. [CrossRef]
36. Günal-Abduljalil, B.; Önöral, Ö.; Ongun, S. Micro-Shear Bond Strengths of Resin-Matrix Ceramics Subjected to Different Surface Conditioning Strategies with or without Coupling Agent Application. *J. Adv. Prosthodont.* **2021**, *13*, 180–190. [CrossRef]
37. Şişmanoğlu, S.; Turunç-oğuzman, R. Microshear Bond Strength of Contemporary Self- Adhesive Resin Cements to CAD/CAM Restorative Materials: Effect of Surface Treatment and Aging. *J. Adhes. Sci. Technol.* **2020**, *34*, 2484–2498. [CrossRef]
38. Yoshihara, K.; Nagaoka, N.; Maruo, Y.; Nishigawa, G.; Irie, M.; Yoshida, Y.; Van Meerbeek, B. Sandblasting May Damage the Surface of Composite CAD—CAM Blocks. *Dent. Mater.* **2017**, *33*, e124–e135. [CrossRef]
39. Reymus, M.; Roos, M.; Eichberger, M.; Edelhoff, D.; Hickel, R.; Stawarczyk, B. Bonding to New CAD/CAM Resin Composites: Influence of Air Abrasion and Conditioning Agents as Pretreatment Strategy. *Clin. Oral Investig.* **2019**, *23*, 529–538. [CrossRef]
40. Zattera, A.C.A.; Morganti, F.A.; de Souza Balbinot, G.; Della Bona, A.; Collares, F.M. The Influence of Filler Load in 3D Printing Resin-Based Composites. *Dent. Mater.* **2024**, *40*, 1041–1046. [CrossRef]
41. Katheng, A.; Kanazawa, M.; Iwaki, M.; Minakuchi, S. Evaluation of Dimensional Accuracy and Degree of Polymerization of Stereolithography Photopolymer Resin under Different Postpolymerization Conditions: An in Vitro Study. *J. Prosthet. Dent.* **2021**, *125*, 695–702. [CrossRef]
42. Tekçe, N.; Tuncer, S.; Demirci, M.; Kara, D.; Baydemir, C. Microtensile Bond Strength of CAD/CAM Resin Blocks to Dual-Cure Adhesive Cement: The Effect of Different sandblasting procedures. *J. Prosthet. Dent.* **2019**, *28*, e485–e490. [CrossRef]
43. Yano, H.T.; Ikeda, H.; Nagamatsu, Y.; Masaki, C.; Hosokawa, R.; Shimizu, H. Correlation between Microstructure of CAD/CAM Composites and the Silanization Effect on Adhesive Bonding. *J. Mech. Behav. Biomed. Mater.* **2020**, *101*, 103441. [CrossRef]
44. Murillo-gomez, F.; Wanderley, R.B.; De Goes, M.F. Impact of Silane-Containing Universal Adhesive on the Biaxial Flexural Strength of a Resin Cement/Glass-Ceramic System. *Oper. Dent.* **2019**, *44*, 200–209. [CrossRef]
45. Braga, R.R.; Meira, J.B.C.; Boaro, L.C.C.; Xavier, T.A. Adhesion to Tooth Structure: A Critical Review of "Macro" Test Methods. *Dent. Mater.* **2010**, *26*, e38–e49. [CrossRef]
46. Mostafavi, D.M.; Methani, M.M.; Piedra-Cascon, W.; Zandinejad, A.; Att, W.; Revilla-León, M. Influence of the Polymerization Postprocessing Procedures on the Accuracy of Additively Manufactured Dental Model Material. *Int. J. Prosthodont.* **2023**, *36*, 479–485. [CrossRef]
47. Kim, M.J.; Kim, Y.K.; Kim, K.H.; Kwon, T.Y. Shear Bond Strengths of Various Luting Cements to Zirconia Ceramic: Surface Chemical Aspects. *J. Dent.* **2011**, *39*, 795–803. [CrossRef]
48. Lüthy, H.; Loeffel, O.; Hammerle, C.H.F. Effect of Thermocycling on Bond Strength of Luting Cements to Zirconia Ceramic. *Dent. Mater.* **2006**, *22*, 195–200. [CrossRef]
49. Barbon, F.J.; Moraes, R.R.; Isolan, C.P.; Spazzin, A.O.; Boscato, N. Influence of Inorganic Filler Content of Resin Luting Agents and Use of Adhesive on the Performance of Bonded Ceramic. *J. Prosthet. Dent.* **2019**, *122*, 566.e1–566.e11. [CrossRef]
50. Chen, Y.; Yao, C.; Huang, C.; Wang, Y. The Effect of Monowave and Polywave Light-Polymerization Units on the Adhesion of Resin Cements to Zirconia. *J. Prosthet. Dent.* **2019**, *121*, 549.e1–549.e7. [CrossRef]

Disclaimer/Publisher's Note: The statements, opinions and data contained in all publications are solely those of the individual author(s) and contributor(s) and not of MDPI and/or the editor(s). MDPI and/or the editor(s) disclaim responsibility for any injury to people or property resulting from any ideas, methods, instructions or products referred to in the content.

Article

Bond Strength of Milled and Printed Zirconia to 10-Methacryloyloxydecyl Dihydrogen Phosphate (10-MDP) Resin Cement as a Function of Ceramic Conditioning, Disinfection and Ageing

Wolfgang Bömicke [1,*], Franz Sebastian Schwindling [2], Peter Rammelsberg [1] and Stefan Rues [1]

1. Department of Prosthetic Dentistry, University of Heidelberg, 69120 Heidelberg, Germany; peter.rammelsberg@med.uni-heidelberg.de (P.R.); stefan.rues@med.uni-heidelberg.de (S.R.)
2. Department of Prosthetic Dentistry, Medical University Innsbruck, 6020 Innsbruck, Austria; sebastian.schwindling@tirol-kliniken.at
* Correspondence: wolfgang.boemicke@med.uni-heidelberg.de

Abstract: This study aimed to assess the suitability of printed zirconia (ZrO_2) for adhesive cementation compared to milled ZrO_2. Surface conditioning protocols and disinfection effects on bond strength were also investigated. ZrO_2 discs (n = 14/group) underwent either alumina (Al_2O_3) airborne particle abrasion (APA; 50 µm, 0.10 MPa) or tribochemical silicatisation (TSC; 110 µm Al_2O_3, 0.28 MPa and 110 µm silica-modified Al_2O_3, 0.28 MPa), followed by disinfection (1 min immersion in 70% isopropanol, 15 s water spray, 10 s drying with oil-free air) for half of the discs. A resin cement containing 10-methacryloyloxydecyl dihydrogen phosphate (10-MDP) was used for bonding (for TSC specimens after application of a primer containing silane and 10-MDP). Tensile bond strength was measured after storage for 24 h at 100% relative humidity or after 30 days in water, including 7500 thermocycles. Surface conditioning significantly affected bond strength, with higher values for TSC specimens. Ageing and the interaction of conditioning, disinfection and ageing also impacted bond strength. Disinfection combined with APA mitigated ageing-related bond strength decrease but exacerbated it for TSC specimens. Despite these effects, high bond strengths were maintained even after disinfection and ageing. Adhesive cementation of printed ZrO_2 restorations exhibited comparable bond strengths to milled ZrO_2, highlighting its feasibility in clinical applications.

Keywords: lithography-based ceramic manufacturing; tribochemical silicatisation; additive manufacturing; adhesive cementation; zirconium dioxide

Citation: Bömicke, W.; Schwindling, F.S.; Rammelsberg, P.; Rues, S. Bond Strength of Milled and Printed Zirconia to 10-Methacryloyloxydecyl Dihydrogen Phosphate (10-MDP) Resin Cement as a Function of Ceramic Conditioning, Disinfection and Ageing. *Materials* **2024**, *17*, 2159. https://doi.org/10.3390/ma17092159

Academic Editor: Josip Kranjčić

Received: 12 April 2024
Revised: 26 April 2024
Accepted: 28 April 2024
Published: 5 May 2024

Copyright: © 2024 by the authors. Licensee MDPI, Basel, Switzerland. This article is an open access article distributed under the terms and conditions of the Creative Commons Attribution (CC BY) license (https://creativecommons.org/licenses/by/4.0/).

1. Introduction

Biological, economic, and esthetic considerations have led to the increasing replacement of traditional metal-ceramics by all-ceramic materials in the fabrication of (in particular fixed) dental prostheses [1,2]. Zirconia (ZrO_2) is playing a leading role in this trend. The reasons for this include the high load-bearing capacity of the material due to its excellent strength [1], superior marginal adaption [3] and the possibility of monolithic processing in reduced thicknesses, which has been made practical by developments in colouring technique and the availability of pre-coloured blanks. All this has led to an expansion of the range of applications of the material to include the realisation of complex restoration geometries and minimally invasive restorations [4].

For ZrO_2 single crowns and fixed partial dentures (FPDs), a recent review of the effect of the luting agent used to seat the restorations concluded that high survival rates can be achieved when conventional cements are used for luting [5]. However, the selected studies suggested even greater success with composite or self-adhesive resin cements [5]. In contrast, adhesive cementation is essential for minimally invasive restorations such as vestibular and occlusal veneers (tabletops) and resin-bonded FPDs, as the aim is to achieve a defect-adapted preparation rather than to generate axially parallel surfaces that create a wedging effect during cementation and thus hold the restoration in place. Instead, the long-term retention of these restorations is based on adhesion, making the quality of the adhesive bond a primary prognostic criterion [6].

In the case of ZrO_2 restorations, there were initial concerns about whether they could be effectively adhesively bonded because the material lacks a glass phase and cannot be etched with hydrofluoric acid, so there was no established method of creating a retentive micro-relief to prepare for a micromechanical bond. Silanisation to create a chemical bond was also ineffective. Today, we have advanced to the point where a permanent bond between a composite cement and ZrO_2 is possible. The prerequisites are (1) an Al_2O_3 airborne particle abrasion process that cleans, roughens and simultaneously enlarges the surface to prepare it for micromechanical bonding and (2) the use of a composite resin or primer containing a functional monomer that enables chemical coupling of the adhesive to the ZrO_2 substrate [7]. The functional phosphate monomer 10-methacryloyloxydecyl dihydrogen phosphate (10-MDP) has been used successfully in this context [7,8]. As an alternative to a pure Al_2O_3 blasting process, tribochemical silicatisation can be used as a surface pretreatment for ZrO_2 bonding [9]. The combination of tribochemical silicatisation of the ZrO_2 surface with a silane and 10-MDP-containing primer and 10-MDP-containing cement proved to be effective in achieving a sufficiently strong long-term bond [10]. There is clinical data to support both approaches [4,7,11]. However, Al_2O_3 blasting is supported by a larger number of cases and a longer observation period.

More recently, ZrO_2 has become available as a material for additive manufacturing of dental restorations using the printing process [12,13]. Compared to subtractive milling, ZrO_2 printing offers material savings/increased cost effectiveness [14] and the ability to create complex geometries with greater accuracy of fit [15] and allows for thinner restorations by eliminating the risk of material damage from the milling process [16]. Overall, these fabrication characteristics support a minimally invasive approach with printed ZrO_2 restorations but only if a bond strength similar to that of milled material can be achieved. However, while more and more studies are focusing on the mechanical strength [17–22], fit [15,23–25] and biocompatibility [26–28] of the printed material, there has been little research into the adhesion of resins with printed ZrO_2 [29–31].

In the meantime, studies have shown very well which cleaning methods work on contaminated ZrO_2 surfaces [32]. However, little is known about the disinfection of uncontaminated but mechanically conditioned surfaces, although this is inevitable under hygienic conditions, so that disinfection is also of interest as a factor possibly influencing bond strength.

Therefore, the aim of the present study was to determine the influence of the ZrO_2 type (milled, printed), ceramic conditioning method (Al_2O_3 blasting, tribochemical silicatisation), disinfection and artificial ageing on the strength of the ZrO_2–resin cement bond. The null hypothesis was that none of these variables would affect the resin bond strength to the ZrO_2.

2. Materials and Methods

The materials used in the study and their specifications are listed in Table 1. All materials were used in accordance with the manufacturer's instructions for use. Test specimen preparation, including all bonding procedures and tensile testing, was performed by one trained person in the position of a physical-technical assistant.

Table 1. Specifications of study materials.

Material	Brand	LOT	Composition (as Disclosed by Manufacturer)	Material
Milled zirconia	IPS e.max ZirCAD LT	X54 580	88–95.5 wt% zirconium oxide (ZrO_2), 4.5–≤6 wt% yttrium oxide (Y_2O_3), ≤5 wt% hafnium oxide (HfO_2), ≤1 wt% aluminium oxide (Al_2O_3), ≤1 wt% other oxides for coloring	Ivoclar Vivadent, Schaan, Liechtenstein
Printed zirconia	LithaCon 3Y 230	N.a.	3 mol% yttria stabilized tetragonal zirconia polycrystal	Lithoz, Vienna, Austria
Multifunctional primer	Clearfil Ceramic Primer Plus	AX0039, 2A0061	>80% ethanol, 3-trimethoxysilylpropyl methacrylate, 10-methacryloyloxydecyl dihydrogen phosphate	Kuraray Europe, Hattersheim, Germany
Adhesive resin cement	Panavia 21	2G0018, 49A0019, 5E0015	Catalyst paste: 10-methacryloyloxydecyl dihydrogen phosphate, hydrophobic aromatic dimethacrylate, hydrophobic aliphatic dimethacrylate, silanated silica filler, colloidal silica, catalysts; Universal paste: hydrophobic aromatic dimethacrylate, hydrophobic aliphatic dimethacrylate, hydrophilic aliphatic dimethacrylate, silanated titanium oxide, silanated barium glass filler, catalysts, accelerators, pigments	Kuraray Europe, Hattersheim, Germany
Oxygen-inhibiting gel	Oxyguard II	480101, 720103, A40106	50–70% glycerol, polyethyleneglycol, catalysts, accelerators, dyes	Kuraray Europe, Hattersheim, Germany
Core build-up resin	Rebilda DC	2133130, 2205471	Catalyst paste: 10–25% urethane dimethacrylate (UDMA), 5–10% 1,12-dodecane dimethacrylate (DDDMA), 2.5–5% bisphenol A-glycidyl methacrylate (BIS GMA), ≤2.5% benzoyl peroxide; Base paste: 10–25% UDMA, 5–10% DDDMA, 2.5–5% BIS GMA	VOCO, Cuxhaven, Germany

17

A total of 224 ZrO$_2$ discs (diameter 8.4 mm, thickness 3.4 mm) were fabricated, 112 from milled ZrO$_2$ (MZ, IPS e. max ZirCAD LT, Ivoclar Vivadent, Schaan, Liechtenstein) and 112 from printed ZrO$_2$ (PZ, LithaCon 3Y 230, Lithoz, Vienna, Austria), and ground to a uniform surface finish using 220-grit diamond discs in a semi-automatic grinding and polishing machine (Tegramin-25, Struers, Willich, Germany).

Half of the discs were subjected to airborne particle abrasion (APA) with 50 μm Al$_2$O$_3$ particles (Alustrahl, Omnident, Rodgau Nieder-Roden, Germany) at 0.10 MPa, while the other half were tribochemically silicatised (TSC) in a two-step blasting process (1. Rocatec Pre: 110 μm Al$_2$O$_3$ particles, 0.28 MPa, 2. Rocatec Plus: 110 μm silica modified Al$_2$O$_3$ particles, 0.28 MPa, 3M Oral Care, Seefeld, Germany). All blasting was performed at 10 mm distance from the surface at a 90-degree angle. The discs were blackened in advance with a felt-tip pen to ensure that the surface treatment was complete. Blasting agent residue was removed with a strong stream of oil-free air.

Half of the ZrO$_2$ discs were then disinfected (D), while the other half were not disinfected (ND). Disinfection consisted of immersion in 70% isopropanol (Carl Roth, Karlsruhe, Germany) for 1 min, followed by a 15 s water spray and drying with a strong stream of oil-free air for 10 s.

Before adhesive cementation, a primer containing silane and 10-MDP (Clearfil Ceramic Primer Plus, Kuraray Europe, Hattersheim, Germany) was applied to the TSC discs.

Autopolymerising 10-MDP-based resin cement (Panavia 21, Kuraray Europe) was used to adhesively cement acrylic tubes filled with dual polymerising core build-up resin (Rebilda DC, VOCO, Cuxhaven, Germany) to the ZrO$_2$ discs. The tubes were filled just prior to adhesive cementation and the core build-up resin light polymerised from four orthogonal positions from the tube surface (40 s per position) using a 1000 mW/cm^2 cordless pen-style, LED light polymerisation device (SmartLite Focus LED, Dentsply Sirona, Bensheim, Germany). The bonding area was defined by the 3.3 mm internal diameter of the tubes. Adhesive cementation was performed under a constant load of 7.5 N in a special cementing device that ensured perpendicular alignment of the acrylic tube with the ZrO$_2$ disc. After 10 min, the test specimens were transferred to an incubator and stored at 37 °C under 100% humidity for 24 h.

Half of the specimens were then subjected to a tensile test to determine the bond strength (initial bond strength). The other half of the specimens were artificially aged prior to the bond strength test. The ageing protocol consisted of water storage at a constant temperature of 37 °C interrupted by 7500 thermocycles at 6.5 °C and 60 °C with a dwell time at each temperature of 45 s and a total transfer time of 7.5 s (Thermocycler TC 1, SD Mechatronik, Feldkirchen-Westerham, Germany). The periods of water storage at 37 °C and the period of thermocycling of the test specimens added up to a total of 30 days of storage of the test specimens in water, and the specimens were alternated between the storage conditions according to the following scheme: 4 days of 37 °C water storage, 9 days of thermocycling, 17 days of 37 °C water storage.

The tensile test was performed in a universal testing machine (Z005, Zwick/Roell, Ulm, Germany) at a crosshead speed of 1 mm/min using a moment-free pull-off device. The bond strength (MPa) was calculated by dividing the force (N) applied when the specimen debonded by the bonding area (8.55 mm^2). It was defined that test specimens which debonded spontaneously prior to tensile testing (pre-test failures) would be included in the statistics at 0 MPa.

Debonded specimens were optically evaluated with a digital microscope (ZEISS Smartzoom 5, Carl Zeiss, Oberkochen, Germany) at 75× magnification for relative adhesive failure (%) in the bonding area using special measurement software (ZEN core 3.2, Carl Zeiss).

Additional ZrO$_2$ discs (not used for bond strength testing) were prepared to evaluate the surface morphology produced by the different ceramic conditioning methods (APA, TSC) qualitatively by scanning electron microscopy (SEM) and quantitatively by surface roughness measurement. SEM (JSM-6510, JEOL, Eching, Germany) was performed with magnifications of 500×, 1000× and 5000× and an acceleration voltage of 5 kV. Average surface roughness R_a and ten-point height R_z ($R_{z(iso)}$) [33]) were measured using a tactile profilometer (MarSurf GD 140, Mahr, Göttingen, Germany). The roughness of the discs was evaluated along 6 measuring tracks for 2 discs of each surface treatment (including the 220-grit diamond polished baseline surface) and ZrO_2 type. Each track had a length of 5.6 mm and was measured 3 times. For two perpendicular directions, each 3 tracks were arranged parallel to each other (1 mm distance). Each track was divided into seven intervals and evaluation of roughness parameters took place on a 4 mm long track without the first and last interval. Gauss-filtering took place for wave lengths above $\lambda_c = 0.25$ mm.

Bond strength data were verified for normal distribution (Shapiro–Wilk test) and homoscedasticity (Levene test). The influence of ZrO_2 type, ceramic conditioning method, disinfection, and ageing on bond strength was analysed by multifactorial analysis of variance (ANOVA). A one-way ANOVA with test group as the independent variable, followed by a post hoc Tukey test, was used to pairwise compare test groups for bond strength. For all tests, a $p < 0.05$ was considered statistically significant.

3. Results
3.1. Bond Strength

All specimens could be tested for tensile bond strength (no pre-test failures occurred). The bond strengths measured in the study groups are shown graphically in Figure 1 and listed in Table 2.

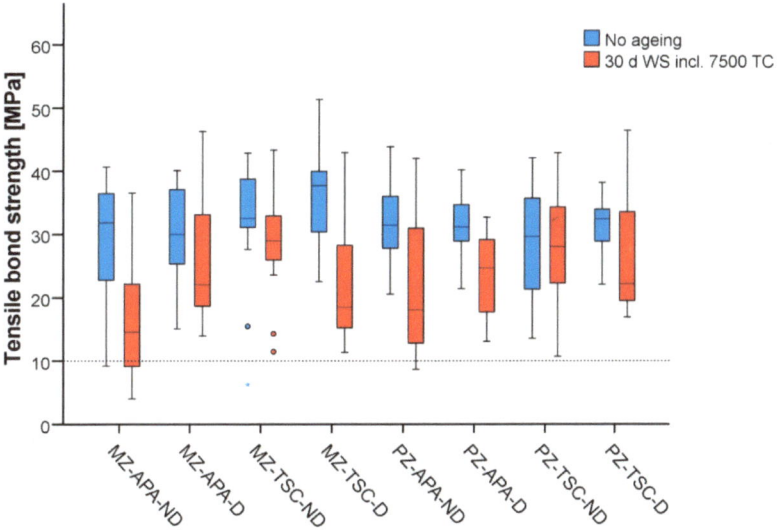

Figure 1. Whisker and box plots of bond strengths in study groups (n = 14 per ageing subgroup). Dotted line marks empirical 10 MPa threshold for clinical recommendation. MZ: milled zirconia, PZ: printed zirconia, APA: airborne particle abrasion, TSC: tribochemical silicatisation, ND: not disinfected, D: disinfected.

Table 2. Tensile bond strength [MPa] in study groups.

Study Groups (n = 14 per Ageing Subgroup)	No Ageing							Ageing						
								30 d Water Storage Incl. 7500 TC						
	Mean	SD	Min	Max	Median	25th Pct	75th Pct	Mean	SD	Min	Max	Median	25th Pct	75th Pct
MZ-APA-ND	29.2 ab	9.3	9.2	40.7	31.9	22.8	36.5	16.6 c	10.3	4.0	36.6	14.6	9.2	22.2
MZ-APA-D	29.7 ab	7.4	15.1	40.1	30.0	25.4	37.1	25.2 abc	9.7	13.9	46.3	22.1	18.7	33.1
MZ-TSC-ND	31.7 ab	10.0	6.3	42.9	32.6	31.1	38.7	28.8 ab	8.9	11.5	43.3	29.0	26.0	33.0
MZ-TSC-D	36.2 a	7.5	22.6	51.4	37.7	30.4	40.0	22.9 bc	10.6	11.3	43.0	18.5	15.2	28.3
PZ-APA-ND	32.1 ab	6.8	20.6	43.9	31.5	27.8	36.0	21.6 bc	11.1	8.7	42.1	18.1	12.8	31.0
PZ-APA-D	31.2 ab	5.2	21.4	40.2	31.2	28.9	34.7	24.0 bc	6.8	13.1	32.7	24.7	17.7	29.2
PZ-TSC-ND	28.7 ab	9.6	13.6	42.1	29.7	21.4	35.7	27.6 abc	8.5	10.7	42.9	28.1	22.3	34.3
PZ-TSC-D	32.0 ab	4.5	22.1	38.2	32.5	28.9	34.0	26.8 abc	9.20	16.9	46.5	22.2	19.5	33.5

Different lowercase letters indicate a statistically significant difference in bond strength in the Tukey post hoc test. SD: standard deviation, Pct: percentile, MZ: milled zirconia, PZ: printed zirconia, APA: airborne particle abrasion, TSC: tribochemical silicatisation, ND: not disinfected, D: disinfected.

A statistically significant effect on bond strength was found for ceramic conditioning method ($p = 0.007$) and ageing ($p < 0.001$) as well es for the interaction of ceramic conditioning method, disinfection and ageing ($p = 0.006$) (Table 3).

Table 3. Multifactorial analysis of variance for effect of zirconia type, ceramic conditioning method, disinfection and ageing on bond strength.

Source	Typ III Sum of Squares	df	Mean Square	F	p
Corrected model	4904.915 [a]	15	326.994	4.359	<0.001
Intercept	172,656.653	1	172,656.653	2301.463	<0.001
Zirconia type	12.946	1	12.946	0.173	0.678
Ceramic conditioning method	549.472	1	549.472	7.324	0.007
Disinfection	118.306	1	118.306	1.577	0.211
Ageing	2859.215	1	2859.215	38.112	<0.001
Zirconia type * ceramic conditioning method	140.891	1	140.891	1.878	0.172
Zirconia type * disinfection	11.653	1	11.653	0.155	0.694
Zirconia type * ageing	76.928	1	76.928	1.025	0.312
Ceramic conditioning method * disinfection	80.197	1	80.197	1.069	0.302
Ceramic conditioning method * ageing	134.556	1	134.556	1.794	0.182
Disinfection * ageing	7.011	1	7.011	0.093	0.760
Zirconia type * ceramic conditioning method * disinfection	116.540	1	116.540	1.553	0.214
Zirconia type * ceramic conditioning method * ageing	96.534	1	96.534	1.287	0.258
Zirconia type * disinfection * ageing	1.948	1	1.948	0.026	0.872
Ceramic conditioning method * disinfection * ageing	588.806	1	588.806	7.849	0.006
Zirconia type * ceramic conditioning method * disinfection * ageing	109.914	1	109.914	1.465	0.227
Error	15,604.245	208	75.020		
Total	193,165.813	224			
Corrected total	20,509.159	223			

[a] R-Squared = 0.239 (Adjusted R-Squared = 0.184).

Mean initial bond strengths ranged from 29.2 MPa to 36.2 MPa for MZ and from 28.7 MPa to 32.1 MPa for PZ. There was no statistically significant difference among the subgroups without ageing ($p \geq 0.643$). Aged specimens had lower mean bond strengths of 16.6 MPa to 28.8 MPa for MZ and 21.6 MPa to 27.6 MPa for PZ. Among the aged subgroups, a statistically significant lower mean bond strength was found for MZ-APA-ND compared to MZ-TSC-ND specimens ($p = 0.021$). The greatest reduction in bond strength due to ageing was observed in APA-ND and TSC-D specimens. This was found to be statistically significant for MZ (MZ-APA-ND: $p = 0.014$, MZ-TSC-D: $p = 0.007$).

3.2. Failure Mode

The failure mode of the specimens was mainly cohesive in all study groups. The proportion of adhesive failure generally increased with ageing and reached a maximum value of a mean of 13.3% for MZ-APA-ND (Figure 2).

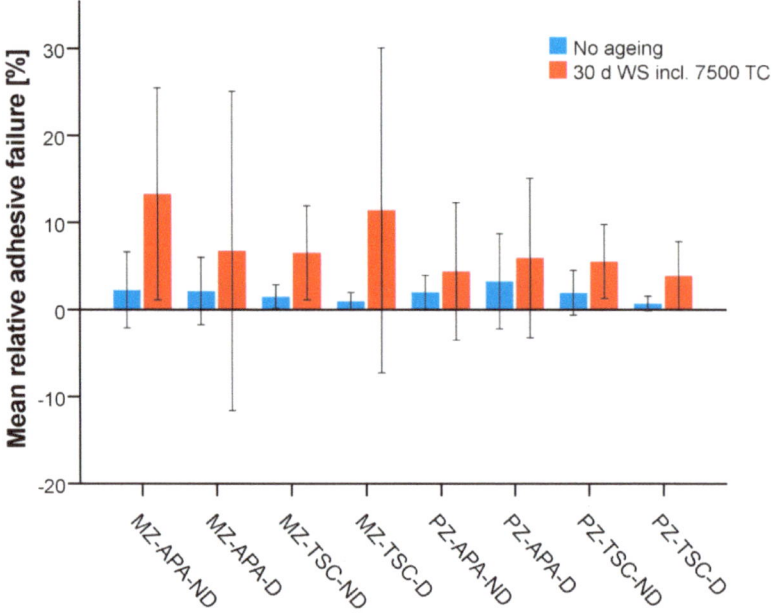

Figure 2. Bar plots of mean relative adhesive failure in study groups (n = 14 per ageing subgroup). Error bars: +/− standard deviation. MZ: milled zirconia, PZ: printed zirconia, APA: airborne particle abrasion, TSC: tribochemical silicatisation, ND: not disinfected, D: disinfected.

3.3. Surface Morphology and Roughness

The SEM analysis showed that the blasting methods used in the study resulted in a comparable surface morphology. The TSC surfaces exhibited a slightly coarser structure compared to the APA surfaces. No differences were observed between milled and printed ZrO_2 at any chosen magnification. Figure 3 shows the different surfaces at 1000X magnification.

APA approximately doubled the roughness of a 220-grit diamond-polished ZrO_2 surface and TSC quadrupled it (Table 4). Comparable values were found for milled and printed ZrO_2 (Table 4).

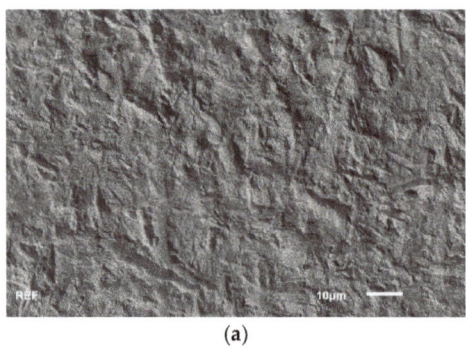

(a)

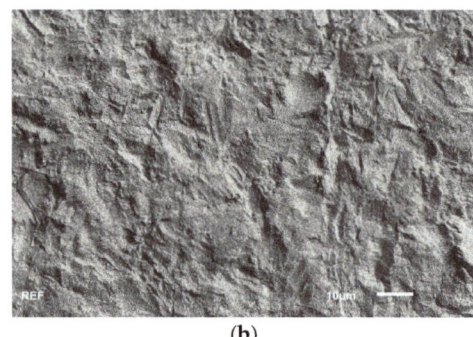

(b)

Figure 3. *Cont.*

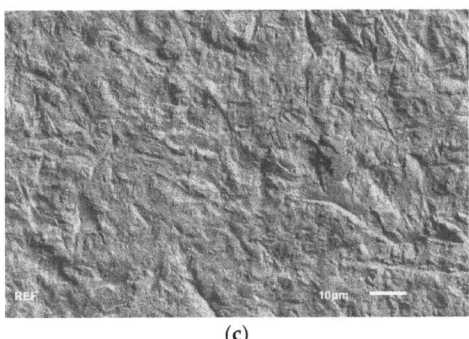 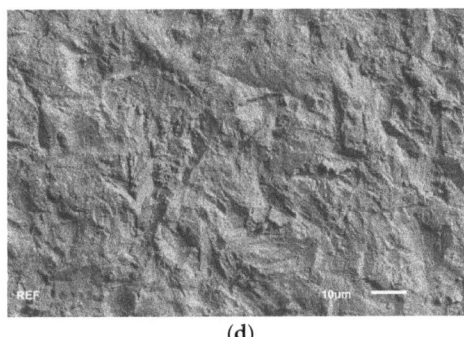

(c)   (d)

Figure 3. Scanning electron microscopic images of surfaces generated on different zirconia types (milled zirconia, MZ/printed zirconia, PZ) by different conditioning methods (airborne particle abrasion, APA/tribochemical silicatisation, TSC) at 1000× magnification: (**a**) MZ-APA; (**b**) MZ-TSC; (**c**) PZ-APA; (**d**) PZ-TSC.

Table 4. Mean values [μm] of zirconia surface roughness measurements for different ceramic conditioning methods.

Ceramic Surface Conditioning Method	MZ		PZ	
	R_a	R_z	R_a	R_z
220-grit diamond disc polishing (starting surface)	0.4763	3.0689	0.4420	2.9333
APA	0.9348	6.2130	0.8377	5.4151
TSC	1.9214	11.0322	1.8998	11.0238

MZ: milled zirconia, PZ: printed zirconia, APA: airborne particle abrasion, TSC: tribochemical silicatization.

4. Discussion

The objective of this study was to investigate the impact of ZrO_2 type, ceramic conditioning method, disinfection and ageing on the bond strength between ZrO_2 and resin. The null hypothesis was that none of these variables would affect the resin bond strength to ZrO_2. Based on the measured data, the hypothesis was partially rejected. Specifically, there was a statistically significant impact on bond strength for different ceramic conditioning methods, ageing and the combined effect of ceramic conditioning method, disinfection and ageing. Within aged subgroups, a statistically significant difference in mean bond strength was observed, with MZ-APA-ND showing lower bond strength compared to MZ-TSC-ND specimens. Finally ageing led to a statistically significant reduction for MZ-APA-ND and MZ-TSC-D specimens.

In this study, APA and TSC were chosen as the ceramic conditioning methods because they could be considered established for preparing the resin bond to ZrO_2, not least because they have the most evidence in the literature [34,35]. They also appeared to be particularly suitable because they are easy to apply under practical conditions [10]. A control group without mechanical surface conditioning was not used in this study because it is well known that omitting mechanical roughening of the ceramic substrate results in significantly lower bond strength [35,36]. Recent reviews have shown TSC to outperform APA in achieving stronger bonds with ZrO_2 [9,34,37,38]. One of these reviews specified, however, that in combination with an MDP resin cement, APA and TSC may be equivalent in terms of achievable bond strength [38]. This well aligns with the present study's findings. However, it is important to consider the entire bonding process, not just the physical conditioning step, including the adhesive used [35,38]. Using TSC without a proper silane afterward may be ineffective [39]. At the same time, primers/adhesives containing 10-MDP can create strong chemical bonds with ZrO_2 [37]. Accordingly, a primer containing both a silane and 10-MDP was used in this study on TSC test specimens. In addition, it has already been shown that such a combination of silane and 10-MDP on TSC ZrO_2 surfaces did result in stable bond strengths [10,40,41].

Irrespective of any possible chemical processes, the higher bond strength of the TSC specimens could have simply been related to the surface morphologies produced by the different blasting processes. In terms of SEM morphology, these were comparable for the printed and milled samples and differed only with respect to the ceramic conditioning method chosen, with the TSC samples having a coarser surface. In the roughness evaluation, the values obtained for R_a and R_z were approximately twice as high for the TSC samples compared to the APA samples. However, there are no studies that could readily substantiate this assumption, as the effects that can be attributed to surface roughness are generally overlaid by other influencing factors, particularly the choice of cement [38]. Studies in which neither increasing Al_2O_3 particle size [42] nor increasing air abrasion pressure [10,36] resulted in increased bond strength when used with an MDP-containing cement or primer provide evidence that absolute roughness might be of minor importance. This assumption is also supported by the results of a recently published study, which showed that not R_a but the presence (area %) of nanoscale surface irregularities was the most predominant factor for the strength of the resin-zirconia bond [43].

Another difference between the APA and TSC specimens was the use of a primer containing silane and MDP in the TSC specimens. As mentioned above, this is necessary for the chemical coupling of the resin cement to the applied silicate layer, but it also increases the wettability of the surface of the coated ZrO_2 substrate [44,45], which in turn may have resulted in improved cement flow onto the ZrO_2 surface and better mechanical interlocking, and thus increased bond strength in the TSC groups.

The chosen combinations of ceramic conditioning methods (APA or TSC) and 10-MDP-based resin cement, as used in this study, are bonding protocols for which data are available from clinical trials [4,7,11]. Therefore, it was considered particularly useful to validate them for printed ZrO_2. In the current study, 10 MPa was used as the threshold for clinically acceptable bond strength. It is assumed that bond strength values above this threshold are sufficient to ensure that, for example, a single-retainer resin-bonded fixed partial denture in the anterior region, for which a minimum bonding area of approximately 30 mm^2 is recommended [46], will not detach under the occlusal forces that may be exerted on it in this position [47]. Overall, it was found that even after ageing, only very few test specimens were below this threshold, and these were almost exclusively APA test specimens of MZ or PZ without disinfection, which in principle qualifies all bonding protocols tested here for clinical use.

Ageing reduced the bond strength of the test specimens; however, a statistically significant reduction was only found for MZ-APA-ND and MZ-TSC-D test specimens. For artificial ageing, a combination of 30 days of water storage including 7500 thermocycles was used, which in accordance with "ISO/TS 4640:2023, Dentistry, Test methods for tensile bond strength to tooth structure" might be considered as medium-term ageing. It should be noted that bond strength tests comparing this ageing protocol with 6 months of water storage or 150 days of water storage including 37500 thermocycles suggest that, with extended ageing, statistically significant effects could also occur in other test groups, which is why conclusive statements on long-term bond strength cannot be made based on this study. On the other hand, with a maximum decrease in bond strength of approximately 37% and 43% (measured for MZ-TSC-D and MZ-APA-ND specimens, respectively), the protocols tested proved to be effective in terms of bond durability [38] and, in view of the clinical threshold defined above, the absolute bond strengths found still contain significant ageing reserves. The ageing resistance of TSC specimens has been attributed to the hydrolytic stability of the siloxane bonds formed between the silanol groups of the silane and the silica layer deposited on the ZrO_2 surface [48]. However, ageing effects must also be expected for TSC ZrO_2 [49]. For 10-MDP, it was shown that it bonds directly to ZrO_2 not only via ionic bonding but also hydrogen bonding [50]. However, it has also been shown that this bond is subject to hydrolytic degradation over longer periods of time [51]. This, in turn, is relativised by the finding that MDP-containing primers, universal adhesives and resin cements create bonds to ZrO_2 with acceptable strength after long-term aging, regardless of such hydrolytic processes [52].

In addition to the effects of surface conditioning and ageing, the influence of disinfection was of interest. This had derived from the fact that, in general, the bonding surface has the highest surface energy after conditioning and any contamination should be avoided to achieve the best possible bond quality with the subsequently applied adhesives [32]. For TSC samples, it was found that the silane should be applied to the freshly silicatised ZrO_2 and that cleaning with water (spray or ultrasonic bath) prior to primer application is not advisable [53]. However, as noted in a recent systematic review, ultrasonic cleaning prior to resin cement application is widely used [37]. Similarly, distilled water, alcohol, acetone, ethanol and isopropanol have been used for 1 to 10 min without consideration of the effect of such cleaning steps on adhesion to ZrO_2, although all were considered beneficial [37]. As the physical conditioning of the ceramic surface often takes place in the dental laboratory, disinfection is essential for further hygienic processing of the restoration. The only way to avoid this is to carry out all ceramic conditioning steps chairside. Technically, this is possible with the appropriate blasting equipment, but the time required, and the increased cleaning requirements of the treatment room associated with the blasting process argue against this procedure. A statistically significant effect of disinfection was found in this study only in the interaction with ageing and conditioning method, which was expressed as a lower sensitivity to ageing of the adhesive bond for APA samples and, in contrast, an increased sensitivity to ageing for TSC samples. The mechanisms underlying this observation cannot be determined at this time. In principle, it is conceivable that disinfection may have interfered with silane coupling, as has already been shown for the effect of water on a silicatised surface [53], and that hydrolytic processes were able to take place to a greater extent, whereas 10-MDP was less affected. The positive effect of disinfection on the APA specimens could be based on a cleaning effect by removing loose abrasive from the surface and increasing the bond quality accordingly.

In the current study, no effect of the ceramic substrate on bond strength was observed. To the best of the authors' knowledge, only three other studies have evaluated resin bond strength to printed ZrO_2 [29–31]. Control groups from milled ZrO_2 were used in two of these studies [29,31]. Zandinejad et al. compared milled ZrO_2 specimens with printed ZrO_2 specimens of increasing porosity (0%, 20%, 40%) [29]. The ZrO_2 specimens were bonded after being wet-polished with 600 grit silicon carbide paper and air-abraded with 50 μm Al_2O_3 particles at 0.2 MPa. Contrary to the results of the present study, a statistically significant higher bond strength was found for the unaged group of milled ZrO_2, whereas for aged (5000 thermocycles) specimens, the bond strength of milled and additive manufactured ZrO_2 with 0% porosity was at the same level. In addition, it was found that increasing porosity was associated with decreasing bond strength for additively manufactured ZrO_2. With reference to Branco et al. [54], the authors attributed the initially higher bond strength of milled zirconia to a lower wettability of additively manufactured nanostructured ZrO_2. Overall, there was a high number of pre-test failures and a predominance of adhesive failure in the specimens, which appears to severely limit the ability to draw conclusions in relation to the ZrO_2 substrate, rather suggesting that an adhesive system was used that appears unsuitable for ZrO_2 bonding. Zhang et al. compared the initial bond strength of milled and printed ZrO_2 with or without airborne particle abrasion using 110 μm Al_2O_3 particles at 0.2 MPa [31]. Additionally, a group of printed ZrO_2 with hexagonal surface microstructures was tested [31]. As expected, APA statistically significantly increased the bond strength of milled and printed specimens, with the printed specimens lagging slightly (but statistically significantly) behind the milled specimens. Interestingly, the establishment of hexagonal microstructures had the same effect on bond strength as APA and ensured that there was no statistically significant difference between APA and microstructured printed ZrO_2. Dai et al. focused exclusively on the possibilities offered by the introduction of microstructures on the surface of printed

ZrO_2 in terms of the bond strength achievable with a resin cement [30]. There was no milled control. Surfaces that were exclusively microstructured (using grooves or a hexagonal grid) did not reach the bond strength that could be achieved as a result of 0.2 MPa 50 µm Al_2O_3 APA after aging with 10,000 thermocycles but exceeded it in the case of the grooved surface when it was additionally subjected to an APA process.

As mentioned above, the study is limited in terms of its predictive value for long-term bond strength. Other limitations include the method of artificial ageing used in this study and the selection of adhesives tested. In terms of simulating the clinical situation, the ageing protocol differed from a clinical application in that, in addition to storage in a humid environment and thermal and mechanical stress on the bond due to thermocycling, direct mechanical forces would act on the bond in the oral cavity, which was not represented in the study and for which anatomical specimens would typically be used. With regard to the adhesive used, the results are only valid for this adhesive. This is a limitation as there are now many adhesives being promoted for bonding ZrO_2, which vary greatly in composition, mode of application, and sensitivity to ageing.

The results of this study, in conjunction with the last two studies discussed, are very useful in formulating the need for further research. In principle, the adhesive bond to printed ZrO_2 seems to be subject to the same factors (in terms of the adhesive used, the influence of surface conditioning and ageing) as to milled ZrO_2. In the future, however, the possibility of microstructuring printed ZrO_2 surfaces may reduce or eliminate the need for separate surface conditioning. However, this is dependent on finding a microstructure that allows bond strengths comparable to those achieved using the current standard, i.e., APA or TSC. The importance of chemical bonding should also be re-evaluated in the context of microstructured surfaces.

5. Conclusions

High bond strengths were achieved with the surface modifications tested, even after disinfection and ageing. While disinfection in combination with Al_2O_3 airborne particle abrasion resulted in a lower loss of bond strength due to ageing, it increased the negative ageing effect for the tribochemically silicatised specimens. Adhesive cementation of printed ZrO_2 resulted in bond strengths that were comparable to those of milled ZrO_2.

Author Contributions: Conceptualization, W.B., S.R. and F.S.S.; methodology, W.B. and S.R.; formal analysis, W.B. and S.R.; resources, P.R. and F.S.S.; data curation, W.B. and S.R.; writing—original draft preparation, W.B. and S.R.; writing—review and editing, P.R. and F.S.S.; supervision, W.B.; project administration, W.B. and S.R. All authors have read and agreed to the published version of the manuscript.

Funding: This research was funded by the Dietmar Hopp Foundation, Germany, grant number 1DH1911472.

Institutional Review Board Statement: Not applicable.

Informed Consent Statement: Not applicable.

Data Availability Statement: The data on which the results of this study are based can be made available upon reasoned request to the corresponding author.

Acknowledgments: The authors would like to thank Clemens Schmitt for test specimen preparation, ageing management and bond strength testing.

Conflicts of Interest: The authors declare no conflicts of interest. The funders had no role in the design of the study; in the collection, analyses, or interpretation of data; in the writing of the manuscript; or in the decision to publish the results.

References

1. Zarone, F.; Di Mauro, M.I.; Ausiello, P.; Ruggiero, G.; Sorrentino, R. Current status on lithium disilicate and zirconia: A narrative review. *BMC Oral Health* **2019**, *19*, 134. [CrossRef] [PubMed]
2. Ghodsi, S.; Jafarian, Z. A Review on Translucent Zirconia. *Eur. J. Prosthodont. Restor. Dent.* **2018**, *26*, 62–74. [CrossRef] [PubMed]

3. Ferrini, F.; Paolone, G.; Di Domenico, G.L.; Pagani, N.; Gherlone, E.F. SEM Evaluation of the Marginal Accuracy of Zirconia, Lithium Disilicate, and Composite Single Crowns Created by CAD/CAM Method: Comparative Analysis of Different Materials. *Materials* **2023**, *16*, 2413. [CrossRef] [PubMed]
4. Bömicke, W.; Rathmann, F.; Pilz, M.; Bermejo, J.L.; Waldecker, M.; Ohlmann, B.; Rammelsberg, P.; Zenthöfer, A. Clinical Performance of Posterior Inlay-Retained and Wing-Retained Monolithic Zirconia Resin-Bonded Fixed Partial Dentures: Stage One Results of a Randomized Controlled Trial. *J. Prosthodont.* **2021**, *30*, 384–393. [CrossRef]
5. Blatz, M.B.; Vonderheide, M.; Conejo, J. The Effect of Resin Bonding on Long-Term Success of High-Strength Ceramics. *J. Dent. Res.* **2018**, *97*, 132–139. [CrossRef]
6. Edelhoff, D.; Ozcan, M. To what extent does the longevity of fixed dental prostheses depend on the function of the cement? Working Group 4 materials: Cementation. *Clin. Oral Implant. Res.* **2007**, *18* (Suppl. S3), 193–204. [CrossRef]
7. Kern, M. Bonding to oxide ceramics—Laboratory testing versus clinical outcome. *Dent. Mater.* **2015**, *31*, 8–14. [CrossRef]
8. Inokoshi, M.; De Munck, J.; Minakuchi, S.; Van Meerbeek, B. Meta-analysis of bonding effectiveness to zirconia ceramics. *J. Dent. Res.* **2014**, *93*, 329–334. [CrossRef] [PubMed]
9. Kumar, R.; Singh, M.D.; Sharma, V.; Madaan, R.; Sareen, K.; Gurjar, B.; Saini, A.K. Effect of Surface Treatment of Zirconia on the Shear Bond Strength of Resin Cement: A Systematic Review and Meta-Analysis. *Cureus* **2023**, *15*, e45045. [CrossRef]
10. Bömicke, W.; Schürz, A.; Krisam, J.; Rammelsberg, P.; Rues, S. Durability of Resin-Zirconia Bonds Produced Using Methods Available in Dental Practice. *J. Adhes. Dent.* **2016**, *18*, 17–27. [CrossRef]
11. Quigley, N.P.; Loo, D.S.S.; Choy, C.; Ha, W.N. Clinical efficacy of methods for bonding to zirconia: A systematic review. *J. Prosthet. Dent.* **2021**, *125*, 231–240. [CrossRef] [PubMed]
12. Revilla-León, M.; Meyer, M.J.; Zandinejad, A.; Özcan, M. Additive manufacturing technologies for processing zirconia in dental applications. *Int. J. Comput. Dent.* **2020**, *23*, 27–37. [PubMed]
13. Methani, M.M.; Revilla-León, M.; Zandinejad, A. The potential of additive manufacturing technologies and their processing parameters for the fabrication of all-ceramic crowns: A review. *J. Esthet. Restor. Dent.* **2020**, *32*, 182–192. [CrossRef] [PubMed]
14. Teegen, I.S.; Schadte, P.; Wille, S.; Adelung, R.; Siebert, L.; Kern, M. Comparison of properties and cost efficiency of zirconia processed by DIW printing, casting and CAD/CAM-milling. *Dent. Mater.* **2023**, *39*, 669–676. [CrossRef]
15. Rues, S.; Zehender, N.; Zenthöfer, A.; Bömicke, W.; Herpel, C.; Ilani, A.; Erber, R.; Roser, C.; Lux, C.J.; Rammelsberg, P.; et al. Fit of anterior restorations made of 3D-printed and milled zirconia: An in-vitro study. *J. Dent.* **2023**, *130*, 104415. [CrossRef] [PubMed]
16. Maeder, M.; Pasic, P.; Ender, A.; Özcan, M.; Benic, G.I.; Ioannidis, A. Load-bearing capacities of ultra-thin occlusal veneers bonded to dentin. *J. Mech. Behav. Biomed. Mater.* **2019**, *95*, 165–171. [CrossRef]
17. Zenthöfer, A.; Ilani, A.; Schmitt, C.; Rammelsberg, P.; Hetzler, S.; Rues, S. Biaxial flexural strength of 3D-printed 3Y-TZP zirconia using a novel ceramic printer. *Clin. Oral Investig.* **2024**, *28*, 145. [CrossRef]
18. Mirt, T.; Kocjan, A.; Hofer, A.K.; Schwentenwein, M.; Iveković, A.; Bermejo, R.; Jevnikar, P. Effect of airborne particle abrasion and regeneration firing on the strength of 3D-printed 3Y and 5Y zirconia ceramics. *Dent. Mater.* **2024**, *40*, 111–117. [CrossRef] [PubMed]
19. Lu, Y.; Wang, L.; Dal Piva, A.M.O.; Tribst, J.P.M.; Čokić, S.M.; Zhang, F.; Werner, A.; Kleverlaan, C.J.; Feilzer, A.J. Effect of printing layer orientation and polishing on the fatigue strength of 3D-printed dental zirconia. *Dent. Mater.* **2024**, *40*, 190–197. [CrossRef]
20. Kyung, K.Y.; Park, J.M.; Heo, S.J.; Koak, J.Y.; Kim, S.K.; Ahn, J.S.; Yi, Y. Comparative analysis of flexural strength of 3D printed and milled 4Y-TZP and 3Y-TZP zirconia. *J. Prosthet. Dent.* **2024**, *131*, 529.e1–529.e9. [CrossRef]
21. Hajjaj, M.S.; Alamoudi, R.A.A.; Babeer, W.A.; Rizg, W.Y.; Basalah, A.A.; Alzahrani, S.J.; Yeslam, H.E. Flexural strength, flexural modulus and microhardness of milled vs. fused deposition modeling printed Zirconia; effect of conventional vs. speed sintering. *BMC Oral Health* **2024**, *24*, 38. [CrossRef] [PubMed]
22. Frąckiewicz, W.; Szymlet, P.; Jedliński, M.; Światłowska-Bajzert, M.; Sobolewska, E. Mechanical characteristics of zirconia produced additively by 3D printing in dentistry—A systematic review with meta-analysis of novel reports. *Dent. Mater.* **2024**, *40*, 124–138. [CrossRef] [PubMed]
23. Toksoy, D.; Önöral, Ö. Influence of glazing and aging on the marginal, axial, axio-occlusal, and occlusal fit of 3-unit monolithic zirconia restorations fabricated using additive and subtractive techniques. *J. Prosthet. Dent.* **2024**, *131*, 658.e1–658.e9. [CrossRef] [PubMed]
24. Lee, H.B.; Noh, M.J.; Bae, E.J.; Lee, W.S.; Kim, J.H. Accuracy of zirconia crown manufactured using stereolithography and digital light processing. *J. Dent.* **2024**, *141*, 104834. [CrossRef] [PubMed]
25. Zhu, H.; Zhou, Y.; Jiang, J.; Wang, Y.; He, F. Accuracy and margin quality of advanced 3D-printed monolithic zirconia crowns. *J. Prosthet. Dent.* **2023**. [CrossRef] [PubMed]
26. Zandinejad, A.; Khurana, S.; Liang, Y.; Liu, X. Comparative evaluation of gingival fibroblast growth on 3D-printed and milled zirconia: An in vitro study. *J. Prosthodont.* **2024**, *33*, 54–60. [CrossRef] [PubMed]
27. Rabel, K.; Nath, A.J.; Nold, J.; Spies, B.C.; Wesemann, C.; Altmann, B.; Adolfsson, E.; Witkowski, S.; Tomakidi, P.; Steinberg, T. Analysis of soft tissue integration-supportive cell functions cultured on 3D printed biomaterials for oral implant-supported prostheses. *J. Biomed. Mater. Res. A* **2024**. [CrossRef] [PubMed]
28. Rodríguez-Lozano, F.J.; López-García, S.; Sánchez-Bautista, S.; Pérez-López, J.; Raigrodski, A.J.; Revilla-León, M. Effect of milled and lithography-based additively manufactured zirconia (3Y-TZP) on the biological properties of human osteoblasts. *J. Prosthet. Dent.* **2023**, *130*, 889–896. [CrossRef] [PubMed]

29. Zandinejad, A.; Khanlar, L.N.; Barmak, A.B.; Tagami, J.; Revilla-León, M. Surface Roughness and Bond Strength of Resin Composite to Additively Manufactured Zirconia with Different Porosities. *J. Prosthodont.* **2022**, *31*, 97–104. [CrossRef]
30. Dai, K.; Wu, J.; Yu, H.; Zhao, Z.; Gao, B. Effects of Surface Textures Created Using Additive Manufacturing on Shear Bond Strength Between Resin and Zirconia. *J. Adhes. Dent.* **2024**, *26*, 79–86. [CrossRef]
31. Zhang, C.; Meng, J.; Zhang, L.; Fan, S.; Yi, Y.; Zhang, J.; Wu, G. Influence of 3D printed surface micro-structures on molding performance and dental bonding properties of zirconia. *J. Dent.* **2024**, *144*, 104937. [CrossRef] [PubMed]
32. Thammajaruk, P.; Guazzato, M.; Naorungroj, S. Cleaning methods of contaminated zirconia: A systematic review and meta-analysis. *Dent. Mater.* **2023**, *39*, 235–245. [CrossRef] [PubMed]
33. Gadelmawla, E.S.; Koura, M.M.; Maksoud, T.M.A.; Elewa, I.M.; Soliman, H.H. Roughness parameters. *J. Mater. Process. Technol.* **2002**, *123*, 133–145. [CrossRef]
34. Scaminaci Russo, D.; Cinelli, F.; Sarti, C.; Giachetti, L. Adhesion to Zirconia: A Systematic Review of Current Conditioning Methods and Bonding Materials. *Dent. J.* **2019**, *7*, 74. [CrossRef] [PubMed]
35. Papia, E.; Larsson, C.; du Toit, M.; Vult von Steyern, P. Bonding between oxide ceramics and adhesive cement systems: A systematic review. *J. Biomed. Mater. Res. B Appl. Biomater.* **2014**, *102*, 395–413. [CrossRef]
36. Yang, B.; Barloi, A.; Kern, M. Influence of air-abrasion on zirconia ceramic bonding using an adhesive composite resin. *Dent. Mater.* **2010**, *26*, 44–50. [CrossRef] [PubMed]
37. Comino-Garayoa, R.; Peláez, J.; Tobar, C.; Rodríguez, V.; Suárez, M.J. Adhesion to Zirconia: A Systematic Review of Surface Pretreatments and Resin Cements. *Materials* **2021**, *14*, 2751. [CrossRef] [PubMed]
38. Rigos, A.E.; Sarafidou, K.; Kontonasaki, E. Zirconia bond strength durability following artificial aging: A systematic review and meta-analysis of in vitro studies. *Jpn. Dent. Sci. Rev.* **2023**, *59*, 138–159. [CrossRef]
39. Ruales-Carrera, E.; Cesar, P.F.; Henriques, B.; Fredel, M.C.; Özcan, M.; Volpato, C.A.M. Adhesion behavior of conventional and high-translucent zirconia: Effect of surface conditioning methods and aging using an experimental methodology. *J. Esthet. Restor. Dent.* **2019**, *31*, 388–397. [CrossRef]
40. Tanaka, R.; Fujishima, A.; Shibata, Y.; Manabe, A.; Miyazaki, T. Cooperation of phosphate monomer and silica modification on zirconia. *J. Dent. Res.* **2008**, *87*, 666–670. [CrossRef]
41. Bielen, V.; Inokoshi, M.; Munck, J.D.; Zhang, F.; Vanmeensel, K.; Minakuchi, S.; Vleugels, J.; Naert, I.; Van Meerbeek, B. Bonding Effectiveness to Differently Sandblasted Dental Zirconia. *J. Adhes. Dent.* **2015**, *17*, 235–242. [CrossRef] [PubMed]
42. Gomes, A.L.; Castillo-Oyagüe, R.; Lynch, C.D.; Montero, J.; Albaladejo, A. Influence of sandblasting granulometry and resin cement composition on microtensile bond strength to zirconia ceramic for dental prosthetic frameworks. *J. Dent.* **2013**, *41*, 31–41. [CrossRef] [PubMed]
43. Wongsue, S.; Thanatvarakorn, O.; Prasansuttiporn, T.; Nimmanpipug, P.; Sastraruji, T.; Hosaka, K.; Foxton, R.M.; Nakajima, M. Effect of surface topography and wettability on shear bond strength of Y-TZP ceramic. *Sci. Rep.* **2023**, *13*, 18249. [CrossRef] [PubMed]
44. Chuang, S.F.; Kang, L.L.; Liu, Y.C.; Lin, J.C.; Wang, C.C.; Chen, H.M.; Tai, C.K. Effects of silane- and MDP-based primers application orders on zirconia-resin adhesion-A ToF-SIMS study. *Dent. Mater.* **2017**, *33*, 923–933. [CrossRef] [PubMed]
45. de Souza, G.; Hennig, D.; Aggarwal, A.; Tam, L.E. The use of MDP-based materials for bonding to zirconia. *J. Prosthet. Dent.* **2014**, *112*, 895–902. [CrossRef]
46. Kern, M. *Resin-Bonded Fixed Dental Prostheses: Minimally Invasive–Esthetic–Reliable*, 1st ed.; Quintessenz Verlag: Berlin, Germany, 2018; p. 264.
47. Waltimo, A.; Könönen, M. Maximal bite force and its association with signs and symptoms of craniomandibular disorders in young Finnish non-patients. *Acta Odontol. Scand.* **1995**, *53*, 254–258. [CrossRef] [PubMed]
48. Oliveira-Ogliari, A.; Collares, F.M.; Feitosa, V.P.; Sauro, S.; Ogliari, F.A.; Moraes, R.R. Methacrylate bonding to zirconia by in situ silica nanoparticle surface deposition. *Dent. Mater.* **2015**, *31*, 68–76. [CrossRef]
49. Ebeid, K.; Wille, S.; Salah, T.; Wahsh, M.; Zohdy, M.; Kern, M. Bond strength of resin cement to zirconia treated in pre-sintered stage. *J. Mech. Behav. Biomed. Mater.* **2018**, *86*, 84–88. [CrossRef] [PubMed]
50. Nagaoka, N.; Yoshihara, K.; Feitosa, V.P.; Tamada, Y.; Irie, M.; Yoshida, Y.; Van Meerbeek, B.; Hayakawa, S. Chemical interaction mechanism of 10-MDP with zirconia. *Sci. Rep.* **2017**, *7*, 45563. [CrossRef]
51. Chen, C.; Chen, Y.; Lu, Z.; Qian, M.; Xie, H.; Tay, F.R. The effects of water on degradation of the zirconia-resin bond. *J. Dent.* **2017**, *64*, 23–29. [CrossRef]
52. Yang, L.; Chen, B.; Xie, H.; Chen, Y.; Chen, Y.; Chen, C. Durability of Resin Bonding to Zirconia Using Products Containing 10-Methacryloyloxydecyl Dihydrogen Phosphate. *J. Adhes. Dent.* **2018**, *20*, 279–287. [CrossRef] [PubMed]
53. Lima, R.B.W.; Barreto, S.C.; Hajhamid, B.; de Souza, G.M.; de Goes, M.F. Effect of cleaning protocol on silica deposition and silica-mediated bonding to Y-TZP. *Dent. Mater.* **2019**, *35*, 1603–1613. [CrossRef] [PubMed]
54. Branco, A.C.; Silva, R.; Santos, T.; Jorge, H.; Rodrigues, A.R.; Fernandes, R.; Bandarra, S.; Barahona, I.; Matos, A.P.A.; Lorenz, K.; et al. Suitability of 3D printed pieces of nanocrystalline zirconia for dental applications. *Dent. Mater.* **2020**, *36*, 442–455. [CrossRef] [PubMed]

Disclaimer/Publisher's Note: The statements, opinions and data contained in all publications are solely those of the individual author(s) and contributor(s) and not of MDPI and/or the editor(s). MDPI and/or the editor(s) disclaim responsibility for any injury to people or property resulting from any ideas, methods, instructions or products referred to in the content.

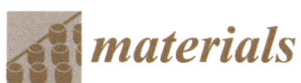

Article

Effect of Luting Materials on the Accuracy of Fit of Zirconia Copings: A Non-Destructive Digital Analysis Method

Lara Berger [1], Ragai-Edward Matta [1,*], Christian Markus Weiß [1], Werner Adler [2], Manfred Wichmann [1] and José Ignacio Zorzin [3]

[1] Department of Prosthodontics, University Hospital Erlangen, Glückstrasse 11, 91054 Erlangen, Germany; lara.berger@uk-erlangen.de (L.B.); weiss_christian_markus@outlook.de (C.M.W.)
[2] Institute of Medical Informatics, Biometry and Epidemiology (IMBE) of the Friedrich-Alexander-University, Erlangen-Nuremberg, Waldstrasse 6, 91054 Erlangen, Germany; werner.adler@fau.de
[3] Dental Clinic 1—Department of Operative Dentistry and Periodontology, Erlangen University Hospital, Glueckstrasse 11, 91054 Erlangen, Germany; jose.zorzin@fau.de
* Correspondence: ragai.matta@uk-erlangen.de; Tel.: +49-9131-8533604

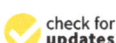

Citation: Berger, L.; Matta, R.-E.; Weiß, C.M.; Adler, W.; Wichmann, M.; Zorzin, J.I. Effect of Luting Materials on the Accuracy of Fit of Zirconia Copings: A Non-Destructive Digital Analysis Method. *Materials* **2024**, *17*, 2130. https://doi.org/10.3390/ma17092130

Academic Editors: Josip Kranjčić and Tina Poklepovic Pericic

Received: 9 April 2024
Revised: 26 April 2024
Accepted: 28 April 2024
Published: 1 May 2024

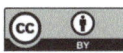

Copyright: © 2024 by the authors. Licensee MDPI, Basel, Switzerland. This article is an open access article distributed under the terms and conditions of the Creative Commons Attribution (CC BY) license (https://creativecommons.org/licenses/by/4.0/).

Abstract: The marginal accuracy of fit between prosthetic restorations and abutment teeth represents an essential aspect with regard to long-term clinical success. Since the final gap is also influenced by the luting techniques and materials applied, this study analyzed the accuracy of the fit of single-tooth zirconia copings before and after cementation using different luting materials. Forty plaster dies with a corresponding zirconia coping were manufactured based on a single tooth chamfer preparation. The copings were luted on the plaster dies ($n = 10$ per luting material) with a zinc phosphate (A), glass–ionomer (B), self-adhesive resin (C), or resin-modified glass–ionomer cement (D). The accuracy of fit for each coping was assessed using a non-destructive digital method. Intragroup statistical analysis was conducted using Wilcoxon signed rank tests and intergroup analysis by Kruskal–Wallis and Mann–Whitney U tests ($\alpha = 0.05$). Accuracy of fit was significantly different before/after cementation within A (0.033/0.110 µm) and B (0.035/0.118 µm; $p = 0.002$). A had a significantly increased marginal gap compared to C and D, and B compared to C and D ($p \leq 0.001$). Significantly increased vertical discrepancies between A and B versus C and D ($p < 0.001$) were assessed. Of the materials under investigation, the zinc phosphate cement led to increased vertical marginal discrepancies, whereas the self-adhesive resin cement did not influence the restoration fit.

Keywords: marginal fit; zirconia; self-adhesive resin cement; glass–ionomer cement; resin-modified glass–ionomer cement; zinc phosphate cement; CAD–CAM technology; ceramics; dental materials; prosthodontics

1. Introduction

Indirect all-ceramic restorations can realistically imitate natural human teeth, and therefore enjoy a very high popularity among dentists as they satisfy the increasing aesthetic demands of patients nowadays [1,2]. In this context, the spectrum of treatment methods and processing technologies must be continuously improved in order to optimally combine optimized functionality, biocompatibility, and the aesthetics of these ceramic materials [3,4].

There is a general digital transformation occurring within everyday dental practice, accompanied by an increasing interest in computer-assisted processes for the fabrication of dental prostheses in order to offer a standardized manufacturing chain with improved technical and biological properties of the component [5]. Considering this, the Computer-Aided Design (CAD)/Computer-Aided Manufacturing (CAM) fabrication of ceramic restorations is usually carried out by subtractive processes in which the workpiece is milled out of an industrially prefabricated blank [3]. The subtractive milling process is an advanced technique for the fabrication of ceramic restorations that has been proven over more than two decades [3,6,7]. CAD/CAM technology was pioneered and introduced to dentistry by François Duret in 1971 with his theoretical and experimental research on the computer-assisted manufacturing crowns. In 1980, Mörmann and Brandestini started with the development of a CAD/CAM system with an intraoral camera, a design computer and a milling unit using a ceramic block for manufacturing inlays at chair-side. Their research led in 1985 to the CEREC system (Dentsply Sirona, Bensheim, Germany). Based on these technologies, further chair- and lab-side dental CAD/CAM systems were developed [8]. The manufacturing of dental prostheses can also be performed using additive processes. In the field of dentistry, there are two main technologies that are widely used. One of them is stereolithography (SLA), which is typically utilized to create models, aligners, and provisional structures. The other is direct metal laser sintering (DMLS), which has the capability to produce metal dental crowns and appliance frames [9].

In contemporary dental practices, silicate and oxide ceramics are the preferred materials for the subtractive milling of crowns and bridges. Due to their superior mechanical stability, oxide ceramics are frequently selected as the material of choice for a wide range of dental applications [10]. Oxide ceramics consist of a pure polycrystalline phase without any glass phase. Today, zirconium oxide (ZrO_2) is predominantly used, to which 3 mol% yttria (Y_2O_3) is added in order to stabilize the crystals in the tetragonal crystal phase at room temperature (yttria-stabilized tetragonal zirconia polycrystals, Y-TZP) [10]. At 3 mol% yttria, dental zirconium oxide ceramics (3Y-TZP) exhibit the highest fracture toughness. However, these ceramics are almost opaque due to the birefringence of the tetragonal crystals and the numerous grain boundaries [10]. They are suitable only as framework structures for single crowns or multi-unit veneered bridges, which must be veneered with silicate ceramics. The aesthetics of these veneered restorations are unrivaled. However, chipping of the veneer often occurs. An alternative to minimize fracture risk is to fabricate the restoration monolithically. Adding 4 and 5 mol% of yttrium oxide (4Y- and 5Y-TZP) decreases the proportion of zirconium oxide crystals in the tetragonal phase, and the proportion of cubic crystals and grain sizes increases. Zirconium oxide becomes translucent and more aesthetic, but fracture toughness decreases [11]. These modern 4Y and 5Y-TZP zirconium oxide ceramics with color gradients in combination with coloring techniques and dental expertise allow for monolithic restorations that are aesthetically more than satisfactory [12].

In this regard, the marginal accuracy of fit between crowns or fixed partial dentures and abutment teeth, which was defined by Holmes et al. [13] as the linear distance from the edge of the restoration to the preparation margin of the die, has been well-known for a long time, and represents an essential aspect with regard to the long-term clinical success of prosthetic restorations. The marginal measuring distance extends 1 mm in the direction of the lumen from the edge of the preparation and restoration, respectively [14,15]. The authors also determined the absolute marginal discrepancy (xyz), which results from the angular combination of the vertical and horizontal marginal discrepancy as the hypotenuse of a right-angled triangle, as the margins of fixed restorations often exhibit over- or under-extension [13]. For milled restorations, the vertical fit is influenced by the number of axes of the milling machine [16]. Inadequate crown margins can lead to gingival inflammation, which results in periodontal disease or secondary caries of the abutment tooth due to the washout of the luting material [1,17–20]. In addition, deviations in fit can cause increased stress within the restorative material, which can reduce the strength of the material and cause failure by fracture [1,21]. In the literature, previously non-evidence-based recommendations of a clinically acceptable marginal gap vary from 50 to maximum tolerance values of 120 µm under clinical conditions [22]. However, a certain amount of space is required during insertion for cementation of the restoration, and this is unavoidable [23]. At the same time, the applied luting technique and the properties of the corresponding luting materials, as well as their flow behavior during the cementation process, can influence the final size of the marginal gap [24–26].

Basically, a distinction can be made between luting cements and composites for the final cementation of restorations; the former can be further divided into conventional and modified luting materials. Common conventional luting materials include phosphate and glass–ionomer cements based on an acid-base reaction in which the bond is reinforced by the retention and resistance of the restorative abutment teeth by means of microretentions [27–30]. As this class of materials has evolved to expand the range of applications and improve properties, modifications have been made, resulting in the introduction of resin-modified, metal-reinforced, and high-viscosity materials. In particular, resin-modified glass–ionomer cements have entered the market as luting cements. The polymerization of these two-component materials, consisting of a photopolymerizable monomer, ionizable glasses, and water, is also based on an acid-base reaction [31–35]. In contrast, composites are used for the adhesive cementation of indirect restorations via both microretentions and chemical bonding. The classic representatives require conditioning of the tooth, whereas the newer, self-adhesive composites interact chemically and physically with the tooth surface [36]. Preheating composite resin for luting procedures is used to reduce material viscosity and improve restoration setting [37].

The final film thickness of the luting material is important, as failure to meet this required standard would result in poor seating of the restoration, disrupting both functional and occlusal relationships [38]. Ideally, the material that is used should be able to flow out to a low film thickness, which is influenced by various factors, such as the size and shape of the filler particles, the viscosity in the uncured state, and the setting rate [39,40]. The International Organization for Standardization (ISO) defines various standards for dental luting materials, such as requirements and test methods for powder/liquid acid-base dental cements [41], water-based resin-modified cements [42], and polymer-based materials with adhesive components [43,44]. The mentioned norms require a maximal film thickness of 25 μm for acid-base dental cements and 50 μm for resin-based luting materials [45].

However, film thickness measurements set up following the aforementioned ISO norms do not consider the effects of the geometry of the abutment and the crown on the material flow. Different studies regarding the internal fit of luted restorations can be found in the literature, but none of them have used non-destructive methods and different classes of luting materials.

Therefore, the present study investigated the extent to which different luting cements and materials influence the resulting marginal accuracies of CAD/CAM-milled zirconia single-tooth restorations after subtractive fabrication using a digital non-destructive method. The first hypothesis was that there is no difference in the fit of a particular zirconia single-tooth restoration before and after cementation. The second hypothesis was that there is no difference in the fit of the different zirconia single-tooth restorations after cementation.

2. Materials and Methods

The measurements carried out in this in vitro investigation were based on a metal master model, which corresponded to an in vivo chamfer preparation of a single tooth to derive an all-ceramic single crown.

Consequently, a total of 40 individual double mix impressions were taken from this master model using an addition-cured polyvinyl siloxane (AFFINIS PRECIOUS light und regular body, Coltène/Whaledent AG, Altstaetten, Switzerland), which were then poured with Class IV super hard stone (GC Fujirock EP Classic, GC, Tokyo, Japan). The individual plaster dies were digitized with a dental model scanner (Dental Wings 3SERIES, Dental Wings Inc., Montréal, QC, Canada) and DWOS 5.0.1.3084 Software (Dental Wings Inc.) used for the further CAD design of anatomically reduced zirconium oxide crown copings. During the manufacturing process, the marginal gap parameter of all crown copings was set to 20 μm, whereas the basic parameters amounted to a minimum layer thickness of 0.5 mm, a margin thickness of 0.25 mm, and vertical and horizontal placeholders for the cement of 40 μm each for all crown copings.

To three-dimensionally (3D) measure the fit between the crown copings and the plaster dies, optical object registration was performed using an ATOS Triple Scan (GOM GmbH, Braunschweig, Germany) non-contact blue-light industrial scanner. For this purpose, the plaster dies were equipped in advance with high-contrast reference points with a diameter of 0.4 mm (GOM GmbH) to enhance the precision of the subsequent scanning process. All scanning procedures were conducted by the same experienced clinician.

In accordance with the triple scan protocol of Holst et al. and Matta et al. [46,47], for each case, four single scans were taken of the corresponding dies and crown copings so that the copings could be positioned correctly on a virtual plane before and after cementation. First, all of the plaster dies and crown copings were optically scanned separately; the crown copings were coated in advance with a thin layer of a mixture of 90% ethanol and pure titanium dioxide powder using an airbrush to reduce possible light reflection, and then fixed in a specially calibrated measuring frame (Reference frame, GOM GmbH).

Subsequently, the copings on the plaster dies, which were fixed in the adapted position with adhesive wax (Supradent-Wax, Anton Gerl GmbH, Munich, Germany) before cementation, were scanned together before and after definitive cementation. The cementation procedures were performed under a constant punch pressure of 10 N in a standardized manner using a rondel construction [48,49]. All cementation procedures were performed by the same experienced clinician who had previously performed the scanning procedures.

As the dependence of the selected luting material on the fit of the crown copings was also investigated in this study, four different luting materials were selected, each cementing 10 crown copings in self-cure mode: a zinc phosphate cement (HOFFMANN'S READY2MIX ZINC PHOSPHATECEMENT NORMAL, Hoffmann Dental Manufaktur, Berlin, Germany—Group A), a glass–ionomer cement (Ketac Cem Aplicap, 3M, St. Paul, MN, USA—Group B), a self-adhesive resin cement (RelyX Unicem 2 Automix, 3M, St. Paul, MN, USA—Group C), and a resin-modified glass–ionomer luting cement (GC FujiCem 2 Automix, GC, Tokyo, Japan—Group D). The luting materials under investigation, batch numbers, composition, filler sizes, and film thickness as disclosed by the manufacturers are listed in Table 1.

Surface Triangulation Language (STL) file formats were generated from the obtained data, which generally exhibited an average measurement error of 3 μm due to the scanning method and virtual object registration [46]. With the aid of the GOM "Inspect Professional" software 2017 (GOM GmbH), a virtual surface and section analysis could be performed. Therefore, the individual scans of the plaster dies and crown copings were virtually superimposed on the jointly digitized dies and copings before and after cementation ("matching") and finally aligned with high precision for data comparisons using the local best-fit function. In the following step, a marginal surface of the copings was defined, which extended 1 mm parallel to the crown margin in the direction of the lumen, so that a 3D surface analysis of the marginal fit accuracies could be performed. Subsequently, discrepancies in this area from the virtual plaster dies as reference models could be calculated by an area comparison and visualized using a color plot. Following this procedure, a surface analysis was performed for the condition before and after cementation so that the respective fits could be compared (Figure 1).

In addition, a two-dimensional (2D) examination of the margin fit of the crown copings was performed, so the matched files before and after cementation were virtually split into 20 sectional images at 18° intervals. By creating a coordinate system, it was possible to calculate the vertical, horizontal, and absolute marginal discrepancies (Figure 2).

In the statistical analysis, the measurements before and after cementation of the crown copings were compared using Wilcoxon signed rank tests. The differences in the situations before and after cementation were calculated and compared between the four groups. For this purpose, a global Kruskal–Wallis test was performed and pairwise group comparisons carried out with Mann–Whitney U tests. The mean values of the 20 repeated measurements were used for the statistical tests of the 2D measurements. The statistical analysis was performed using statistical software R 4.0.3 [50] with a significance level of 0.05.

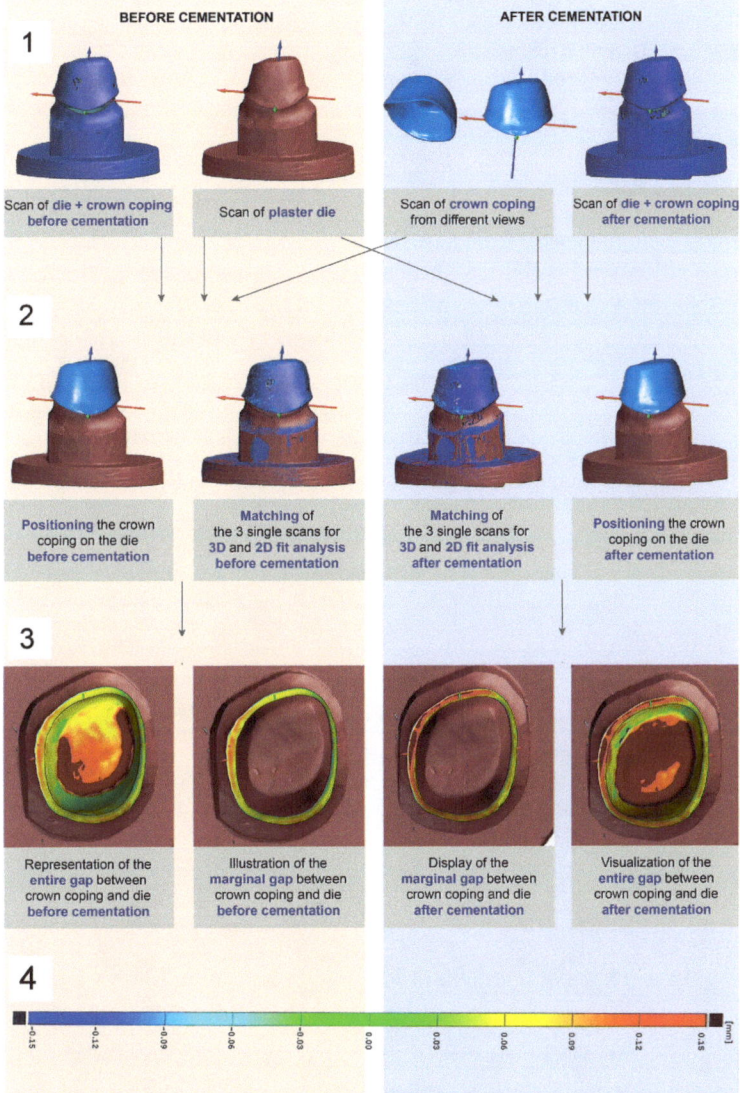

Figure 1. (**1**) Analytical protocol consisting of four scans in each case: single scan of the plaster die, single scan of the ceramic crown coping, scan of the adapted coping on the die in its final position before cementation, and scan of definitively cemented coping on the die. (**2**) Virtual superimposition of the individual scans (plaster dies, crown copings) with the situations before and after cementation. (**3**) Surface analysis of the entire and the marginal gap between the crown coping and the plaster die before and after cementation. (**4**) False color scale to visualize the discrepancies (mm) as color-coded distance maps. Green areas indicate deviations between 0 and 50 µm, yellow areas show deviations from 50 to 100 µm, and red areas highlight deviations of more than 100 µm.

Table 1. Manufacturer's specifications of the luting materials investigated.

Luting Material	HOFFMANN'S READY2MIX NORMAL	Ketac Cem Aplicap	RelyX Unicem 2 Automix	GC Fuji-Cem 2
Material type	Zinc phosphate	Glass-ionomer	Self-adhesive resin	Resin-modified glass–ionomer
Manufacturer	Hoffmann Dental Manufaktur GmbH, Berlin, Germany	3M, St. Paul, MN, USA	3M, St. Paul, MN, USA	GC, Tokyo, Japan
Shade	Yellow	Yellow	A2	Light Yellow
Lot number	N.A.	529059	574731	141211A
Composition	Powder: Zinc oxide, magnesium oxide Liquid: Ortho-phosphoric acid	Powder: Glass powder, pigments Liquid: Water, Acrylic acid/Maleic acid copolymer, tartaric acid, preservative	Base paste: Phosphorylated methacrylate monomers, methacrylate monomers, silanized fillers, initiators, stabilizers, rheology additive Catalyst paste: Methacrylate monomers, basic and silanized fillers, initiators, stabilizers, pigments, rheology additive	Paste A: Fluoroalumino-silicate glass, initiator, UDMA, dimethacrylate, pigments, silicon dioxide, inhibitor Paste B: Silicon dioxide, UDMA, dimethacrylate, initiator, inhibitor
Filler particle size	N.A.	≤12 µm	<9.5 µm	N.A.
Film thickness	N.A.	16 ± 1 µm	13 µm	N.A.

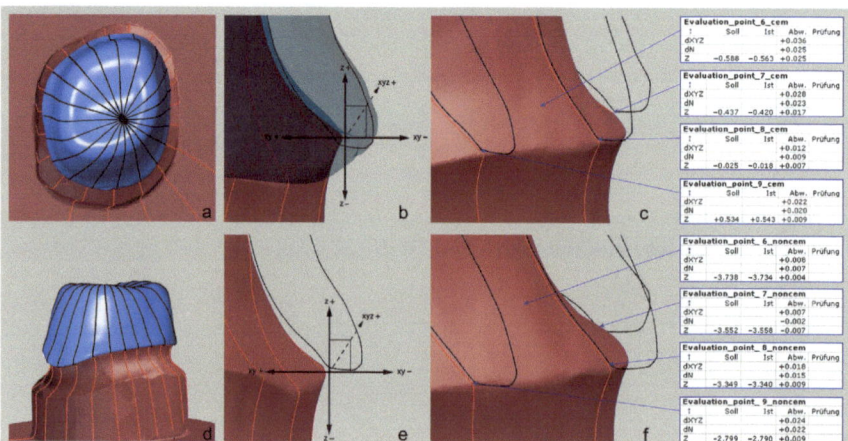

Figure 2. Visualization of the 2D sectional examination through the die with the 20 virtually positioned sections (**a**,**d**) and representation of the constructed coordinate system between coping and preparation margin of the plaster die (**b**,**e**). z = vertical marginal discrepancy from the most inferior edge of the coping to the outermost edge of the die, n = horizontal marginal discrepancy from the determined perpendiculars of the most inferior edge of the coping as well as the outermost edge of the die, xyz = absolute marginal discrepancy as a 2D vector of the vertical (z) and horizontal (n) discrepancy. An illustration of the 2D marginal deviations (**c**,**f**) of the coping before (**d**–**f**) and after cementation (**a**–**c**) is also provided.

3. Results

The 3D measurements of the crown copings before and after cementation (Table 2), compared by Wilcoxon signed rank tests, illustrate significant differences within Group A (deviation in µm: 0.033 ± 0.004 before vs. 0.110 ± 0.049 after cementation, $p = 0.002$) and Group B (deviation in µm: 0.035 ± 0.005 before vs. 0.118 ± 0.048 after cementation, $p = 0.002$). To determine the influence of the selected luting material on the resulting fit, and thus the discrepancies between the four groups, the differences in the respective situations were calculated and compared between the groups using the global Kruskal–Wallis test and pairwise group comparisons with Mann–Whitney U tests. Group A (difference in µm: 0.077 ± 0.049) exhibited a significantly larger marginal gap ($p < 0.001$) than Group C (difference in µm: 0.001 ± 0.008), and Group D (difference in µm: 0.001 ± 0.012). In addition, a significantly larger deviation was observed in Group B (difference in µm: 0.083 ± 0.046) compared to Group C ($p < 0.001$) and Group D ($p = 0.001$; Figure 3).

Table 2. Descriptive statistics of the 3D measured values of the marginal fit in µm, the corresponding standard deviations (SD), the maximum and minimum values (Max, Min) and the *p*-values when comparing the two time points before and after cementation for all groups (Group A–D).

3D Analysis of the Marginal Fit (µm) before and after Cementation						
Group		Mean	SD	Min	Max	*p*-Value
Group A	before cem	0.033	0.004	0.028	0.038	0.002
	after cem	0.110	0.049	0.059	0.210	
Group B	before cem	0.035	0.005	0.031	0.043	0.002
	after cem	0.118	0.048	0.039	0.188	
Group C	before cem	0.042	0.005	0.035	0.053	1.0
	after cem	0.042	0.007	0.033	0.058	
Group D	before cem	0.038	0.003	0.035	0.042	0.722
	after cem	0.040	0.012	0.027	0.067	

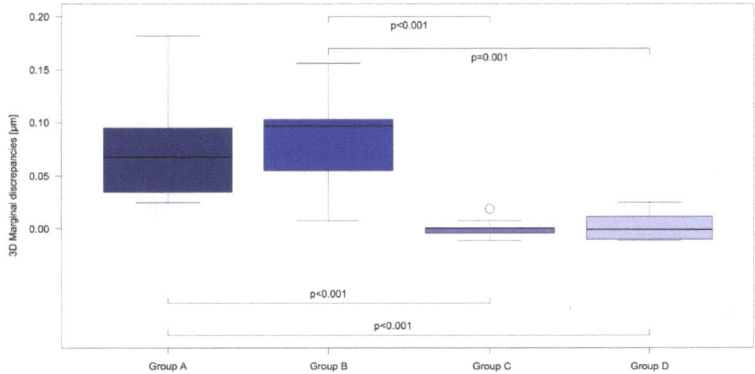

Figure 3. Comparison of marginal 3D differences between the four study groups (A–D) using boxplot diagrams.

In the course of the 2D examinations (Table 3) of the marginal fit at the two time points before and after cementation of the copings, significant differences were elicited in the vertical dimensions within Group A (deviation in µm: 0.030 ± 0.015 before vs.

0.193 ± 0.146 after cementation, $p = 0.002$) and Group B (deviation in μm: $-0.004 ± 0.015$ before vs. 0.164 ± 0.092 after cementation, $p = 0.002$). In contrast, the horizontal marginal discrepancies differed significantly only within Group B (discrepancy in μm: 0.010 ± 0.006 before vs. 0.020 ± 0.009 after cementation, $p = 0.002$).

Table 3. Mean values of the data of the 2D virtual analysis of the vertical, horizontal and absolute marginal discrepancy in μm before and after cementation for all groups (Group A–D). Furthermore, representation of the calculated standard deviations (SD), the maximum and minimum values (Max, Min) and the p-values when comparing the respective data series.

2D Analysis of the Marginal Fit (μm) before and after Cementation							
Parameter	Group		Mean	SD	Min	Max	p-Value
Vertical marginal discrepancy	A	before cem	0.030	0.015	−0.002	0.052	0.002
		after cem	0.193	0.146	0.051	0.551	
	B	before cem	−0.004	0.015	−0.025	0.017	0.002
		after cem	0.164	0.092	0.011	0.291	
	C	before cem	0.018	0.007	0.008	0.031	0.322
		after cem	0.026	0.020	−0.003	0.064	
	D	before cem	0.011	0.002	0.007	0.014	0.846
		after cem	0.013	0.025	−0.014	0.057	
Horizontal marginal discrepancy	A	before cem	−0.021	0.014	−0.049	0.002	0.232
		after cem	−0.017	0.019	−0.046	0.015	
	B	before cem	0.010	0.006	0.003	0.024	0.002
		after cem	0.020	0.009	0.006	0.038	
	C	before cem	0.018	0.005	0.009	0.026	0.126
		after cem	0.014	0.006	0.008	0.026	
	D	before cem	0.012	0.003	0.009	0.017	0.922
		after cem	0.013	0.006	0.006	0.023	
Absolute marginal discrepancy	A	before cem	0.045	0.014	0.031	0.076	0.002
		after cem	0.207	0.148	0.076	0.570	
	B	before cem	0.031	0.005	0.026	0.042	0.002
		after cem	0.187	0.094	0.048	0.319	
	C	before cem	0.028	0.009	0.014	0.041	0.131
		after cem	0.037	0.016	0.021	0.070	
	D	before cem	0.017	0.003	0.012	0.023	0.002
		after cem	0.038	0.016	0.021	0.075	

Regarding the absolute marginal discrepancy, significant differences were established not only within Group A (deviation in μm: 0.045 ± 0.014 before vs. 0.207 ± 0.148 after cementation, $p = 0.002$) and B (deviation in μm: 0.031 ± 0.005 before vs. 0.187 ± 0.094 after cementation, $p = 0.002$), but also within Group D (deviation in μm: 0.017 ± 0.003 before vs. 0.038 ± 0.016 after cementation, $p = 0.002$).

For the statistical comparison of the 2D measurements between the respective groups, the differences in the averaged values were used. Groups A (difference in μm: 0.164 ± 0.146) and B (difference in μm: 0.169 ± 0.087) showed significantly larger vertical marginal deviations ($p < 0.001$) than Groups C (difference in μm: 0.009 ± 0.018) and D (difference in μm: 0.002 ± 0.025). Concerning the horizontal deviations, significant differences ($p = 0.038$) were observed when comparing Groups A (difference in μm: 0.004 ± 0.008) and C (difference in μm: −0.004 ± 0.007). In addition, Group B (difference in μm: 0.009 ± 0.006) exhibited significantly larger horizontal discrepancies than Groups C ($p < 0.001$) and D (difference in μm: 0.001 ± 0.006, $p = 0.004$). With regard to the comparison of absolute marginal discrepancies between all groups, significantly larger discrepancies were found for Groups A (difference in μm: 0.162 ± 0.150) and B (difference in μm: 0.155 ± 0.095) compared to Groups C (difference in µm: 0.009 ± 0.017, $p < 0.001$) and D (difference in µm: 0.022 ± 0.017, $p < 0.001$ and $p = 0.002$, Figure 4).

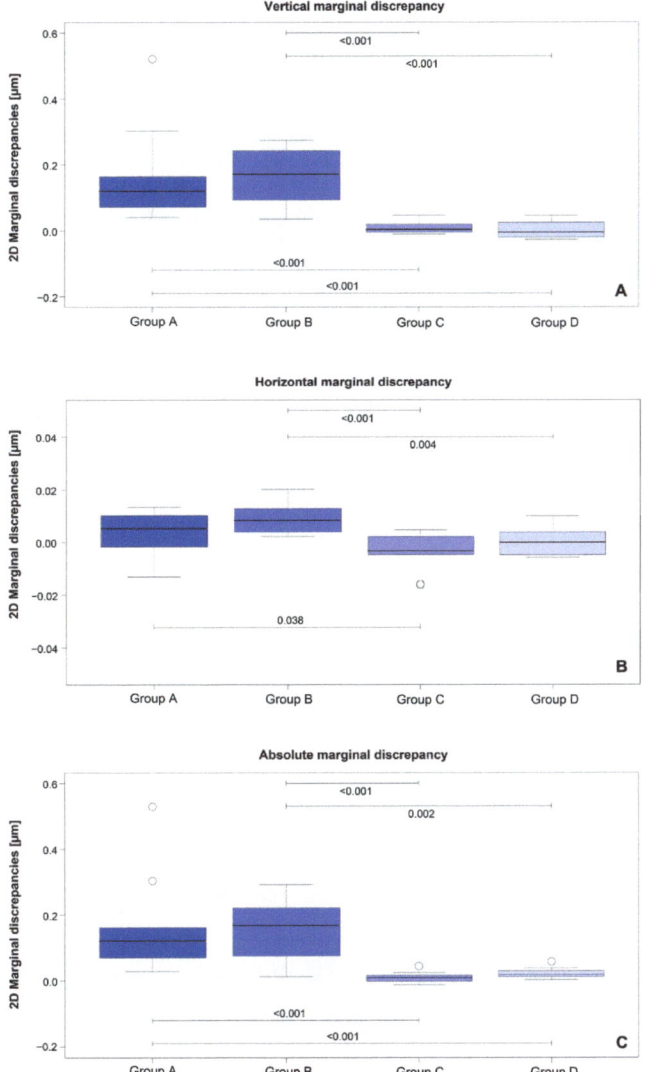

Figure 4. Comparison of marginal 2D differences with regard to the vertical (**A**), horizontal (**B**) and absolute marginal discrepancies (**C**) between the four study groups (A–D) using boxplot diagrams.

4. Discussion

This study aimed to identify the most commonly used materials for luting macroretentive zirconia restorations in dental practice. It selected different representative materials and mixing modes for the applications. Group A involved hand-mixing zinc phosphate cement, which is widely used in dental practices due to its cost-effectiveness and long shelf life. Group B included glass–ionomer as a capsule mix material. Group C investigated the effectiveness of a gold standard self-adhesive automix resin cement, and Group D evaluated a representative resin-modified glass–ionomer cement (RMGIC). A laboratory scanner was employed to standardize the models' digitization and produce the crowns. Using natural teeth as die material would have complicated the repeatability of preparing the same die. Therefore, gypsum replicas were manufactured instead. The laboratory scanner yielded more reproducible scan results compared to an intraoral scanner due to standardized scan paths. Conversely, the paths with the intraoral scanner can exhibit greater variability from one scan to another.

The measurement technology applied in this study was based on the virtual superimposition of STL data sets for the corresponding crown copings with the plaster dies before and after cementation as a result of optical data generation, and this enabled quantitative, non-destructive marginal 3D fitting, as well as 2D section analysis. The triple scan protocol described by Holst et al. [46] enabled a large number of measurement points to be generated, and the marginal fit could also be evaluated based on the horizontal marginal, vertical marginal, and absolute marginal fit discrepancies, ensuring reliable results of increased significance. Nevertheless, optical scanning and evaluation systems may be influenced by system-related or external aspects, such as the surface quality or the scan depth of the objects, and no absolute accuracy of the measurements can be achieved [46].

The first hypothesis was that there is no difference in the fit of a zirconia single-tooth restoration from before to after cementation within the same luting material. This hypothesis has to be partially rejected, as Group A (zinc phosphate cement) and Group B (glass–ionomer cement) had significantly increased 2D and 3D marginal fit discrepancies after cementation. As stated by Jorgensen, the thickness of zinc phosphate cement between restoration and tooth and, thus, the marginal fit of crowns is influenced by cementation pressure and duration, cement viscosity, temperature, and preparation taper influence [51]. Among all of the materials under investigation, the luting material of Group A was mixed by hand. Following the manufacturer's recommendations, a determined powder-to-liquid ratio was mixed to obtain the cement. Despite the use of measuring aids such as scoops and dropper bottles, hand mixing has been repeatedly reported to lead to improper mixing ratios, which influences different material properties, including cement viscosity and working time [52,53]. Walton reported that significantly different film thicknesses were measured, even by experienced clinicians under standardized ambient conditions and mixing instruments, and pre-weighted liquid and powder [54]. For Group A, the measured vertical marginal discrepancy increased by 0.163 µm after cementation. Considering that the actual minimum thickness detected between teeth during occlusion (minimal interdental threshold) is 17 µm, the increase in vertical marginal discrepancy for Group A would represent significant occlusal interference [55]. Under clinical circumstances, a time-consuming occlusal adjustment would be necessary. Furthermore, a marginal gap wider than 120 µm is not recommended [22]. It is very likely that, in Group A, the problems resulting from suboptimal mixing combined with the relatively low cement gap of the restorations (40 µm) led to increased 3D, 2D vertical (z), and absolute margin discrepancies (xyz). This lack of marginal fit calls into question the suitability of zinc phosphate cement with modern high-fit CAD/CAM restorations when other luting materials are easier to apply, and achieve a better fit after cementation under the same conditions. However, in contrast to Group A, this is a glass–ionomer cement in capsule mix form. In this case, mixing-induced problems in viscosity and setting properties cannot be responsible for the increased marginal discrepancies. The restorations in the present study have a relatively narrow cement gap, resulting in a tight fit (between 0.033 and 0.042 µm 3D marginal fit). The literature shows that tighter-fitting restorations will have increased vertical lift; in the present case, there was an increased vertical marginal discrepancy (0.160 µm for Group B) [56]. The tighter fit, in combination with the probably too-high viscosity of the glass–ionomer, may have reduced the material's outflow and led to the restoration tilting, resulting in the significantly increased horizontal marginal discrepancy.

Only Group C (self-adhesive resin cement) and Group D (resin-modified glass–ionomer cement, except for the absolute marginal discrepancy) had any influence on the marginal fit. Both materials are delivered in automix canulae, where the catalyst and base paste are mixed. Mixing the pastes in an automix syringe requires optimized rheology, which results in cementation without affecting the marginal fit [57]. The self-adhesive resin luting material can be recommended for clinical use in terms of marginal fit. In addition, the self-adhesive cement generated the most robust adhesion to zirconia among all of the luting materials under investigation due to chemical bonds between its phosphomethacrylates and the zirconia and tooth substrates [58–60]. The investigated resin-modified glass–ionomer was superior to the zinc phosphate and glass–ionomer cement in regard to marginal fit. However, some older resin-modified glass–ionomers were prone to swelling and hydrolytic degradation due to their hydrophilic monomer content [61,62]. Whether this applies to the modern representatives of this material class needs to be investigated.

Despite the productive and interesting findings, it is imperative to acknowledge the limitations of the current study. Although a representative selection of fastening materials was made, incorporating a substantial portion of those currently available, it only encompasses a fraction of the variety accessible today. Additionally, factors such as the geometry of the tooth die, i.e., the convergence angle, the inner transitions, and the design of the preparation margin, may influence cement flow behavior. Consequently, while the study's results remain valid, they should be interpreted in light of these considerations.

The results of the present study suggest that the influence of luting materials on the fit of restorations is a complex issue. All investigated materials meet their respective ISO norms, especially for film thickness. However, the ISO method does not seem to be able to offer absolute conclusions about how the fit of the restoration is ultimately influenced. As can be seen from the literature, a large number of factors, in addition to the film layer thickness, are involved. Investigating and standardizing these influencing factors (convergence angle, preparation margin, cement, and margin gap) should be the subject of further investigations to precisely match the properties of the luting materials and thus achieve a perfect fit. The method used here may be helpful for this purpose.

5. Conclusions

Within the limitations of the present study, the authors drew the following conclusions:
- The digital non-destructive method was able to detect the influence of the luting material on the fit of a zirconia single-tooth restoration before and after cementation;
- The zinc phosphate cement led to increased vertical marginal discrepancies;
- Only the self-adhesive luting resin did not influence the fit of the restoration after cementation, and can be clinically recommended.

Author Contributions: Conceptualization, L.B., R.-E.M., M.W. and J.I.Z.; methodology, L.B., R.-E.M., C.M.W. and J.I.Z.; software, L.B., R.-E.M. and C.M.W.; validation, R.-E.M., C.M.W. and M.W.; formal analysis, L.B., C.M.W., W.A. and J.I.Z.; investigation, C.M.W.; resources, R.-E.M., W.A. and M.W.; data curation, L.B., C.M.W., W.A. and J.I.Z.; writing—original draft preparation, L.B. and J.I.Z.; writing—review and editing, L.B., R.-E.M. and J.I.Z.; visualization, L.B., R.-E.M. and C.M.W. and J.I.Z.; supervision, R.-E.M. and M.W.; project administration, R.-E.M. and M.W.; funding acquisition, R.-E.M. and M.W. All authors have read and agreed to the published version of the manuscript.

Funding: The materials and statistical analysis of the study's data were funded by the ELAN Foundation of the FAU Erlangen-Nuremberg.

Institutional Review Board Statement: Not applicable.

Informed Consent Statement: Not applicable.

Data Availability Statement: The data sets used and/or analyzed during the current study are available from the corresponding author upon reasonable request.

Acknowledgments: The authors gratefully acknowledge the ELAN Foundation of the FAU Erlangen-Nuremberg for funding the materials used for this investigation and the statistical analysis of the data collected.

Conflicts of Interest: The authors declare no conflicts of interest. The funders had no role in the design of the study; in the collection, analyses, or interpretation of data; in the writing of the manuscript; or in the decision to publish the results.

Abbreviations

CAD	Computer-Aided Design
CAM	Computer-Aided Manufacturing
3D	Three-dimensional
2D	Two-dimensional
STL	Standard Transformation Language
Mean	Mean distance
SD	Standard deviation
Min	Minimum distance
Max	Maximum distance

References

1. Pak, H.S.; Han, J.S.; Lee, J.B.; Kim, S.H.; Yang, J.H. Influence of porcelain veneering on the marginal fit of Digident and Lava CAD/CAM zirconia ceramic crowns. *J. Adv. Prosthodont.* **2010**, *2*, 33–38. [CrossRef] [PubMed]
2. Takeichi, T.; Katsoulis, J.; Blatz, M.B. Clinical outcome of single porcelain-fused-to-zirconium dioxide crowns: A systematic review. *J. Prosthet. Dent.* **2013**, *110*, 455–461. [CrossRef] [PubMed]
3. Silva, L.H.D.; Lima, E.; Miranda, R.B.P.; Favero, S.S.; Lohbauer, U.; Cesar, P.F. Dental ceramics: A review of new materials and processing methods. *Braz. Oral Res.* **2017**, *31*, e58. [CrossRef] [PubMed]
4. Zhang, Y.; Lawn, B.R. Novel Zirconia Materials in Dentistry. *J. Dent. Res.* **2018**, *97*, 140–147. [CrossRef] [PubMed]
5. Beuer, F.; Schweiger, J.; Edelhoff, D. Digital dentistry: An overview of recent developments for CAD/CAM generated restorations. *Br. Dent. J.* **2008**, *204*, 505–511. [CrossRef] [PubMed]
6. Duret, F.; Blouin, J.L.; Duret, B. CAD-CAM in dentistry. *J. Am. Dent. Assoc.* **1988**, *117*, 715–720. [CrossRef] [PubMed]
7. Methani, M.M.; Revilla-León, M.; Zandinejad, A. The potential of additive manufacturing technologies and their processing parameters for the fabrication of all-ceramic crowns: A review. *J. Esthet. Restor. Dent.* **2020**, *32*, 182–192. [CrossRef] [PubMed]
8. Miyazaki, T.; Hotta, Y.; Kunii, J.; Kuriyama, S.; Tamaki, Y. A review of dental CAD/CAM: Current status and future perspectives from 20 years of experience. *Dent. Mater. J.* **2009**, *28*, 44–56. [CrossRef] [PubMed]
9. Javaid, M.; Haleem, A. Current status and applications of additive manufacturing in dentistry: A literature-based review. *J. Oral Biol. Craniofacial Res.* **2019**, *9*, 179–185. [CrossRef]
10. Cesar, P.F.; Miranda, R.B.P.; Santos, K.F.; Scherrer, S.S.; Zhang, Y. Recent advances in dental zirconia: 15 years of material and processing evolution. *Dent. Mater.* **2024**, *in press*. [CrossRef]
11. Belli, R.; Hurle, K.; Schürrlein, J.; Petschelt, A.; Werbach, K.; Peterlik, H.; Rabe, T.; Mieller, B.; Lohbauer, U. Relationships between fracture toughness, Y_2O_3 fraction and phases content in modern dental Yttria-doped zirconias. *J. Eur. Ceram. Soc.* **2021**, *41*, 7771–7782. [CrossRef]
12. Jurado, C.A.; Villalobos-Tinoco, J.; Watanabe, H.; Sanchez-Hernandez, R.; Tsujimoto, A. Novel translucent monolithic zirconia fixed restorations in the esthetic zone. *Clin. Case Rep.* **2022**, *10*, e05499. [CrossRef] [PubMed]
13. Holmes, J.R.; Bayne, S.C.; Holland, G.A.; Sulik, W.D. Considerations in measurement of marginal fit. *J. Prosthet. Dent.* **1989**, *62*, 405–408. [CrossRef] [PubMed]
14. Abbate, M.F.; Tjan, A.H.; Fox, W.M. Comparison of the marginal fit of various ceramic crown systems. *J. Prosthet. Dent.* **1989**, *61*, 527–531. [CrossRef]
15. Vasiliu, R.D.; Porojan, S.D.; Porojan, L. In Vitro Study of Comparative Evaluation of Marginal and Internal Fit between Heat-Pressed and CAD-CAM Monolithic Glass-Ceramic Restorations after Thermal Aging. *Materials* **2020**, *13*, 4239. [CrossRef]
16. Padrós, R.; Giner, L.; Herrero-Climent, M.; Falcao-Costa, C.; Ríos-Santos, J.V.; Gil, F.J. Influence of the CAD-CAM Systems on the Marginal Accuracy and Mechanical Properties of Dental Restorations. *Int. J. Environ. Res. Public Health* **2020**, *17*, 4276. [CrossRef] [PubMed]
17. Demir, N.; Ozturk, A.N.; Malkoc, M.A. Evaluation of the marginal fit of full ceramic crowns by the microcomputed tomography (micro-CT) technique. *Eur. J. Dent.* **2014**, *8*, 437–444. [CrossRef]
18. Felton, D.A.; Kanoy, B.E.; Bayne, S.C.; Wirthman, G.P. Effect of in vivo crown margin discrepancies on periodontal health. *J. Prosthet. Dent.* **1991**, *65*, 357–364. [CrossRef] [PubMed]
19. Jacobs, M.S.; Windeler, A.S. An investigation of dental luting cement solubility as a function of the marginal gap. *J. Prosthet. Dent.* **1991**, *65*, 436–442. [CrossRef]
20. Tan, P.L.; Gratton, D.G.; Diaz-Arnold, A.M.; Holmes, D.C. An in vitro comparison of vertical marginal gaps of CAD/CAM titanium and conventional cast restorations. *J. Prosthodont.* **2008**, *17*, 378–383. [CrossRef]
21. Balkaya, M.C.; Cinar, A.; Pamuk, S. Influence of firing cycles on the margin distortion of 3 all-ceramic crown systems. *J. Prosthet. Dent.* **2005**, *93*, 346–355. [CrossRef] [PubMed]

22. McLean, J.W.; von Fraunhofer, J.A. The estimation of cement film thickness by an in vivo technique. *Br. Dent. J.* **1971**, *131*, 107–111. [CrossRef] [PubMed]
23. Christensen, G.J. Marginal fit of gold inlay castings. *J. Prosthet. Dent.* **1966**, *16*, 297–305. [CrossRef] [PubMed]
24. Gavelis, J.R.; Morency, J.D.; Riley, E.D.; Sozio, R.B. The effect of various finish line preparations on the marginal seal and occlusal seat of full crown preparations. *J. Prosthet. Dent.* **1981**, *45*, 138–145. [CrossRef] [PubMed]
25. Gu, X.H.; Kern, M. Marginal discrepancies and leakage of all-ceramic crowns: Influence of luting agents and aging conditions. *Int. J. Prosthodont.* **2003**, *16*, 109–116. [PubMed]
26. Kokubo, Y.; Ohkubo, C.; Tsumita, M.; Miyashita, A.; Vult von Steyern, P.; Fukushima, S. Clinical marginal and internal gaps of Procera AllCeram crowns. *J. Oral Rehabil.* **2005**, *32*, 526–530. [CrossRef] [PubMed]
27. Donovan, T.E.; Cho, G.C. Contemporary evaluation of dental cements. *Compend. Contin. Educ. Dent.* **1999**, *20*, 197–199.
28. Goodacre, C.J.; Campagni, W.V.; Aquilino, S.A. Tooth preparations for complete crowns: An art form based on scientific principles. *J. Prosthet. Dent.* **2001**, *85*, 363–376. [CrossRef]
29. Hill, E.E. Dental cements for definitive luting: A review and practical clinical considerations. *Dent. Clin. North. Am.* **2007**, *51*, 643–658. [CrossRef]
30. Lad, P.P.; Kamath, M.; Tarale, K.; Kusugal, P.B. Practical clinical considerations of luting cements: A review. *J. Int. Oral Health* **2014**, *6*, 116–120.
31. Attin, T.; Vataschki, M.; Hellwig, E. Properties of resin-modified glass-ionomer restorative materials and two polyacid-modified resin composite materials. *Quintessence Int.* **1996**, *27*, 203–209. [PubMed]
32. Berzins, D.W.; Abey, S.; Costache, M.C.; Wilkie, C.A.; Roberts, H.W. Resin-modified glass-ionomer setting reaction competition. *J. Dent. Res.* **2010**, *89*, 82–86. [CrossRef] [PubMed]
33. Coutinho, E.; Yoshida, Y.; Inoue, S.; Fukuda, R.; Snauwaert, J.; Nakayama, Y.; De Munck, J.; Lambrechts, P.; Suzuki, K.; Van Meerbeek, B. Gel phase formation at resin-modified glass-ionomer/tooth interfaces. *J. Dent. Res.* **2007**, *86*, 656–661. [CrossRef] [PubMed]
34. Leyhausen, G.; Abtahi, M.; Karbakhsch, M.; Sapotnick, A.; Geurtsen, W. Biocompatibility of various light-curing and one conventional glass-ionomer cement. *Biomaterials* **1998**, *19*, 559–564. [CrossRef] [PubMed]
35. Nagaraja Upadhya, P.; Kishore, G. Glass ionomer cement: The different generations. *Trends Biomater. Artif. Organs* **2005**, *18*, 158–165.
36. Ferracane, J.L.; Stansbury, J.W.; Burke, F.J. Self-adhesive resin cements—Chemistry, properties and clinical considerations. *J. Oral Rehabil.* **2011**, *38*, 295–314. [CrossRef]
37. Goulart, M.; Borges Veleda, B.; Damin, D.; Bovi Ambrosano, G.M.; Coelho de Souza, F.H.; Erhardt, M.C.G. Preheated composite resin used as a luting agent for indirect restorations: Effects on bond strength and resin-dentin interfaces. *Int. J. Esthet. Dent.* **2018**, *13*, 86–97.
38. Gupta, A.A.; Mulay, S.; Mahajan, P.; Raj, A.T. Assessing the effect of ceramic additives on the physical, rheological and mechanical properties of conventional glass ionomer luting cement—An in-vitro study. *Heliyon* **2019**, *5*, e02094. [CrossRef]
39. Sita Ramaraju, D.; Alla, R.K.; Alluri, V.R.; Raju, M. A review of conventional and contemporary luting agents used in dentistry. *Am. J. Mater. Sci. Eng.* **2014**, *2*, 28–35.
40. White, S.N.; Yu, Z. Film thickness of new adhesive luting agents. *J. Prosthet. Dent.* **1992**, *67*, 782–785. [CrossRef]
41. International Organization for Standardization. Water-Based Cements—Part 1: Powder/Liquid Acid-Base Cements. 2016. Available online: https://www.iso.org/standard/45818.html (accessed on 30 April 2024).
42. International Organization for Standardization. Water-Based Cements—Part 2: Resin-Modified Cements. 2017. Available online: https://www.iso.org/standard/69901.html (accessed on 30 April 2024).
43. International Organization for Standardization. Polymer-Based Luting Materials Containing Adhesive Components. 2021. Available online: https://www.iso.org/standard/56898.html (accessed on 30 April 2024).
44. Zorzin, J.; Petschelt, A.; Ebert, J.; Lohbauer, U. pH neutralization and influence on mechanical strength in self-adhesive resin luting agents. *Dent. Mater.* **2012**, *28*, 672–679. [CrossRef] [PubMed]
45. Kious, A.R.; Roberts, H.W.; Brackett, W.W. Film thicknesses of recently introduced luting cements. *J. Prosthet. Dent.* **2009**, *101*, 189–192. [CrossRef] [PubMed]
46. Holst, S.; Karl, M.; Wichmann, M.; Matta, R.E. A new triple-scan protocol for 3D fit assessment of dental restorations. *Quintessence Int.* **2011**, *42*, 651–657. [PubMed]
47. Matta, R.E.; Schmitt, J.; Wichmann, M.; Holst, S. Circumferential fit assessment of CAD/CAM single crowns—A pilot investigation on a new virtual analytical protocol. *Quintessence Int.* **2012**, *43*, 801–809. [PubMed]
48. Sakrana, A.A.; Al-Zordk, W.; El-Sebaey, H.; Elsherbini, A.; Özcan, M. Does Preheating Resin Cements Affect Fracture Resistance of Lithium Disilicate and Zirconia Restorations? *Materials* **2021**, *14*, 5603. [CrossRef] [PubMed]
49. Tyor, S.; Al-Zordk, W.; Sakrana, A.A. Fracture resistance of monolithic translucent zirconia crown bonded with different self-adhesive resin cement: Influence of MDP-containing zirconia primer after aging. *BMC Oral Health* **2023**, *23*, 636. [CrossRef] [PubMed]
50. The R Project for Statistical Computing. A Language and Environment for Statistical Computing. 2017. Available online: https://www.r-project.org/ (accessed on 20 January 2023).
51. Jørgensen, K.D. Factors affecting the film thickness of zinc phosphate cements. *Acta Odontol. Scand.* **1960**, *18*, 479–490. [CrossRef]

52. Fleming, G.J.; Marquis, P.M.; Shortall, A.C. The influence of clinically induced variability on the distribution of compressive fracture strengths of a hand-mixed zinc phosphate dental cement. *Dent. Mater.* **1999**, *15*, 87–97. [CrossRef]
53. McKenna, J.E.; Ray, N.J.; McKenna, G.; Burke, F.M. The effect of variability in the powder/liquid ratio on the strength of zinc phosphate cement. *Int. J. Dent.* **2011**, *2011*, 679315. [CrossRef]
54. Walton, T.R. The flow properties of zinc phosphate cement: An argument for changing the standard. *Aust. Dent. J.* **1980**, *25*, 215–218. [CrossRef]
55. Kogawa, E.M.; Calderon, P.D.; Lauris, J.R.; Pegoraro, L.F.; Conti, P.C. Evaluation of minimum interdental threshold ability in dentate female temporomandibular disorder patients. *J. Oral Rehabil.* **2010**, *37*, 322–328. [CrossRef] [PubMed]
56. Kern, M.; Schaller, H.G.; Strub, J.R. Marginal fit of restorations before and after cementation in vivo. *Int. J. Prosthodont.* **1993**, *6*, 585–591. [PubMed]
57. Zeller, D.K.; Fischer, J.; Rohr, N. Viscous behavior of resin composite cements. *Dent. Mater. J.* **2021**, *40*, 253–259. [CrossRef] [PubMed]
58. Giannini, M.; Takagaki, T.; Bacelar-Sá, R.; Vermelho, P.M.; Ambrosano, G.M.; Sadr, A.; Nikaido, T.; Tagami, J. Influence of resin coating on bond strength of self-adhesive resin cements to dentin. *Dent. Mater. J.* **2015**, *34*, 822–827. [CrossRef] [PubMed]
59. Lubauer, J.; Belli, R.; Lorey, T.; Max, S.; Lohbauer, U.; Zorzin, J.I. A split-Chevron-Notched-Beam sandwich specimen for fracture toughness testing of bonded interfaces. *J. Mech. Behav. Biomed. Mater.* **2022**, *131*, 105236. [CrossRef] [PubMed]
60. Zorzin, J.; Belli, R.; Wagner, A.; Petschelt, A.; Lohbauer, U. Self-adhesive resin cements: Adhesive performance to indirect restorative ceramics. *J. Adhes. Dent.* **2014**, *16*, 541–546. [CrossRef] [PubMed]
61. Attin, T.; Buchalla, W.; Kielbassa, A.M.; Helwig, E. Curing shrinkage and volumetric changes of resin-modified glass ionomer restorative materials. *Dent. Mater.* **1995**, *11*, 359–362. [CrossRef]
62. Feilzer, A.J.; Kakaboura, A.I.; de Gee, A.J.; Davidson, C.L. The influence of water sorption on the development of setting shrinkage stress in traditional and resin-modified glass ionomer cements. *Dent. Mater.* **1995**, *11*, 186–190. [CrossRef]

Disclaimer/Publisher's Note: The statements, opinions and data contained in all publications are solely those of the individual author(s) and contributor(s) and not of MDPI and/or the editor(s). MDPI and/or the editor(s) disclaim responsibility for any injury to people or property resulting from any ideas, methods, instructions or products referred to in the content.

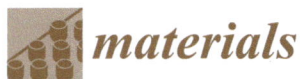

Article

The Influence of Contemporary Denture Base Fabrication Methods on Residual Monomer Content, Flexural Strength and Microhardness

Josip Vuksic [1,2], Ana Pilipovic [3], Tina Poklepovic Pericic [4] and Josip Kranjcic [2,5,*]

1. Department of Removable Prosthodontics, University of Zagreb School of Dental Medicine, Gunduliceva 5, 10000 Zagreb, Croatia; jvuksic@sfzg.unizg.hr
2. Department of Prosthodontics, University Hospital Dubrava, Av. Gojka Šuška 6, 10000 Zagreb, Croatia
3. University of Zagreb Faculty of Mechanical Engineering and Naval Architecture, Ivana Lučića 5, 10000 Zagreb, Croatia; ana.pilipovic@fsb.unizg.hr
4. School of Medicine, University of Split, Šoltanska 2, 21000 Split, Croatia; tinapoklepovic@gmail.com
5. Department of Fixed Prosthodontics, University of Zagreb School of Dental Medicine, Gunduliceva 5, 10000 Zagreb, Croatia
* Correspondence: kranjcic@sfzg.unizg.hr

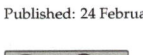

Citation: Vuksic, J.; Pilipovic, A.; Poklepovic Pericic, T.; Kranjcic, J. The Influence of Contemporary Denture Base Fabrication Methods on Residual Monomer Content, Flexural Strength and Microhardness. *Materials* 2024, 17, 1052. https://doi.org/10.3390/ma17051052

Academic Editor: Marco Annunziata

Received: 29 January 2024
Revised: 19 February 2024
Accepted: 22 February 2024
Published: 24 February 2024

Copyright: © 2024 by the authors. Licensee MDPI, Basel, Switzerland. This article is an open access article distributed under the terms and conditions of the Creative Commons Attribution (CC BY) license (https://creativecommons.org/licenses/by/4.0/).

Abstract: (1) Background: Digital technologies are available for denture base fabrication, but there is a lack of scientific data on the mechanical and chemical properties of the materials produced in this way. Therefore, the aim of this study was to investigate the residual monomer content, flexural strength and microhardness of denture base materials as well as correlations between investigated parameters. (2) Methods: Seven denture base materials were used: one conventional heat cured polymethyl methacrylate, one polyamide, three subtractive manufactured materials and two additive manufactured materials. High-performance liquid chromatography was used to determine residual monomer content and the test was carried out in accordance with the specification ISO No. 20795-1:2013. Flexural strength was also determined according to the specification ISO No. 20795-1:2013. The Vickers method was used to investigate microhardness. A one-way ANOVA with a Bonferroni post-hoc test was used for the statistical analysis. The Pearson correlation test was used for the correlation analysis. (3) Results: There was a statistically significant difference between the values of residual monomer content of the different denture base materials ($p < 0.05$). Anaxdent pink blank showed the highest value of 3.2% mass fraction, while Polident pink CAD-CAM showed the lowest value of 0.05% mass fraction. The difference between the flexural strength values of the different denture base materials was statistically significant ($p < 0.05$), with values ranging from 62.57 megapascals (MPa) to 103.33 MPa. The difference between the microhardness values for the different denture base materials was statistically significant ($p < 0.05$), and the values obtained ranged from 10.61 to 22.86 Vickers hardness number (VHN). A correlation was found between some results for the material properties investigated ($p < 0.05$). (4) Conclusions: The selection of contemporary digital denture base manufacturing techniques may affect residual monomer content, flexural strength and microhardness but is not the only criterion for achieving favourable properties.

Keywords: denture bases; hardness; flexural strength; computer-aided design; computer-aided manufacturing

1. Introduction

Rehabilitation of edentulous patients with conventional removable dentures is a standard treatment protocol [1,2], and polymethyl methacrylate (PMMA) remains the most commonly used material for the fabrication of denture bases [3–7]. In addition to the well-known analogue techniques for the fabrication of denture bases, contemporary digital technologies are also available today and are used in everyday dental practise. The application of computer-aided design-computer-aided manufacturing technology (CAD-CAM) for complete dentures holds significant potential for patient care, public health, education and research [8]. CAD-CAM technologies include subtractive and additive manufacturing. Digital technologies have been introduced in the manufacture of prosthetic base parts to overcome shortcomings in the properties of prosthetic base materials and to enable faster, more accurate and more cost-effective manufacturing processes. CAD-CAM technology simplifies the laboratory effort [9] and allows for greater automation of procedures, which could result in better denture quality when compared with standard heat-cured PMMA materials [10], less technician time, shorter clinical protocols [8,11,12] and fewer patient visits [9,10].

In addition to procedural advantages [9], it has been hypothesised that CAD-CAM procedures could provide better material properties [10]. The industrial preparation of pre-polymerised discs for subtractive manufacturing is intended to improve material quality by reducing operator dependency [13]. In the industrial polymerisation of pre-polymerised discs for the production of denture bases, polymerisation shrinkage is also no longer an issue [4,12–14].

Three-dimensional printing technology is also becoming popular in denture base fabrication and brings additional advantages: it is more economical, there is no wear of rotary instruments, there is less waste of raw materials and it enables the simultaneous manufacture of several products [5,6,15–19]. However, evidence on biocompatibility, mechanical properties, clinical performance and long-term patient follow-up is still lacking [9].

Higher residual monomer concentrations in the denture base material have both mechanical and biological consequences [20]. Residual monomer has a negative effect on the mechanical properties of the denture base material [20–27]. In addition, residual monomer that is leaking in the oral cavity can cause biological reactions in the form of inflammation, irritation and allergic reactions [21,22,24,25,27–29]. Residual monomers not only pose a potential risk to the patient but can also pose an occupational risk to the clinician and technician [30]. For this reason, the concentration of residual monomer in the denture base material is one of the most important properties that should be considered.

High flexural strength is required to prevent catastrophic failure of the denture under load [31]. The three-point bending test used to investigate flexural strength simulates the type of load applied to the denture during mastication [26,31,32]. It has been reported that the flexural strength of the denture base material is related to the residual monomer content [10,32].

Microhardness is an important property that is related to the material's resistance to surface abrasion caused by occlusion and mechanical denture cleaning [23] and to the longevity of the denture [26]. Microhardness is thought to be sensitive to residual monomer content and is a simple way to assess the degree of conversion of the monomer [21,23,33]. There is some evidence of a correlation between microhardness testing and flexural properties [34].

The aim of this study was to investigate the residual monomer content, flexural strength and microhardness of denture base materials fabricated using different manufacturing methods, with a focus on CAD-CAM technology. The aim was also to investigate whether correlations exist between the investigated material properties.

The null hypothesis was that there is no difference in residual monomer content, flexural strength and microhardness between different denture base materials and that there are no correlations between the investigated properties.

2. Materials and Methods

The residual monomer content, flexural strength and microhardness of denture base materials were investigated. Seven different denture base materials were used (Table 1). All specimens were prepared according to the manufacturer's instructions.

Table 1. List of the materials used in the study.

Name of the Material	Manufacturer	Description and Purpose of the Material
Meliodent heat cure	Kulzer, Hanau, Germany	Denture base material, PMMA, heat cured
Vertex Thermosens	Vetex Dental, Soesterberg, The Netherlands	Denture base material, polyamide, injection technique
Ivobase CAD pink V	Ivoclar Vivadent, Schaan, Liechtenstein	CAD-CAM denture base material, subtractive manufacturing
Polident pink CAD-CAM disc basic	Polident d.o.o., Volčja draga, Slovenia	CAD-CAM denture base material, subtractive manufacturing
Anaxdent pink blank U medium pink	Anaxdent GmbH, Stuttgart, Germany	CAD-CAM denture base material, subtractive manufacturing
Freeprint denture	Detax, Ettlingen, Germany	CAD-CAM denture base material, additive manufacturing
Imprimo LC denture	Scheu, Iserlohn, Germany	CAD-CAM denture base material, additive manufacturing

CAD-CAM: computer-aided design-computer-aided manufacturing, PMMA: polymethyl methacrylate.

Residual monomer

All materials from Table 1 were used in the analysis of residual monomers, with the exception of polyamide, which does not contain methyl methacrylate (MMA) due to its different chemical composition. In accordance with ISO 20795-1:2013 [35], high-performance liquid chromatography (HPLC) was used for the analysis. The specimens were discs with a diameter of 50 mm and a thickness of 3 ± 0.1 mm. All specimens were slightly oversized and were wet-ground with metallographic grinding papers with a grain size of approximately 30 µm (P 500) and 15 µm (P 1200) until the final dimensions were reached. Water was used during the grinding process to avoid any frictional heat that could lead to monomer loss or depolymerisation. To keep the monomer content constant, the specimens were stored in the freezer after preparation until HPLC. For each denture base material, three specimens were prepared and three measurements were performed for each specimen, totalling 54 measurements. The sample size was determined according to ISO 20795-1:2013 [35].

The list of chemicals used in HPLC are shown in Table 2.

Table 2. List of chemicals used in residual monomer investigation.

Chemical Name	Manufacturer	Purity
Acetone	Acros Organics, Geel, Belgium	99.8%
Diclofenac sodium	Sigma Aldrich, St. Louis, MO, USA	≥98%
Hydroquinone	Fluka, Gillingham, UK	≥99%
Methanol	J.T. Baker, Phillipsburg, NJ, USA	≥99.9%
Methil methacrylate, stabilized	Acros Organics, Geel, Belgium	≥99%
Formic acid	Fischer Scientific, Waltham, MA, USA	≥99%

Three solutions were prepared with the aforementioned chemicals: solution A, B and C. Solution A was 20 mg L^{-1} mass concentration of hydroquinone in acetone. Solution B was 20 mg L^{-1} mass concentration of hydroquinone in methanol. Solution C was a mixture of one part of solution A and four parts by volume of solution B.

Prior to chromatography, extraction of the monomer was performed (Figure 1). First, each specimen disc was broken into small pieces, which were additionally ground using a universal laboratory mill with water cooling (M 20, IKA, Aachen, Germany). Grinding was carried out in 3 s pulses with 20 s pauses to avoid frictional heat and monomer losses.

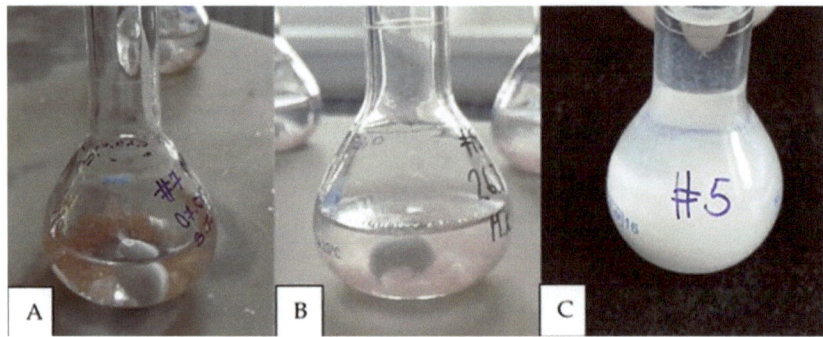

Figure 1. Sample placed in solution A (**A**), after 72 h of dissolving in solution A (**B**), and sample in solution B (**C**).

A sample of approximately 650 mg was placed in a 25 mL glass volumetric flask and 10 mL of solution A was added. Each sample was weighed using an analytical balance and the mass was recorded. Acetone in solution A was used to dissolve the sample and hydroquinone in the same solution to avoid the polymerisation of the dissolved residual methyl methacrylate. After 72 h, 2 mL of the sample solution was transferred to a one-mark 10 mL volumetric glass flask, 10 µL of the internal standard was added and solution B was added to a total volume of 10 mL. Solution B consisted of methanol to precipitate the dissolved polymer and hydroquinone to prevent polymerisation of the dissolved methyl methacrylate. To enhance the precipitation of the polymer, the solution was centrifuged for 15 min (EBA-21, Hettich Zentrifugen, Tuttlingen, Germany). The sample solution was additionally filtered through a syringe filter with a pore size of 0.45 µm (Acrodisc, Pall, Ann Arbor, MI, USA) to remove the remaining dissolved macromolecules that could degrade and clog the HPLC columns.

Immediately after extraction of the monomer, HPLC was performed.

Solution C was used to prepare the calibration diagram. It was additionally diluted with ultrapure water prepared with the Direct-Q 3 UV water purification system (Millipore SAS, Molsheim, France). The mixing ratio was solution C/ultrapure water = 66:34. The dilution of solution C was used to improve the separation of the analytes on the chromatograph. Four different concentrations of MMA were used to generate the calibration curve: 0.5, 1, 1.5 and 3 mg/L (Figure 2). Diclofenac at a concentration of 3 mg/L was used for the internal standard.

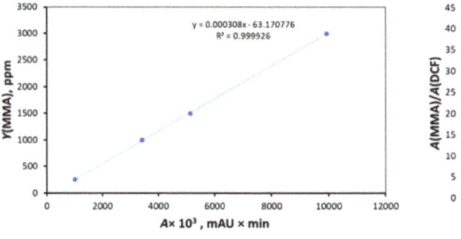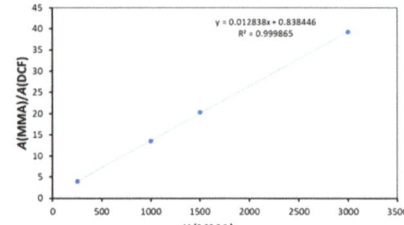

Figure 2. Calibration curve.

The concentration of the residual monomer was determined by HPLC with an internal standard. The Shimadzu LC-10 chromatographic system was used (Shimadzu, Kyoto, Japan), which consisted of an SCL-10AVP controller, two LC-10ADvp pumps, a DGU-20AR degasser and an SPD-M10ADvp UV/DAD detector. A Nucleosil C18 RP column (Macherey Nagel, Dueren, Germany) with a length of 250 mm, an inner diameter of 4.6 mm and a pore size of 5 μm was used for the chromatographic separation of the analytes. The mobile phase consisted of two components: the organic component was methanol and the aqueous component was 0.2% formic acid. Each component was pumped individually, and the components were mixed at a ratio of 0.66 parts organic component and 0.34 parts aqueous component with isocratic elution. The total flow rate was 1.0 mL min^{-1} and the volume of the sample solution was 20 μL. Methyl methacrylate was detected at a wavelength of 235 nm and the internal standard at 276 nm.

The concentration of methyl methacrylate was determined using Class VP v6.14 software (Shimadzu, Kyoto, Japan). The mass of MMA in the sample solution, m_{MMA}, was calculated using the following Equation:

$$m_{MMA} = \gamma_{MMA} \times V_e \times \frac{V_p}{V_a}$$

where γ_{MMA} [mg L^{-1}] represented MMA concentration, V_e [mL] was solution A volume, V_a [mL] was a part of the sample solution transferred after dissolving of the sample, and V_p [mL] was total volume of the sample solution mixed with solution B and the internal standard. Since V_e (10 mL), V_p (10 mL) and V_a (2 mL) were constant, the Equation was simplified as follows:

$$m_{MMA} = \gamma_{MMA} \times 0.05$$

The results of the analysis were calculated according to the following Equation:

$$w = \frac{m_{MMA}}{m_{SAMPLE}} \times 100$$

where w [%] represented the mass fraction of MMA in the sample, m_{MMA} [mg] was the mass of MMA in the sample solution and m_{SAMPLE} [mg] was the mass of the sample.

Flexural strength

The flexural strength analysis was performed according to the specifications of ISO 20795-1:2013 [35] and all seven denture base materials from Table 1 were analysed. Five specimen strips were prepared for each denture base material, totalling 35 specimens. They were 64 mm long, 10.0 ± 0.2 mm wide and 3.3 ± 0.2 mm high. All specimen strips were slightly oversized and were wet-ground with metallographic grinding paper with a grain size of approximately 30 μm (P500), 18 μm (P1000) and 15 μm (P1200) until the final dimensions were reached. The prepared specimens were stored in a water bath at a temperature of 37 ± 1 °C for 50 ± 2 h. After removing the specimens from the water bath, flexural testing was immediately performed.

Flexural testing was conducted with a universal testing machine (Autograph AGS-X, Shimadzu, Kyoto, Japan). A metal flexural test rig was prepared, consisting of a central loading plunger and two polished cylindrical supports with a diameter of 3.2 mm and a length of 10.5 mm. The supports were arranged parallel and perpendicular to the longitudinal centreline. The distance between the centres of the supports was 50 ± 0.1 mm and the loading plunger was located in the centre between the supports. The displacement rate was 5 mm/min and the test was performed until the specimen broke. The maximum load during the test was recorded (Figure 3).

Flexural strength σ [MPa] was calculated using the following Equation:

$$\sigma = \frac{3 * F * l}{2 * b * h * h}$$

where F [N] was the recorded maximum load, l [mm] was the distance between the supports, b [mm] was the width of the specimen strip and h [mm] was the height of the specimen strip.

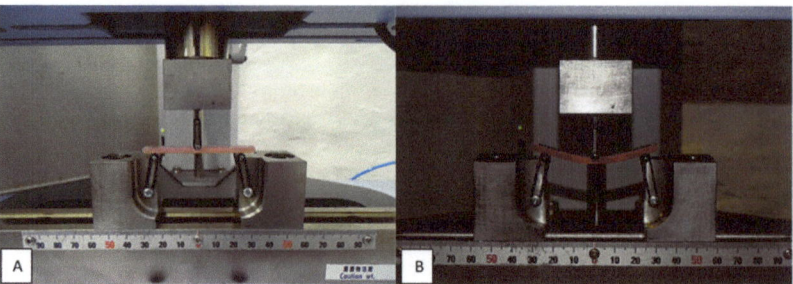

Figure 3. Flexural strength testing: specimen placed in the universal testing machine (**A**), and during the testing (**B**).

Microhardness

Microhardness analysis was performed using the Vickers method and all materials from Table 1 were analysed. The specimens were 25 × 25 mm plates with a thickness of 3 mm. The specimen plates were wet-ground with P500, P1000 or P4000 metallographic grinding paper and polished with a 0.05 μm aluminium oxide suspension and polishing cloth. The Vickers CSV-10 hardness testing machine (ESI Pruftechnik GmbH, Wendlingen, Germany) was used. The load was 100 g with a dwell time of 15 s. For each denture base material, eight specimens were prepared. Five measurements were performed on each specimen, the Vickers hardness value obtained was recorded and the mean value was calculated for each specimen (Figure 4).

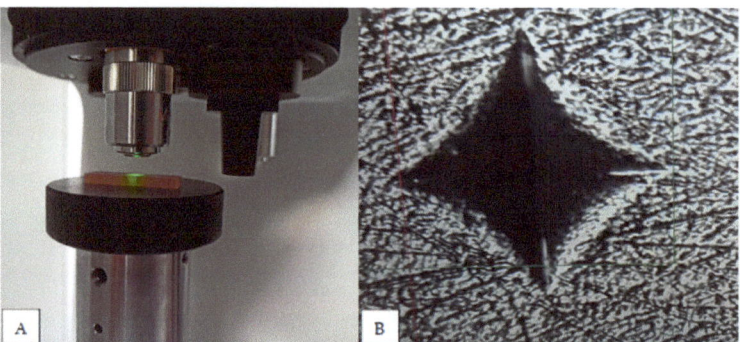

Figure 4. Microhardness testing: specimen placed in the testing machine (**A**), indentation visible on the screen (**B**).

The IBM SPSS software for Windows, version 29.0.1, was used for the statistical analysis. The one-way ANOVA test with a Bonferroni post-hoc test was used for the analysis. Pearson's correlation coefficient r was used to analyse the correlation between the examined properties. p values < 0.05 were considered statistically significant.

3. Results

The results of residual monomer content, flexural strength and microhardness are shown in Table 3. A graph presenting flexural stress as a function of strain for flexural strength testing is shown in Figure 5.

Table 3. Residual monomer, flexural strength and microhardness results.

	Residual Monomer [% Mass Fraction]		Flexural Strength [MPa]		Microhardness [VHN]	
	Mean	SD	Mean	SD	Mean	SD
1. Meliodent Heat Cure	0.53 [3,5]	0.07	97.06 [2,3,7]	6.25	20.58 [2,3,4,5,7]	0.52
2. Vertex Thermosens			62.57 [1,4,5,6]	5.69	10.61 [1,3,4,5,6,7]	0.24
3. Ivobase CAD Pink	3.05 [1,4,6,7]	0.58	79.06 [1,6]	4.65	17.23 [1,2,4,5,6]	0.99
4. Polident Pink CAD-CAM	0.05 [3,5]	0.03	96.27 [2,7]	5.81	22.86 [1,2,3,4,6,7]	0.72
5. Anaxdent Pink Blank	3.20 [1,4,6,7]	1.14	83.31 [2,6]	3.21	18.83 [1,2,3,4,6,7]	0.48
6. Freeprint Denture	0.36 [3,5]	0.16	103.33 [2,3,5,7]	16.71	21.30 [2,3,4,5,7]	0.45
7. Imprimo LC Denture	0.34 [3,5]	0.13	69.75 [1,4,6]	7.63	16.55 [1,2,4,5,6]	0.81

Mpa = megapascal, VHN = Vickers hardness number, SD = standard deviation. Superscripted numbers indicate a statistically significant difference between materials, $p < 0.05$.

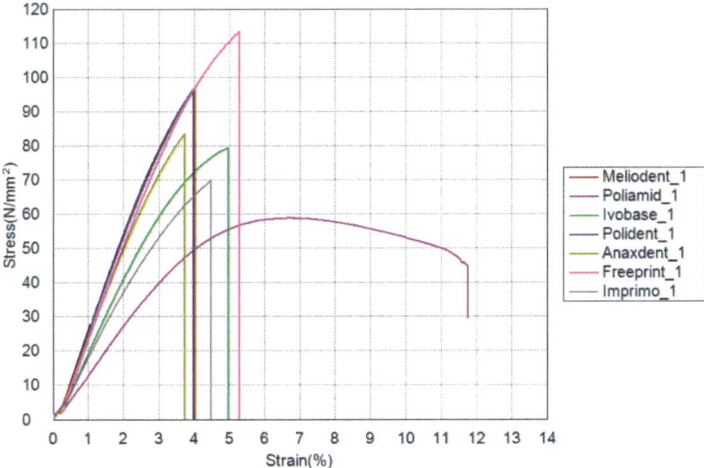

Figure 5. Graph showing flexural stress as a function of strain with average values obtained for each material.

The highest value for residual monomer content was obtained for the denture base material Anaxdent pink blank (3.2% mass fraction), while the lowest value was obtained for Polident pink CAD-CAM (0.05% mass fraction). Anaxdent pink blank and Ivobase CAD pink showed statistically significantly higher values for residual monomer than Meliodent heat cure ($p < 0.001$). Polident pink CAD-CAM showed lower values for residual monomer than Meliodent heat cure, but this was not statistically significant ($p = 0.624$). There was no statistically significant difference in the residual monomer content between Meliodent heat cure and additive manufactured materials (Freeprint denture and Imprimo LC denture) ($p = 1$).

For flexural strength, the highest value was obtained for Freeprint denture (103.33 MPa) and the lowest value for Vertex Thermosens (62.57 MPa). Ivobase CAD pink ($p = 0.037$), Imprimo LC denture ($p < 0.001$) and Vertex Thermosens ($p < 0.001$) showed statistically significantly lower values for flexural strength than Meliodent heat cure, while the highest value for Freeprint denture was not statistically significantly different compared to Meliodent heat cure ($p = 1$). There was no statistically significant difference in flexural strength values between three denture base materials for subtractive manufacturing (p from 0.055 to 1), while there was a statistically significant difference between two denture base materials for additive manufacturing in terms of flexural strength values ($p < 0.001$).

In terms of microhardness, the highest value was obtained for Polident pink CAD-CAM (22.86 VHN) and the lowest value for Vertex Thermosens (10.61 VHN). Polident pink CAD-CAM showed statistically significantly different results compared to all other materials ($p < 0.001$). Vertex Thermosens also showed statistically significantly different results compared to all other materials ($p < 0.001$). All materials examined, with the exception of Freeprint denture, showed statistically significantly different results for microhardness compared to Meliodent heat cure ($p < 0.001$). When comparing the microhardness values of all three denture base materials for subtractive manufacturing, there was a statistically significant difference between all materials ($p < 0.001$), and there was a statistically significant difference in microhardness between two denture base materials for additive manufacturing ($p < 0.001$).

The analysis of the correlation is shown in Table 4. When analysing the correlation, a statistically significant negative correlation was found between residual monomer content and the flexural strength value for conventional heat-cured PMMA material ($p = 0.004$). For polyamide denture base material, no statistically significant correlation was found between the investigated properties ($p = 0.878$). For subtractive manufactured materials, a statistically significant negative correlation was found between the residual monomer content and flexural strength ($p < 0.001$) and between the residual monomer content and microhardness ($p < 0.001$). A statistically significant positive correlation between flexural strength and microhardness was also found in the group of subtractive manufactured materials ($p = 0.001$). A statistically significant positive correlation between flexural strength and microhardness was found for additive manufactured materials ($p = 0.01$).

Table 4. The results for correlation analysis.

		Microhardness (VHN)	Residual Monomer (% Mass Fraction)	Flexural Strength (Mpa)
MELIODENT				
MICROHARDNESS (VHN)	Pearson Correlation	1.000	0.655	−0.822
	P		0.078	0.088
RESIDUAL MONOMER (% mass fraction)	Pearson Correlation	0.655	1.000	−0.976
	P	0.078		0.004 *
FLEXURAL STRENGTH (MPa)	Pearson Correlation	−0.822	−0.976	1.000
	P	0.088	0.004 *	
VERTEX THERMOSENS				
MICROHARDNESS (VHN)	Pearson Correlation	1.000	/	−0.096
	P		/	0.878
RESIDUAL MONOMER (% mass fraction)	Pearson Correlation	/	/	/
	P	/		/
FLEXURAL STRENGTH (MPa)	Pearson Correlation	−0.096	/	1.000
	P	0.878	/	
SUBTRACTIVE MANUFACTURED MATERIALS				
MICROHARDNESS (VHN)	Pearson Correlation	1	−0.815	0.826
	P		0.000 *	0.000 *
RESIDUAL MONOMER (% mass fraction)	Pearson Correlation	−0.815	1	−0.756
	P	0.000 *		0.001 *
FLEXURAL STRENGTH (MPa)	Pearson Correlation	0.826	−0.756	1
	P	0.000 *	0.001 *	
ADDITIVE MANUFACTURED MATERIALS				
MICROHARDNESS (VHN)	Pearson Correlation	1	0.074	0.765
	P		0.786	0.010 *
RESIDUAL MONOMER (% mass fraction)	Pearson Correlation	0.074	1	0.215
	P	0.786		0.551
FLEXURAL STRENGTH (MPa)	Pearson Correlation	0.765	0.215	1
	P	0.010 *	0.551	

* indicates statistically significant correlation between investigated properties ($p < 0.05$). Mpa = megapascal, VHN = Vickers hardness number.

4. Discussion

Residual monomer

Since the conventional heat-curing method for MMA polymerisation is widely known, it represents the best reference system for comparison purposes [36], which is why a conventional heat-cured PMMA material (Meliodent heat cure) was included in this study as a control group. The polymerisation reaction and the conversion of MMA is never complete [37], it is unavoidable and zero content cannot be achieved [20,30].

Higher concentrations of residual monomer in denture base materials have both mechanical and biological consequences [20]. Residual monomer acts as a plasticiser by reducing the forces between the chains, so that it negatively influences the mechanical properties of the denture base material [10,20–27,38,39]. Residual monomer that is leaking in the oral cavity can also cause biological reactions in the form of inflammation, irritation and allergic reactions [21,22,24,25,27–29]. Various signs and symptoms have been reported in patients as a result of exposure to residual monomer: local chemical irritation, hypersensitivity, mucosal inflammation and ulceration, a burning sensation in the mouth, pain, oedema, swelling and respiratory tract irritation [3,30,40–43]. Residual monomer is not only a potential risk for the patient but could also represent an occupational risk for the doctor and the technician [30].

To increase the biocompatibility of the denture base material and to achieve optimal material properties, maximum reduction of residual monomer content is desirable [10]. There are a number of factors that can influence the residual monomer content: the mixing ratio of powder and liquid, polymerisation method [30,38], thickness of the denture [44,45], polishing of the surface [3], alternative methods of polymerisation using autoclaves [21], high pressure [32,46] or prolonged curing time [20], post-polymerisation treatments [21,23,40], storage time and storage conditions after fabrication [25,41,45]. It was found that the residual monomer content tends to be lower in dentures that have been used for a longer period of time, but small amounts could still be found in dentures older than 15 years [28].

High pressure and high temperatures are used in the production of pre-polymerised PMMA blocks for subtractive manufacturing, and the process is strictly controlled in the factory [37]. This process promotes the formation of longer polymer chains and should favour a higher degree of monomer conversion and a lower residual monomer content [2,10,14,24,25,46]. As the residual monomer acts as a plasticiser in PMMA material, it is expected that its lower concentration will also improve the mechanical properties [32].

According to ISO 20795-1 [35], various methods can be used to determine the residual monomer content in denture base materials: gas chromatography, high-performance liquid chromatography or any other chromatographic method that gives the same results as the aforementioned methods. Various laboratory techniques for determining residual monomer content can be found in the literature, including UV spectrophotometry [3]. Two different types of residual monomer investigations can also be found in the literature, one is the determination of the amount of residual monomer in the denture base material sample and the other is the determination of the amount of residual monomer released in the water in which the denture base material samples were stored. ISO 20795-1 only proposes analysis of the residual monomer content in the denture base material sample. The requirement of ISO 20795-1 that the upper limit for residual monomer should be 2.2% mass fraction addresses residual monomer content and not residual monomer elution. In our study, we used HPLC to determine the residual monomer content in samples of denture base material as described in ISO 20795-1.

Kedjarune et al. [43] investigated both residual monomer content and residual monomer release in saliva and found that the material with the lowest content has the lowest release, but a higher content does not necessarily mean a higher release.

Ayman et al. [24] showed lower values of residual monomer content in denture base materials for subtractive manufacturing compared to conventional heat-cured PMMA. On the other hand, Steinmassl et al. [10] found no statistical difference in residual monomer release between denture base materials for subtractive manufacturing and conventional PMMA material.

In our study, the results showed that two materials for subtractive manufacturing (Ivobase CAD pink and Anaxdent pink blank) had a statistically significantly higher residual monomer content compared to Meliodent, the standard material for heat-curing PMMA dentures. In addition, the results for Ivobase CAD pink and Anaxdent pink blank did not meet the requirements for residual monomer content specified in ISO 20795-1 (upper limit of 2.2% mass fraction). Ivoclar CAD pink showed the highest value, while the third material for subtractive manufacturing, Polident pink CAD-CAM, showed the lowest value. These differences in the results for the three materials for subtractive manufacturing could indicate that the technology for the production of denture bases is not the only factor relevant for achieving the expected residual monomer content, but that there are also some differences in the composition of the material and probably different industrial procedures for the production of pre-polymerised discs.

The two materials for additive manufacturing showed lower values compared to Meliodent heat cure, but these were not statistically significantly lower. These results were also well below the upper limit specified in ISO 20795-1. The materials for additive manufacturing differ greatly in composition compared to the heat-cured PMMA materials (the manufacturer stated for Imprimo LC denture that the main component, more than 95%, is bisphenol A polyethylene glycol diether dimethacrylate, and another manufacturer stated for Freeprint denture that the material is MMA-free). There are several explanations for the presence of residual monomer in additive manufactured materials: some amount of MMA could be present in the resin, or it could be a by-product of the photopolymerisation process. It is also possible that a component is present in the material that causes the same reaction as MMA in HPLC on the detector.

Flexural strength

High flexural strength is required to prevent catastrophic failure of the denture under load [4,31]. The three-point bending test used to investigate flexural strength simulates the type of load applied to the denture during mastication [26,31,32,37,47]. Flexural strength is the most commonly used test for dental materials, along with impact strength and microhardness [4,47].

When comparing denture base materials for subtractive manufacturing with conventional PMMA material, recent studies have shown that denture base materials for subtractive manufacturing have statistically significantly higher values for flexural strength [4,12,13,24,31,32,48–51], while some authors showed similar results for milled denture base materials and conventional PMMA materials [2,4,51]. The results of other authors showed statistically significantly lower measured values for subtractive manufactured denture bases [13,51].

When comparing the flexural strength of additive manufactured materials with conventional heat-cured PMMA material, additive manufactured materials showed statistically significantly lower flexural strength values [4,15,47,51,52], while some authors showed similar results for heat-cured PMMA material [4,53] or even statistically significantly higher values [4].

When comparing subtractive with additive manufactured materials, subtractive manufactured materials showed better results [1,6].

In our study, both subtractive and additive manufactured materials showed statistically significantly lower or similar flexural strength values compared to conventional heat-cured PMMA material. When comparing subtractive manufactured materials with additive manufactured materials, the subtractive manufactured materials showed statistically significantly lower, similar or even higher values. All materials, with the exception of Vertex thermosens, met the criterion of a minimum value of 65 MPa for flexural strength proposed by ISO 20795-1 [35]. It can be concluded that the flexural strength value depends on the specific choice of material and not on the choice of manufacturing process.

The chemical composition of additive manufactured materials is not yet fully provided by the manufacturers, and it seems that the chemical composition of resins for additive manufacturing differs significantly [11,18], so the comparison of different studies could be considered difficult [54].

In the production of pre-polymerised blocks for subtractive manufacturing, the details of the production process are trade secrets [38], but the observed differences in the mechanical properties of the milled denture base materials could also indicate different industrial procedures [32,55].

In order to take full advantage of digital denture manufacturing, it is recommended to further improve resins for additive manufacturing by changing the composition and reinforcement and to optimise processing techniques [2,17,37]. The addition of nanoparticles and nanocomposites [11,18,56,57], build-up orientation, polymerisation technique of the 3D printer, post-curing process, and the number and thickness of the layers can influence the mechanical properties of additive manufactured denture base materials [1,17,47,52,58,59].

Microhardness

Microhardness is an important property of denture base materials that indicates the resistance of the material to surface wear [5,21], which means that loss of smoothness is avoided, and plaque retention and pigmentation are reduced, resulting in a longer useful life of the denture [23]. Microhardness is a measure of resistance to local plastic deformation caused by mechanical indentation or abrasion [1,51]. It is one of the most frequently performed tests on materials. Several different methods are used: Vickers, Brinell and Knoop. The Vickers method is considered a valid tool for microhardness testing [21,23] and is most commonly used for microhardness testing of denture base materials. However, the Vickers method also has some limitations: measurements can be limited by the resolution of the optical system, the operator's perception and the elastic recovery of the material [23].

Regarding microhardness, recent studies for subtractive manufactured denture base materials found results similar to conventional PMMA materials [2,13], while several authors reported higher [24,32,60] or even lower values of microhardness [12]. For additive manufactured materials, data from recent studies generally showed the lowest values for microhardness compared to conventional PMMA materials [5,18,47,51,57].

In this study, when comparing three subtractive manufactured materials with conventional heat-cured PMMA, one material showed statistically significantly higher values, while the other two materials showed statistically significantly lower values. For the additive manufactured materials, one material showed a statistically significantly lower value, while the other material showed similar values when compared to the conventional heat-cured PMMA material. All of these results are consistent with the findings of previous studies and may indicate that the choice of manufacturing process alone is not the only criterion for achieving the expected microhardness values.

It is assumed that microhardness is sensitive to residual monomer content and is a simple way to evaluate the degree of conversion of the monomer [21,23,26,32–34]. The hardness values are directly proportional to the amount of residual monomer [23]. Similarly, flexural strength is also proposed as a simple way to indicate the conversion of the monomer, as it is also sensitive to residual monomer content [32,37,55]. Lee et al. [34] investigated the correlation between the different mechanical properties and showed a high positive correlation between the microhardness test and flexural properties.

Our study also investigated the correlation between the properties of the materials. Our results are partly consistent with previous studies [23,34]. A statistically significant positive correlation between microhardness and flexural strength was found for additive and subtractive manufactured materials, but no statistically significant correlation was found for conventionally heat-cured and polyamide materials. As there is no statistically significant correlation between residual monomer content and other properties investigated for additively manufactured materials, the above suggestions (by other authors) for using microhardness and flexural strength values to determine the monomer are not considered.

5. Conclusions

The choice of manufacturing process is not a suitable criterion for achieving desirable values of residual monomer content, flexural strength and microhardness. According to results from this study, it can be concluded that differences between investigated parameters exist, and therefore the null hypothesis is rejected.

The values for residual monomer content are different for the materials tested. The highest values are found in the group of subtractive manufactured materials, but at the same time, the lowest value was also found in the same group of materials (Polident pink material).

The highest value of flexural strength was found in the group of additive manufactured materials, followed by heat-cured PMMA material and a material from the subtractive manufactured group of materials.

The microhardness values differed between the materials tested, even between materials in the same material group (additive and subtractive manufactured materials).

The lowest values for flexural strength and microhardness are obtained for the material Vertex thermosens.

The values of residual monomer influence flexural strength in a group of subtractive manufactured materials (higher residual monomer with lower values for microhardness and flexural strength) and for conventionally heat-cured PMMA (higher residual monomer with lower values for flexural strength).

Author Contributions: Conceptualization, J.V., J.K. and A.P.; methodology, J.V., J.K. and A.P.; software, J.V.; validation, J.V., J.K. and A.P.; formal analysis, J.V., J.K. and A.P.; investigation, J.V. and A.P.; resources, J.V. and T.P.P.; data curation, J.V. and T.P.P.; writing—original draft preparation, J.V. and J.K.; writing—review and editing, J.V. and J.K.; visualization, J.V. and T.P.P.; supervision, J.K.; project administration, J.V., J.K. and A.P.; funding acquisition, J.V., J.K. and A.P. All authors have read and agreed to the published version of the manuscript.

Funding: This research received no external funding.

Institutional Review Board Statement: Not applicable.

Informed Consent Statement: Not applicable.

Data Availability Statement: Data are contained within the article.

Conflicts of Interest: The authors declare no conflicts of interest.

References

1. Srinivasan, M.; Kamnoedboon, P.; McKenna, G.; Angst, L.; Schimmel, M.; Özcan, M.; Müller, F. CAD-CAM Removable Complete Dentures: A Systematic Review and Meta-Analysis of Trueness of Fit, Biocompatibility, Mechanical Properties, Surface Characteristics, Color Stability, Time-Cost Analysis, Clinical and Patient-Reported Outcomes. *J. Dent.* **2021**, *113*, 103777. [CrossRef] [PubMed]
2. Perea-Lowery, L.; Gibreel, M.; Vallittu, P.K.; Lassila, L.V. 3D-Printed vs. Heat-Polymerizing and Autopolymerizing Denture Base Acrylic Resins. *Materials* **2021**, *14*, 5781. [CrossRef]
3. Keul, C.; Seidl, J.; Güth, J.-F.; Liebermann, A. Impact of Fabrication Procedures on Residual Monomer Elution of Conventional Polymethyl Methacrylate (PMMA)—A Measurement Approach by UV/Vis Spectrophotometry. *Clin. Oral Investig.* **2020**, *24*, 4519–4530. [CrossRef] [PubMed]
4. Casucci, A.; Verniani, G.; Barbieri, A.L.; Ricci, N.M.; Ferrari Cagidiaco, E.; Ferrari, M. Flexural Strength Analysis of Different Complete Denture Resin-Based Materials Obtained by Conventional and Digital Manufacturing. *Materials* **2023**, *16*, 6559. [CrossRef] [PubMed]
5. Al-Dulaijan, Y.A.; Alsulaimi, L.; Alotaibi, R.; Alboainain, A.; Alalawi, H.; Alshehri, S.; Khan, S.Q.; Alsaloum, M.; AlRumaih, H.S.; Alhumaidan, A.A.; et al. Comparative Evaluation of Surface Roughness and Hardness of 3D Printed Resins. *Materials* **2022**, *15*, 6822. [CrossRef]
6. Alharethi, N.A. Evaluation of the Influence of Build Orientation on the Surface Roughness and Flexural Strength of 3D-Printed Denture Base Resin and Its Comparison with CAD-CAM Milled Denture Base Resin. *Eur. J. Dent.* **2023**, s-0043-1768972. [CrossRef]
7. Alqutaibi, A.Y.; Baik, A.; Almuzaini, S.A.; Farghal, A.E.; Alnazzawi, A.A.; Borzangy, S.; Aboalrejal, A.N.; AbdElaziz, M.H.; Mahmoud, I.I.; Zafar, M.S. Polymeric Denture Base Materials: A Review. *Polymers* **2023**, *15*, 3258. [CrossRef]
8. Bidra, A.S.; Taylor, T.D.; Agar, J.R. Computer-Aided Technology for Fabricating Complete Dentures: Systematic Review of Historical Background, Current Status, and Future Perspectives. *J. Prosthet. Dent.* **2013**, *109*, 361–366. [CrossRef]

9. Mubaraki, M.Q.; Moaleem, M.M.A.; Alzahrani, A.H.; Shariff, M.; Alqahtani, S.M.; Porwal, A.; Al-Sanabani, F.A.; Bhandi, S.; Tribst, J.P.M.; Heboyan, A.; et al. Assessment of Conventionally and Digitally Fabricated Complete Dentures: A Comprehensive Review. *Materials* **2022**, *15*, 3868. [CrossRef]
10. Steinmassl, P.-A.; Wiedemair, V.; Huck, C.; Klaunzer, F.; Steinmassl, O.; Grunert, I.; Dumfahrt, H. Do CAD/CAM Dentures Really Release Less Monomer than Conventional Dentures? *Clin. Oral Investig.* **2017**, *21*, 1697–1705. [CrossRef]
11. Altarazi, A.; Haider, J.; Alhotan, A.; Silikas, N.; Devlin, H. 3D Printed Denture Base Material: The Effect of Incorporating TiO_2 Nanoparticles and Artificial Ageing on the Physical and Mechanical Properties. *Dent. Mater. J.* **2023**, *39*, 1122–1136. [CrossRef]
12. Becerra, J.; Mainjot, A.; Hüe, O.; Sadoun, M.; Nguyen, J. Influence of High-Pressure Polymerization on Mechanical Properties of Denture Base Resins. *J. Prosthodont.* **2021**, *30*, 128–134. [CrossRef]
13. Pacquet, W.; Benoit, A.; Hatège-Kimana, C.; Wulfman, C. Mechanical Properties of CAD/CAM Denture Base Resins. *Int. J. Prosthodont.* **2018**, *32*, 104–106. [CrossRef]
14. Baba, N.Z.; Goodacre, B.J.; Goodacre, C.J.; Müller, F.; Wagner, S. CAD/CAM Complete Denture Systems and Physical Properties: A Review of the Literature. *J. Prosthodont.* **2021**, *30*, 113–124. [CrossRef]
15. Gad, M.M.; Fouda, S.M.; Abualsaud, R.; Alshahrani, F.A.; Al-Thobity, A.M.; Khan, S.Q.; Akhtar, S.; Ateeq, I.S.; Helal, M.A.; Al-Harbi, F.A. Strength and Surface Properties of a 3D-Printed Denture Base Polymer. *J. Prosthodont.* **2022**, *31*, 412–418. [CrossRef] [PubMed]
16. Kattadiyil, M.T.; AlHelal, A. An Update on Computer-Engineered Complete Dentures: A Systematic Review on Clinical Outcomes. *J. Prosthet. Dent.* **2017**, *117*, 478–485. [CrossRef] [PubMed]
17. Shim, J.S.; Kim, J.-E.; Jeong, S.H.; Choi, Y.J.; Ryu, J.J. Printing Accuracy, Mechanical Properties, Surface Characteristics, and Microbial Adhesion of 3D-Printed Resins with Various Printing Orientations. *J. Prosthet. Dent.* **2020**, *124*, 468–475. [CrossRef] [PubMed]
18. AlGhamdi, M.A.; Fouda, S.M.; Taymour, N.; Akhtar, S.; Khan, S.Q.; Ali, M.S.; Elakel, A.M.; Nassar, E.A.; Gad, M.M. Comparative Evaluation of TiO_2 Nanoparticle Addition and Postcuring Time on the Flexural Properties and Hardness of Additively Fabricated Denture Base Resins. *Nanomaterials* **2023**, *13*, 3061. [CrossRef] [PubMed]
19. Lee, H.-E.; Alauddin, M.S.; Mohd Ghazali, M.I.; Said, Z.; Mohamad Zol, S. Effect of Different Vat Polymerization Techniques on Mechanical and Biological Properties of 3D-Printed Denture Base. *Polymers* **2023**, *15*, 1463. [CrossRef] [PubMed]
20. Lung, C.Y.K.; Darvell, B.W. Minimization of the Inevitable Residual Monomer in Denture Base Acrylic. *Dent. Mater.* **2005**, *21*, 1119–1128. [CrossRef] [PubMed]
21. Ayaz, E.A.; Durkan, R.; Koroglu, A.; Bagis, B. Comparative Effect of Different Polymerization Techniques on Residual Monomer and Hardness Properties of PMMA-Based Denture Resins. *J. Appl. Biomater. Funct. Mater.* **2014**, *12*, 228–233. [CrossRef]
22. Bartoloni, J.A.; Murchison, D.F.; Wofford, D.T.; Sarkar, N.K. Degree of Conversion in Denture Base Materials for Varied Polymerization Techniques 1. *J. Oral Rehabil.* **2000**, *27*, 488–493. [CrossRef]
23. Farina, A.P.; Cecchin, D.; Soares, R.G.; Botelho, A.L.; Takahashi, J.M.F.K.; Mazzetto, M.O.; Mesquita, M.F. Evaluation of Vickers Hardness of Different Types of Acrylic Denture Base Resins with and without Glass Fibre Reinforcement. *Gerodontology* **2012**, *29*, e155–e160. [CrossRef]
24. Ayman, A.-D. The Residual Monomer Content and Mechanical Properties of CAD\CAM Resins Used in the Fabrication of Complete Dentures as Compared to Heat Cured Resins. *Electron. Physician* **2017**, *9*, 4766–4772. [CrossRef]
25. Engler, M.L.P.D.; Güth, J.-F.; Keul, C.; Erdelt, K.; Edelhoff, D.; Liebermann, A. Residual Monomer Elution from Different Conventional and CAD/CAM Dental Polymers during Artificial Aging. *Clin. Oral Investig.* **2020**, *24*, 277–284. [CrossRef] [PubMed]
26. Gungor, H.; Gundogdu, M.; Alkurt, M.; Yesil Duymus, Z. Effect of Polymerization Cycles on Flexural Strengths and Microhardness of Different Denture Base Materials. *Dent. Mater. J.* **2017**, *36*, 168–173. [CrossRef] [PubMed]
27. Seo, R.S.; Vergani, C.E.; Giampaolo, E.T.; Pavarina, A.C.; Machado, A.L. Effect of post-polymerization treatments on the flexural strength and vickers hardness of reline and acrylic denture base resins. *J. Appl. Oral Sci.* **2007**, *15*, 506–511. [CrossRef] [PubMed]
28. Sadamori, S.; Kotani, H.; Hamada, T. The Usage Period of Dentures and Their Residual Monomer Contents. *J. Prosthet. Dent.* **1992**, *68*, 374–376. [CrossRef] [PubMed]
29. De Andrade Lima Chaves, C.; Machado, A.L.; Vergani, C.E.; De Souza, R.F.; Giampaolo, E.T. Cytotoxicity of Denture Base and Hard Chairside Reline Materials: A Systematic Review. *J. Prosthet. Dent.* **2012**, *107*, 114–127. [CrossRef] [PubMed]
30. Rashid, H.; Sheikh, Z.; Vohra, F. Allergic Effects of the Residual Monomer Used in Denture Base Acrylic Resins. *Eur. J. Dent.* **2015**, *9*, 614–619. [CrossRef] [PubMed]
31. Aguirre, B.C.; Chen, J.-H.; Kontogiorgos, E.D.; Murchison, D.F.; Nagy, W.W. Flexural Strength of Denture Base Acrylic Resins Processed by Conventional and CAD-CAM Methods. *J. Prosthet. Dent.* **2020**, *123*, 641–646. [CrossRef]
32. Al-Dwairi, Z.N.; Tahboub, K.Y.; Baba, N.Z.; Goodacre, C.J. A Comparison of the Flexural and Impact Strengths and Flexural Modulus of CAD/CAM and Conventional Heat-Cured Polymethyl Methacrylate (PMMA). *J. Prosthodont.* **2020**, *29*, 341–349. [CrossRef] [PubMed]
33. Rueggeberg, F.A.; Craig, R.G. Correlation of Parameters Used to Estimate Monomer Conversion in a Light-Cured Composite. *J. Dent. Res.* **1988**, *67*, 932–937. [CrossRef]
34. Lee, H.-H.; Lee, C.-J.; Asaoka, K. Correlation in the Mechanical Properties of Acrylic Denture Base Resins. *Dent. Mater. J.* **2012**, *31*, 157–164. [CrossRef] [PubMed]

35. ISO 20795-1:2013; Dentistry—Base Polymers—Part 1: Denture Base Polymers. International Organisation for Standardization: Geneva, Switzerland, 2013.
36. Blagojevic, V.; Murphy, V.M. Microwave Polymerization of Denture Base Materials. A Comparative Study. *J. Oral Rehabil.* **1999**, *26*, 804–808. [CrossRef]
37. Abualsaud, R.; Gad, M. Flexural Strength of CAD/CAM Denture Base Materials: Systematic Review and Meta-Analysis of in-Vitro Studies. *J. Int. Soc. Prevent Communit Dent.* **2022**, *12*, 160. [CrossRef] [PubMed]
38. Raszewski, Z. Acrylic Resins in the CAD/CAM Technology: A Systematic Literature Review. *Dent. Med. Probl.* **2020**, *57*, 449–454. [CrossRef]
39. Bayraktar, G.; Duran, O.; Guvener, B. Effect of Glass Fibre Reinforcement on Residual Methyl Methacrylate Content of Denture Base Polymers. *J. Dent.* **2003**, *31*, 297–302. [CrossRef]
40. Goiato, M.; Freitas, E.; Dos Santos, D.; De Medeiros, R.; Sonego, M. Acrylic Resin Cytotoxicity for Denture Base: Literature Review. *Adv. Clin. Exp. Med.* **2015**, *24*, 679–686. [CrossRef]
41. Bural, C.; AktaŞ, E.; Deniz, G.; Ünlüçerçi, Y.; Bayraktar, G. Effect of Leaching Residual Methyl Methacrylate Concentrations on in Vitro Cytotoxicity of Heat Polymerized Denture Base Acrylic Resin Processed with Different Polymerization Cycles. *J. Appl. Oral. Sci.* **2011**, *19*, 306–312. [CrossRef]
42. Borak, J.; Fields, C.; Andrews, L.S.; Pemberton, M.A. Methyl Methacrylate and Respiratory Sensitization: A Critical Review. *Crit. Rev. Toxicol.* **2011**, *41*, 230–268. [CrossRef]
43. Kedjarune, U.; Charoenworaluk, N.; Koontongkaew, S. Release of Methyl Methacrylate from Heat-curved and Autopolymerized Resins: Cytotoxicity Testing Related to Residual Monomer. *Aust. Dent. J.* **1999**, *44*, 25–30. [CrossRef]
44. Sadamori, S.; Ganefiyanti, T.; Hamada, T.; Arima, T. Influence of Thickness and Location on the Residual Monomer Content of Denture Base Cured by Three Processing Methods. *J. Prosthet. Dent.* **1994**, *72*, 19–22. [CrossRef]
45. Vallittu, P.K.; Miettinen, V.; Alakuijala, P. Residual Monomer Content and Its Release into Water from Denture Base Materials. *Dent. Mater.* **1995**, *11*, 338–342. [CrossRef]
46. Murakami, N.; Wakabayashi, N.; Matsushima, R.; Kishida, A.; Igarashi, Y. Effect of High-Pressure Polymerization on Mechanical Properties of PMMA Denture Base Resin. *J. Mech. Behav. Biomed. Mater.* **2013**, *20*, 98–104. [CrossRef]
47. Lourinho, C.; Salgado, H.; Correia, A.; Fonseca, P. Mechanical Properties of Polymethyl Methacrylate as Denture Base Material: Heat-Polymerized vs. 3D-Printed—Systematic Review and Meta-Analysis of In Vitro Studies. *Biomedicines* **2022**, *10*, 2565. [CrossRef]
48. Iwaki, M.; Kanazawa, M.; Arakida, T.; Minakuchi, S. Mechanical Properties of a Polymethyl Methacrylate Block for CAD/CAM Dentures. *J. Oral. Sci.* **2020**, *62*, 420–422. [CrossRef] [PubMed]
49. Alp, G.; Murat, S.; Yilmaz, B. Comparison of Flexural Strength of Different CAD/CAM PMMA-Based Polymers. *J. Prosthodont.* **2019**, *28*, e491–e495. [CrossRef] [PubMed]
50. Chhabra, M.; Nanditha Kumar, M.; RaghavendraSwamy, K.N.; Thippeswamy, H.M. Flexural Strength and Impact Strength of Heat-Cured Acrylic and 3D Printed Denture Base Resins- A Comparative in Vitro Study. *J. Oral Biol. Craniofac Res.* **2022**, *12*, 1–3. [CrossRef] [PubMed]
51. Prpić, V.; Schauperl, Z.; Ćatić, A.; Dulčić, N.; Čimić, S. Comparison of Mechanical Properties of 3D-Printed, CAD/CAM, and Conventional Denture Base Materials. *J. Prosthodont.* **2020**, *29*, 524–528. [CrossRef] [PubMed]
52. al-Qarni, F.D.; Gad, M.M. Printing Accuracy and Flexural Properties of Different 3D-Printed Denture Base Resins. *Materials* **2022**, *15*, 2410. [CrossRef]
53. Fiore, A.D.; Meneghello, R.; Brun, P.; Rosso, S.; Gattazzo, A.; Stellini, E.; Yilmaz, B. Comparison of the Flexural and Surface Properties of Milled, 3D-Printed, and Heat Polymerized PMMA Resins for Denture Bases: An In Vitro Study. *J. Prosthodont. Res.* **2022**, *66*, 502–508. [CrossRef] [PubMed]
54. Pituru, S.M.; Greabu, M.; Totan, A.; Imre, M.; Pantea, M.; Spinu, T.; Tancu, A.M.C.; Popoviciu, N.O.; Stanescu, I.-I.; Ionescu, E. A Review on the Biocompatibility of PMMA-Based Dental Materials for Interim Prosthetic Restorations with a Glimpse into Their Modern Manufacturing Techniques. *Materials* **2020**, *13*, 2894. [CrossRef] [PubMed]
55. Steinmassl, O.; Offermanns, V.; Stöckl, W.; Dumfahrt, H.; Grunert, I.; Steinmassl, P.-A. In Vitro Analysis of the Fracture Resistance of CAD/CAM Denture Base Resins. *Materials* **2018**, *11*, 401. [CrossRef] [PubMed]
56. Li, M.; Wang, S.; Li, R.; Wang, Y.; Fan, X.; Gong, W.; Ma, Y. The Mechanical and Antibacterial Properties of Boron Nitride/Silver Nanocomposite Enhanced Polymethyl Methacrylate Resin for Application in Oral Denture Bases. *Biomimetics* **2022**, *7*, 138. [CrossRef]
57. Alshaikh, A.A.; Khattar, A.; Almindil, I.A.; Alsaif, M.H.; Akhtar, S.; Khan, S.Q.; Gad, M.M. 3D-Printed Nanocomposite Denture-Base Resins: Effect of ZrO_2 Nanoparticles on the Mechanical and Surface Properties In Vitro. *Nanomaterials* **2022**, *12*, 2451. [CrossRef] [PubMed]
58. Unkovskiy, A.; Bui, P.H.-B.; Schille, C.; Geis-Gerstorfer, J.; Huettig, F.; Spintzyk, S. Objects Build Orientation, Positioning, and Curing Influence Dimensional Accuracy and Flexural Properties of Stereolithographically Printed Resin. *Dent. Mater.* **2018**, *34*, e324–e333. [CrossRef] [PubMed]

59. Altarazi, A.; Haider, J.; Alhotan, A.; Silikas, N.; Devlin, H. Assessing the Physical and Mechanical Properties of 3D Printed Acrylic Material for Denture Base Application. *Dent. Mater.* **2022**, *38*, 1841–1854. [CrossRef]
60. Zeidan, A.E.; Abd Elrahim, R.; Abd El Hakim, A.; Harby, N.; Helal, M. Evaluation of Surface Properties and Elastic Modulus of CAD-CAM Milled, 3D Printed, and Compression Moulded Denture Base Resins: An in Vitro Study. *J. Int. Soc. Prevent Communit Dent.* **2022**, *12*, 630. [CrossRef]

Disclaimer/Publisher's Note: The statements, opinions and data contained in all publications are solely those of the individual author(s) and contributor(s) and not of MDPI and/or the editor(s). MDPI and/or the editor(s) disclaim responsibility for any injury to people or property resulting from any ideas, methods, instructions or products referred to in the content.

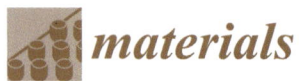 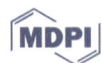

Article

Tensile Bond Strength between Different Denture Base Materials and Soft Denture Liners

Josip Vuksic [1,2], Ana Pilipovic [3], Tina Poklepovic Pericic [4] and Josip Kranjcic [1,5,*]

1. Department of Removable Prosthodontics, School of Dental Medicine, University of Zagreb, Gunduliceva 5, 10000 Zagreb, Croatia; jvuksic@sfzg.hr
2. Department of Prosthodontics, University Hospital Dubrava, Av. Gojka Šuška 6, 10000 Zagreb, Croatia
3. Department of Technology, Faculty of Mechanical Engineering and Naval Architecture, University of Zagreb, Ivana Lučića 5, 10000 Zagreb, Croatia; ana.pilipovic@fsb.hr
4. Department of Prosthodontics, School of Medicine, University of Split, Šoltanska 2, 21000 Split, Croatia; tinapoklepovic@gmail.com
5. Department of Fixed Prosthodontics, School of Dental Medicine, University of Zagreb, Gunduliceva 5, 10000 Zagreb, Croatia
* Correspondence: kranjcic@sfzg.hr

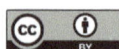

Citation: Vuksic, J.; Pilipovic, A.; Poklepovic Pericic, T.; Kranjcic, J. Tensile Bond Strength between Different Denture Base Materials and Soft Denture Liners. *Materials* **2023**, *16*, 4615. https://doi.org/10.3390/ma16134615

Academic Editor: Bongju Kim

Received: 2 June 2023
Revised: 19 June 2023
Accepted: 21 June 2023
Published: 26 June 2023

Copyright: © 2023 by the authors. Licensee MDPI, Basel, Switzerland. This article is an open access article distributed under the terms and conditions of the Creative Commons Attribution (CC BY) license (https://creativecommons.org/licenses/by/4.0/).

Abstract: (1) Background: Various materials are available for CAD-CAM denture base fabrication, for both additive and subtractive manufacturing. However, little has been reported on bond strength to soft denture liners. Therefore, the aim of this study was to investigate tensile bond strength, comparing between different denture base materials and soft denture liners. (2) Methods: Seven different materials were used for denture base fabrication: one heat-polymerized polymethyl methacrylate, three materials for subtractive manufacturing, two materials for additive manufacturing and one polyamide. Two materials were used for soft denture lining: one silicone-based and one acrylate-based. The study was conducted according to the specification ISO No. 10139-2:2016, and the type of failure was determined. The Kruskal–Wallis test with Dunn's post hoc test was used to analyse the values of tensile bond strength, and Fisher's exact test was used to analyse the type of failure. p Values < 0.05 were considered statistically significant. (3) Results: The tensile bond strength values were not statistically significantly different combining all the materials used for denture base fabrication with the acrylate-based soft denture liner ($p > 0.05$), and the average values ranged between 0.19 and 0.25 Mpa. The tensile bond strength values of the different denture base materials and silicone-based denture liner were statistically significantly different ($p < 0.05$), and the average values ranged between 1.49 and 3.07 Mpa. The type of failure was predominantly adhesive between polyamide and both additive-manufactured denture base materials in combination with the acrylate-based soft liner ($p < 0.05$). (4) Conclusions: The use of digital technologies in denture base fabrication can have an influence on different tensile bond strength values for soft denture liners, with different types of failure when compared with heat-cured PMMA. Similar tensile bond strength values were found between the acrylate-based soft denture liner and denture base materials. Significant differences in tensile bond strength values were found between the silicone-based soft denture liner and denture base materials, where the additive-manufactured and polyamide denture base materials showed lower values than heat-cured PMMA and subtractive-manufactured denture base materials.

Keywords: denture liners; CAD-CAM; denture base

1. Introduction

Among the various materials used for denture base fabrication, polymethyl methacrylate (PMMA) became the gold standard soon after its introduction into clinical use [1,2]. It has many advantageous properties, including a low cost, ease of handling, a light weight, low water solubility and water sorption, stability in oral environments and high aesthetic results, but also has some shortcomings, including a residual monomer, brittleness, poor mechanical properties, high polymerization shrinkage and a lack of radiopacity [1,3–5]. For this reason, there is an ongoing search for a better material. One direction is to chemically modify PMMA using monomers, oligomers, copolymers and cross-linking agents [6–9]. Investigations were also performed with the incorporation of filler particles and fibres into the PMMA, with recent trends towards nanoparticle incorporation (zirconium dioxide nanoparticles, silicone dioxide nanoparticles, diamond nanoparticles) [5,9]. Different processing techniques were also proposed (injection moulding, microwave, heat polymerization under high pressure, autoclave) [9]. The other direction is the use of materials with a completely different chemical formula from PMMA, such as polyamide, polycarbonate and polyester [10,11]. When compared with PMMA, these materials have a lower elastic modulus, lower surface roughness, lower allergenic risk and higher resistance to acids, but also have some other disadvantages, including complicated manipulation and different processing and polishing methods, the fact that special and more expensive equipment is required, higher water sorption, a higher risk of fracture and lower colour stability [10,11]. Recently, polyetheretherketone (PEEK) and a high-performance polymer based on polyether ketone (BioHPP) were also proposed for denture base fabrication [9].

Recently, new digital technologies have increasingly been used in dentistry and are also available for denture base fabrication, both subtractive and additive [3,6,12–15]. When compared with heat-cured PMMA, digital technologies can theoretically accelerate the fabrication of the denture, reduce the possibility of errors, improve precision and achieve better material properties. It is also possible to reduce the number of patient visits to the dental office and reduce the dental technician's working time [1,16–18]. With stored computer data, it is easy to reproduce the same denture if necessary [19,20]. However, there is a lack of scientific data for these types of materials, especially for additive technologies.

The denture base should be meticulously fitted to the residual ridge after its fabrication. Due to the resorption of the alveolar bone, which is a chronic, progressive and irreversible process, the shape of the residual ridge changes. Denture relining, as a common clinical procedure in dentistry, can prolong the use of the existing denture by adapting the denture base to the changes in soft and hard tissues. This procedure is much faster and less expensive than fabricating a new denture. Hard and soft denture liners can be used. Soft denture liners can be used for both short- and long-term use, and they can be silicone- and acrylate-based [21,22].

Soft denture liners have a cushioning effect and can contribute to an even distribution of functional loads on the denture-bearing area and improve patient comfort, especially in cases of undercuts, sensitive mucosa, and bruxomania [22–24]. They may also be helpful after surgical procedures and for immediate dentures. It is proven that soft denture lining can improve oral-health-related quality of life, masticatory function, and overall patient satisfaction with the denture [25–27].

Bond strength between the denture base material and soft denture liner is considered as one of the key factors for the long-term success of the relining procedure [23,28–33]. However, the bond strength values between denture base materials (especially in additive and subtractive manufacturing) and soft denture liners are poorly studied, and standardised tests are rarely used. Therefore, the aim of this study was to investigate the tensile bond strength values between denture base materials and soft denture liners using the method described in specification ISO No. 10139-2:2016 [34], with an emphasis on denture base materials for computer-aided design–computer-aided manufacturing (CAD-CAM) technology. Additionally, the type of failure was investigated. The null hypothesis was stated: There is no difference in tensile bond strength between the different denture base materials and soft denture liners, and there is no difference in the type of failure between the different denture base materials and soft denture liners.

2. Materials and Methods

Seven different denture base materials and two different soft denture liners were used in this study. The materials used are shown in Table 1.

Table 1. Materials used in this study.

Name of the Material	Manufacturer	Description and Purpose of the Material
Meliodent heat cure	Kulzer, Hanau, Germany	Denture base material, PMMA, heat-cured
Vertex Thermosens	Vetex Dental, Soesterberg, Netherlands	Denture base material, polyamide, injection technique
Ivobase CAD pink V	Ivoclar Vivadent, Schaan, Liechtenstein	CAD CAM denture base material, subtractive manufacturing
Polident pink CAD/CAM disc basic	Polident d.o.o., Volčja draga, Slovenia	CAD CAM denture base material, subtractive manufacturing
Anaxdent pink blank U medium pink	Anaxdent GmbH, Stuttgart, Germany	CAD CAM denture base material, subtractive manufacturing
Freeprint denture	Detax, Ettlingen, Germany	CAD CAM denture base material, additive manufacturing
Imprimo LC denture	Scheu, Iserlohn, Germany	CAD CAM denture base material, additive manufacturing
Soft liner	GC Europe, Leuven, Belgium	Soft denture liner, acrylate-based, direct relining method
Reline II soft	GC Europe, Leuven, Belgium	Soft denture liner, silicone-based, direct relining method

This study was performed according to the specification ISO No. 10139-2:2016 [34]. Plates with dimensions of 25 ± 3 mm $\times$ 25 ± 3 mm and a thickness of 3 ± 0.5 mm, composed of denture base material, were the basis for specimen preparation. The flat surfaces of the plates were kept plane-parallel and wet-ground with standard P500 metallographic grinding paper. After the preparation of the plates, they were stored in a water bath at 37 ± 1 °C for 30 ± 2 days.

Two plates, a polytetrafluoroethylene (PTFE) collar and a PMMA rod, were needed for one specimen. The PTFE collar had an inner diameter of 10 ± 0.5 mm and a height of 3 ± 0.25 mm. The PMMA rod had an outer diameter of 10 mm and a height of 20 mm.

After the plates were removed from the water bath, they were dried, and for the silicone-based liner, adhesive was applied to the adhesive surface of the plate. The PTFE collar was placed in the centre of the plate, and the prepared soft liner material was applied with slight excess while being confined within the PTFE collar and closed with the second plate. The specimen was clamped for 1 h. Then, the PMMA rod was attached to the top of the second plate using cyanoacrylate cement. A custom-made template was used to assemble the specimen and to maintain the vertical alignment of the specimen.

The specimens were again stored in a water bath at 37 ± 1 °C for 23 ± 1 h. Immediately after removal from the water bath, the specimens were placed in the universal testing machine (Autograph AGS-X, Shimadzu, Kyoto, Japan). To ensure the vertical alignment of the specimen in the testing machine, a custom-made loading assembly was used. The tensile test was performed at a displacement rate of 10 mm/min (Figure 1). The maximum load (F) during debonding was recorded. The sample size was determined using the specification ISO No. 10139-2:2016 [34]. For each denture base material in combination with one soft liner, 10 specimens were prepared, and 140 measurements were performed in total.

The tensile bond strength B (MPa) was calculated according to the formula $B = F/A$, where F (N) is the maximum load recorded and A (mm^2) is the adhesive area. The adhesive area was defined according to the inner diameter of the PTFE collar.

The type of failure was determined visually according to the instructions of specification ISO 10365:2022 [35]. High-resolution photographs were taken using a digital single-lens reflex camera EOS 250D (Canon, Ota City, Tokio, Japan) with a macro-objective at a $10\times$ magnification. A distinction was made between adhesive, cohesive and mixed types of failure.

MedCalc® Statistical Software v20.010 was used for the statistical analysis. The Kruskal–Wallis test with Dunn's post hoc test was used to analyse the values of tensile bond strength, and Fisher's exact test was used to analyse the type of failure. p Values < 0.05 were considered statistically significant.

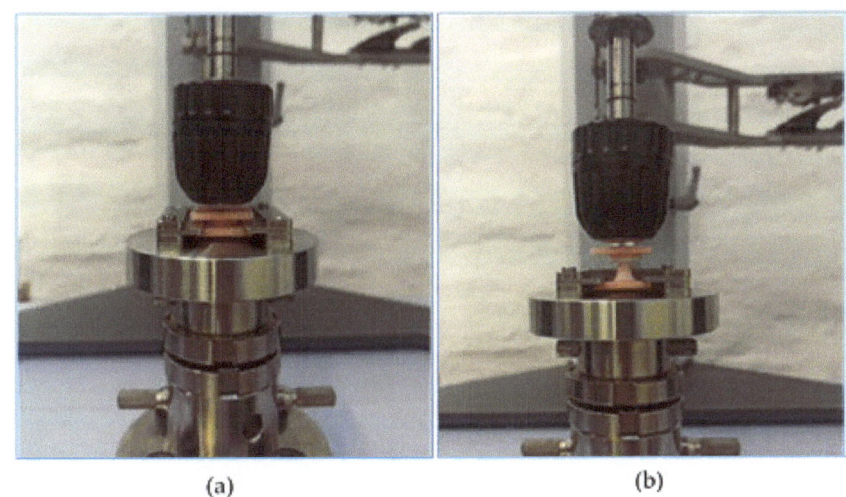

Figure 1. Specimen placed in the universal testing machine at the beginning of testing (**a**) and during testing (**b**).

3. Results

The results of tensile bond strength for both soft denture liners are shown in Table 2 and in Figures 2 and 3. Two graphs presenting tensile stress as a function of strain for both soft denture liners used in this study are shown in Figures 4 and 5.

Table 2. Tensile bond strength between denture base materials and soft liners.

		GC Soft Liner		GC Reline II Soft	
		Mean (MPa)	SD	Mean (MPa)	SD
1.	meliodent heat cure	0.23	0.07	2.84 [2, 6, 7]	0.33
2.	vertex thermosens	0.23	0.06	1.49 [1, 3, 4, 5]	0.47
3.	ivobase cad pink	0.24	0.08	2.85 [2, 6, 7]	0.23
4.	polident pink cad/cam	0.25	0.08	3.07 [2, 5, 6, 7]	0.23
5.	anaxdent pink blank	0.24	0.08	2.74 [2, 4, 6, 7]	0.27
6.	freeprint denture	0.20	0.07	1.89 [1, 3, 4, 5]	0.47
7.	imprimo lc denture	0.19	0.09	1.80 [1, 3, 4, 5]	0.50

MPa = megapascal, SD = standard deviation. Superscripted numbers indicate a statistical difference between the groups of denture base materials, $p < 0.05$.

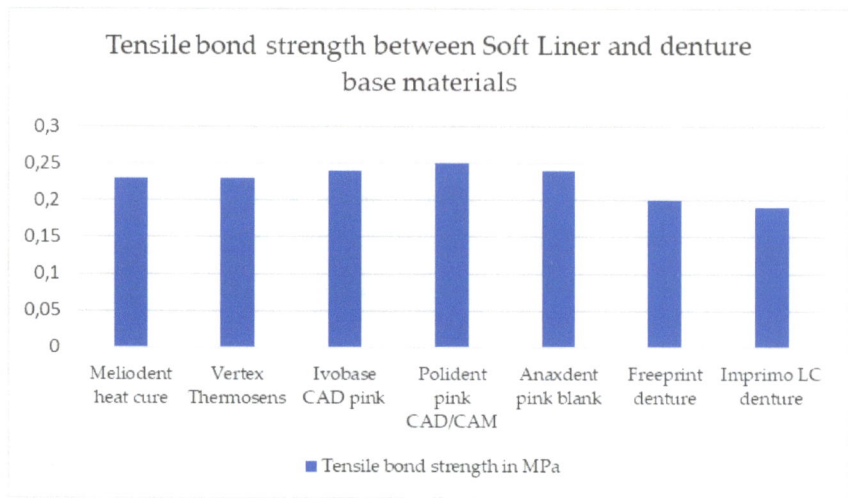

Figure 2. Tensile bond strength results between soft liner and different denture base materials.

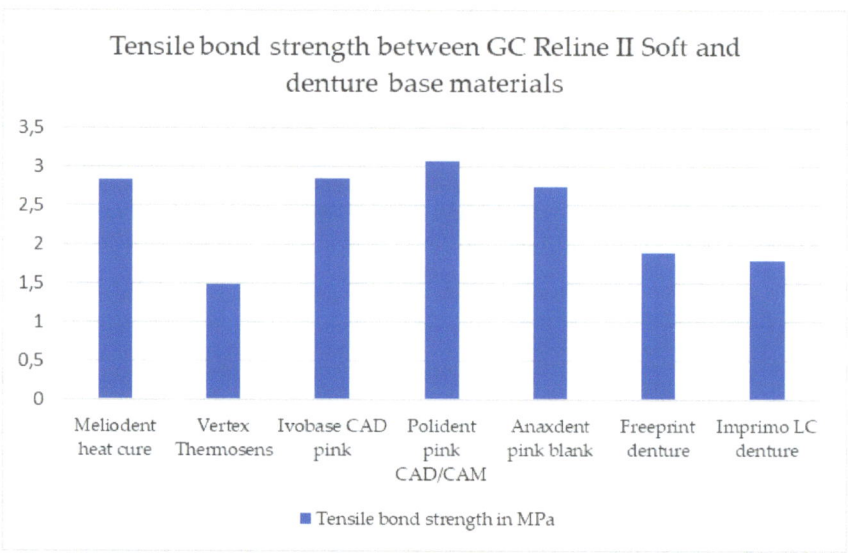

Figure 3. Tensile bond strength results between GC Reline II Soft and different denture base materials.

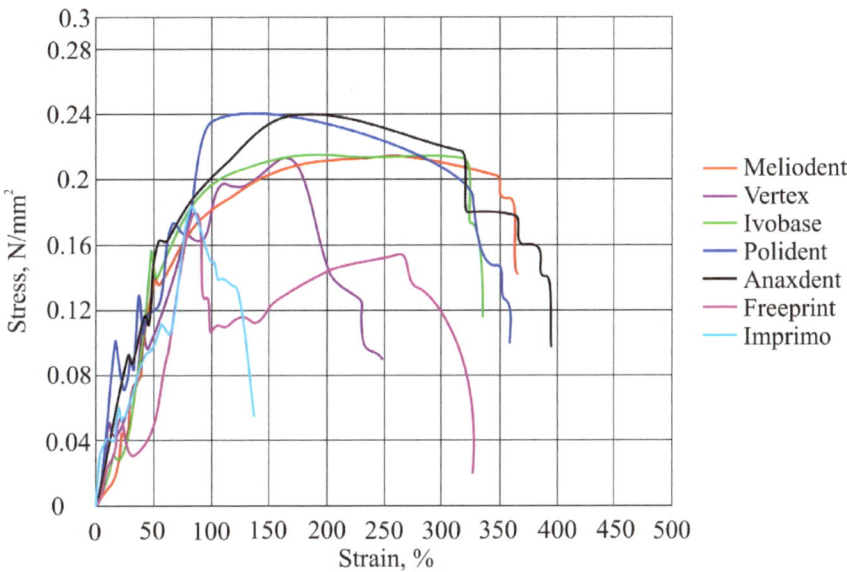

Figure 4. Graph showing tensile stress as a function of strain with average values obtained for the soft liner.

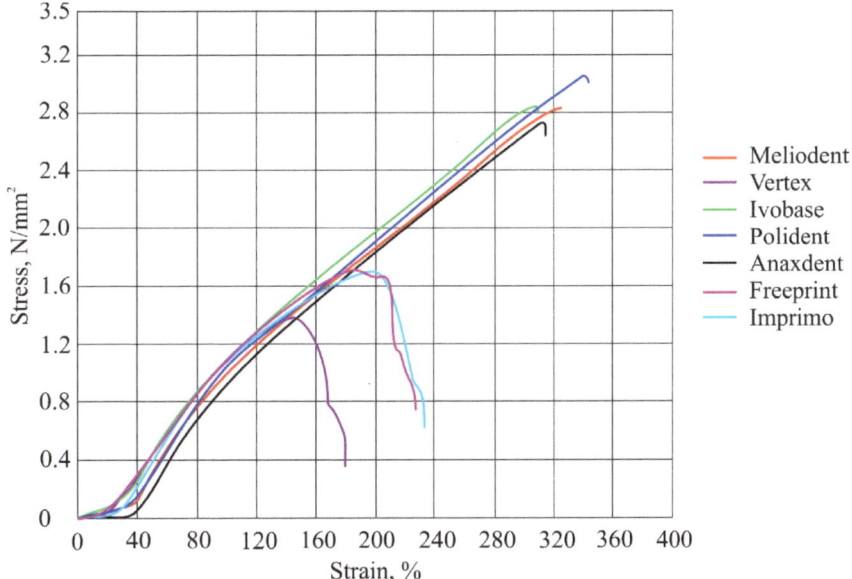

Figure 5. Graph showing tensile stress as a function of strain with average values obtained for the for Reline II Soft.

There was no statistically significant difference in the tensile bond strength values between the GC Soft Liner and different denture base materials ($p > 0.05$) (Table 2).

Statistically significantly different values of tensile bond strength were found between the GC Reline II Soft and different denture base materials ($p < 0.05$) (Table 2).

The tensile bond strength value between the heat-cured PMMA denture base material and GC Reline II Soft was statistically significantly higher ($p < 0.05$) than the bond strength values between the GC Reline II Soft and both additive-manufactured materials (Table 2).

The bond strength value between the poliamide denture base material and GC Reline II Soft was statistically significantly lower ($p < 0.05$) than the bond strength values measured between the GC Reline II Soft and all three materials used for subtractive denture fabrication and between the GC Reline II Soft and heat-cured PMMA material (Table 2).

The tensile bond strength values between all three subtractive-manufactured denture base materials and the GC Reline II Soft were statistically significantly higher ($p < 0.05$) than the tensile bond strength values between the GC Reline II Soft and poliamide, as well as both additive-manufactured denture base materials (Table 2).

In addition, a statistically significantly higher tensile bond strength value was found between the Polident pink CAD-CAM and GC Reline II Soft compared to the tensile bond strength value between the Anaxdent pink blank and GC Reline II Soft ($p < 0.05$) (Table 2).

Both additive-manufactured denture base materials showed statistically significantly lower tensile bond strength values ($p < 0.05$) in combination with GC Reline II Soft compared to the combination of GC Reline II Soft with all three subtractive-manufactured denture base materials and with heat-cured PMMA (Table 2).

The results for the type of failure for both soft denture liners are shown in Table 3. Representative photographs of the fracture modes are shown in Figure 6.

Table 3. Type of failure.

	Soft Liner			GC Reline II Soft		
	Type of Failure			Type of Failure		
	Adhesive	Cohesive	Mixed	Adhesive	Cohesive	Mixed
meliodent	1	9	0	4	6	0
vertex thermosens	7 *	3 *	0 *	6	1	3
ivobase cad pink	0	9	1	8 *	2 *	0 *
polident pink cad/cam	0	10	0	3	6	1
anaxdent pink blank	0	10	0	6	4	0
freeprint denture	7 *	3 *	1 *	0 *	5 *	5 *
imprimo lc denture	9 *	1 *	0 *	0	8	2

* indicates statistical difference between groups ($p < 0.05$).

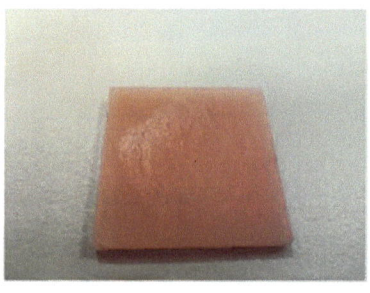
(a)

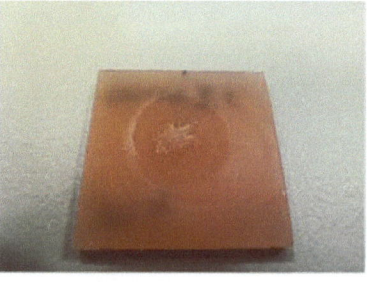
(b)

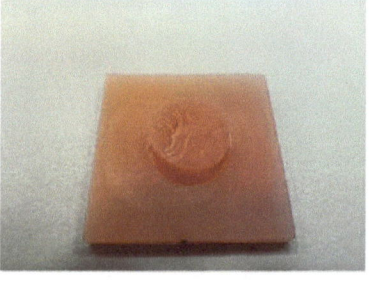
(c)

Figure 6. Representative photographs of failure types: adhesive type of failure (**a**), mixed type of failure (**b**) and cohesive type of failure (**c**).

For the GC Soft Liner, there was a statistically significant difference in the results for the type of failure between different denture base materials ($p < 0.05$). When the GC Soft

Liner was combined with polyamide and both additive denture base materials, the type of failure was predominantly adhesive, whereas when the GC Soft Liner was combined with all other denture base materials, the type of failure was predominantly or exclusively cohesive (Table 3).

For the GC Reline II Soft, there was also a statistically significant difference between the results for the type of failure for different denture base materials ($p < 0.05$). For the combination of GC Reline II Soft and Ivobase CAD pink, the type of failure was dominantly adhesive, and for the combination of GC Reline II Soft and the Imprimo LC denture, the type of failure was predominantly cohesive (Table 3).

4. Discussion

Denture relining is a clinical procedure used to adjust the denture base to soft and hard tissue changes. It extends the use of the existing denture, is less expensive and faster than fabricating a new denture and improves the patient's oral-health-related quality of life, masticatory function and overall satisfaction with their denture. The bond strength values between denture base materials manufactured with digital technologies (especially additive manufacturing) and denture liners are poorly studied.

Therefore, the aim of this study was to investigate tensile bond strength values between denture base materials and soft denture liners, with an emphasis on denture base materials for CAD-CAM technology. Three different materials for subtractive manufacturing and two for additive manufacturing were included in our study. In addition, a polyamide denture base material was included, because it is used as an alternative to PMMA in standard analogue processes for denture base fabrication. Heat-cured PMMA was included as the gold standard among the materials used for denture base fabrication.

According to the results, there was no statistically significant difference in the tensile bond strength values between the different denture base materials and soft liner, but there was a statistically significant difference in the tensile bond strength values between the different denture base materials and Reline II Soft. The polyamide and both additive-manufactured denture base materials showed statistically lower tensile bond strength values when combined with the GC Reline II Soft compared to the heat-cured PMMA and all three subtractive-manufactured denture base materials. There was also a statistically significant difference in the tensile bond strength values between the Polident pink CAD/CAM and Anaxdent pink blank in combination with the Reline II Soft. Therefore, for the results of tensile bond strength between the GC Soft Liner and different denture base materials, the null hypothesis was accepted. For the tensile bond strength results between the Reline II Soft and different denture base materials, the null hypothesis was rejected.

In terms of the type of failure, both the additive-manufactured and polyamide denture base materials showed statistically significantly different values for the GC Soft Liner, with the adhesive type dominating. Therefore, the null hypothesis for the results regarding the type of failure between the GC Soft Liner and different denture base materials was rejected. The GC Soft Liner is acrylate-based and used without adhesive, because it is considered that the monomer of the liner causes the swelling of the surface of the denture base material and the chemical bond between the two materials. Polyamide materials have a different chemical composition from PMMA, also being additive-manufactured materials that are not pure PMMA materials in terms of composition, and they have many other additives. Therefore, it can be concluded that there was no chemical bonding, which was the cause of the predominantly adhesive type of failure [33].

In our study, a statistically significant difference in the type of failure was found between the GC Reline II Soft and the different denture base materials. For the combination of GC Reline II Soft and Ivobase CAD pink, the type of failure was predominantly adhesive, and for the combination of GC Reline II Soft and the Imprimo LC denture, the type of failure was predominantly cohesive. No dominant or exclusive type of failure was observed for the combination of GC Reline II Soft and all other denture base materials. The null hypothesis for the failure type between GC Reline II Soft and the different denture base materials was rejected.

In the study conducted by Awad et al. [36], the tensile bond strength between denture base materials and denture liners was investigated. The tensile bond strength values varied between different material combinations, and the type of failure between the denture base materials and soft liners was predominantly adhesive. Wemken et al. [37] found no statistically significant difference in the tensile bond strength values between different denture base materials (heat-cured PMMA, subtractive and additive manufacturing) and a soft liner, while the type of failure was exclusively adhesive. Azpiazu-Flores et al. [38] described the lowest tensile bond strength values between additive-manufactured denture base materials and long-term soft liners. In contrast, Choi et al. [31] described the lowest tensile bond strength values between subtractive-manufactured denture base materials and a soft liner, with most cases showing the adhesive type of failure.

Our results for the type of failure are partially in accordance with the results obtained by Awad et al. [36]. In their study, they included two soft denture liners, both acrylate-based. For one, the results were similar, while for the other, the results differed. Wemken et al. [37] included just one soft denture liner, which was silicone-based, in their study and observed an exclusively adhesive type of failure for all the denture base materials, in contrast with our results. Choi et al. [31] included one acrylate-based and two silicone-based soft denture liners in their study and observed an exclusively or predominantly adhesive type of failure in all combinations of the materials, again in contrast with our results. When comparing our study with the aforementioned studies, it can be noted that the materials used were from the same groups of materials but not from the same manufacturers. Additionally, the preparation of the samples and testing methods differed greatly, which could be the reason for such a discrepancy in the results for the type of failure. No firm conclusions can be drawn at this point, and further investigations are required considering the type of failure.

A polyamide denture base material was included in this study because it is used as an alternative to PMMA in the standard fabrication of analogue denture bases. It has a crystalline structure, making it a more chemical-resistant material that does not react with adhesives and monomers, in contrast to PMMA [39,40]. Therefore, it is more difficult to achieve a satisfactory bond strength with soft denture liners, and it is recommended that one uses additional surface preparation methods for polyamide materials [41,42].

In ISO 10139-2:2016 [34], it is stated that it is important to achieve a vertical alignment of the specimen in the testing machine to avoid torsional forces acting on the specimen. For this reason, we used a custom-made loading assembly with a flexible connection in the upper part of the assembly. Another way to achieve vertical alignment was demonstrated by Kim et al. [21], using a ball-and-socket joint in the lower part of the assembly.

ISO 10139-2:2016 [34] also states that the minimum bond strength required for soft long-term denture liners should be at least 1.0 MPa for soft materials and at least 0.5 MPa for extra-soft materials for at least 8 of the 10 specimens tested. The GC Reline II Soft, which we used in our study, met the minimum requirements for all denture base materials. The GC Soft Liner, on the other hand, had results all below 0.3 MPa, but according to the manufacturer, it is a short-term soft liner; thus, it does not need to meet the minimum requirement of 1.0 MPa. For short-term soft liners, ISO 10139-2:2016 does not specify minimum bond strength requirements. It should also be mentioned that some authors have cited 0.44 MPa as a minimum requirement for soft liners in previous studies [23,31,43,44].

It is stated in the literature that acrylate-based soft liners have a higher bond strength than silicone-based materials. This is due to the similar chemical compositions of the denture base material and the soft liner, which allow for a chemical bond between the two materials and better adhesion. When using silicone-based soft liners, it is important to use a suitable adhesive; otherwise, no chemical bond between the two materials will be established [28]. In our study, the silicone-based soft liner showed statistically significantly higher values for tensile bond strength than the acrylate-based one, but since the acrylate-based material in our study is intended for short-term use and the silicone-based one is intended for long-term use, they cannot be directly compared.

It was observed that during the mixing of the GC Soft Liner, there were many air inclusions inside the material, and these inclusions were also observed on the contact surface of the denture base material and soft liner. This material is mixed by hand, and these air inclusions reduce the contact area between the two materials and decrease the bond strength. The GC Reline II Soft is mixed using mixing tips, so that there are no visible air inclusions inside the mixed material, and with careful application, air inclusion on the contact surface of the two materials can be avoided. Kim et al. [21] pointed out this problem in their study.

In previous studies [31,45], micropores and air inclusions were found on the contact surface of a denture base material and silicone-based soft liner using a scanning electron microscope (SEM), which were not visible to the naked eye. Since the primer is used to ensure the adhesion of the silicone-based material, it is assumed that either the chemical reaction between the solvent in the primer (ethyl acetate) and the denture base material or the evaporation of the solvent is the cause of these air inclusions, and they may act as the fracture initiation site and reduce the contact area and the bond strength.

According to data from the available literature, it can be observed that in previous studies, different investigation methods were used for bond strength tests, including shear bond, peel bond and tensile bond strength tests, while the tensile bond strength test was most commonly used [37]. Tensile strength testing was also performed in different ways, with different specimen preparation methods, different specimen surface preparation techniques and different displacement rates. It can be concluded that the main problem in tensile bond strength testing was the control of the adhesive surface. Therefore, different specimen preparation methods were used. Some authors used the method with a metal flask and specimen invested in putty silicone impression material. The specimens were usually rod-shaped, with free space for the soft liner between two parts. The vertical orientation of the specimen was also controlled in this way. After the soft liner hardened, the specimens could be easily removed from the dental flask. Other authors used the method described in ISO 10139-2:2016 [34], but it was usually modified. In this method, the bonding surface is controlled with a PTFE or PE collar between the two plates of the denture base material. Since different examination methods were used in previous studies, it is difficult or not possible to compare different studies. It is only possible to draw certain conclusions within a single investigation. Therefore, in our investigation, we aimed to follow the instructions of the specification ISO 10139-2:2016 in full [34].

A general statement about the bond strength between additive and subtractive denture base materials, on the one hand, and soft denture liners, on the other, is currently not possible for several reasons. First, there are only a few studies that have been conducted on this topic. Second, different test methods were used in these studies. Third, different materials were used as a control group (heat-cured, injection-moulded PMMA from different manufacturers). Fourth, the research results vary between different studies; thus, the results cannot be summarised, and no clear conclusions can be drawn.

The limitation of this study is the fact that only one acrylate-based and one silicone-based soft denture liner were used, and for more firm conclusions to be obtained, more soft lining materials should be included in future investigations.

Our proposition for future investigations is to include more different soft denture lining materials from all categories, including those for short-term and long-term use, both acrylate-based and silicone-based, so that more firm conclusions could be obtained. Additionally, it should be investigated whether different types of surface pretreatments for additive-manufactured dentures could improve the tensile bond strength values when soft denture liners are used.

5. Conclusions

The use of digital technologies in denture base fabrication may influence the tensile bond strength values between denture base materials and soft denture liners (with different types of failure) when compared with heat-cured PMMA denture base materials.

There is no significant difference in tensile bond strength between the acrylate-based soft denture liner and denture base materials, which is not the case for the silicone-based soft denture liner. For the silicone-based soft denture liner used in combination with both additive-manufactured denture base materials, the values of tensile bond strength were statistically significantly lower than those for the same material used in combination with heat-cured PMMA and all three subtractive-manufactured denture base materials. The basic Polident pink CAD-CAM disc showed the highest tensile bond strength value in combination with the silicone-based soft liner.

Based on the higher values of tensile bond strength between subtractive-manufactured denture bases and PMMA denture bases with silicone-based soft liners, it can be suggested that practitioners use this combination of materials more frequently. All the investigated denture base materials can be combined well with acrylate soft denture liners.

Author Contributions: Conceptualization, J.V., J.K. and A.P.; methodology, J.V., J.K. and A.P.; software, J.V.; validation, J.V., J.K. and A.P.; formal analysis, J.V., J.K. and A.P.; investigation, J.V. and A.P.; resources, J.V. and T.P.P.; data curation, J.V. and T.P.P.; writing—original draft preparation, J.V. and J.K.; writing—review and editing, J.V. and J.K.; visualization, J.V. and T.P.P.; supervision, J.K.; project administration, J.V., J.K. and A.P.; funding acquisition, J.V., J.K. and A.P. All authors have read and agreed to the published version of the manuscript.

Funding: This research received no external funding.

Institutional Review Board Statement: Not applicable.

Informed Consent Statement: Not applicable.

Data Availability Statement: Not applicable.

Conflicts of Interest: The authors declare no conflict of interest.

References

1. Al-Dwairi, Z.N.; Tahboub, K.Y.; Baba, N.Z.; Goodacre, C.J.; Özcan, M. A Comparison of the Surface Properties of CAD/CAM and Conventional Polymethylmethacrylate (PMMA). *J. Prosthodont.* **2019**, *28*, 452–457. [CrossRef] [PubMed]
2. Aguirre, B.C.; Chen, J.H.; Kontogiorgos, E.D.; Murchison, D.F.; Nagy, W.W. Flexural Strength of Denture Base Acrylic Resins Processed by Conventional and CAD-CAM Methods. *J. Prosthet. Dent.* **2020**, *123*, 641–646. [CrossRef] [PubMed]
3. Anadioti, E.; Musharbash, L.; Blatz, M.B.; Papavasiliou, G.; Kamposiora, P. 3D Printed Complete Removable Dental Prostheses: A Narrative Review. *BMC Oral Health* **2020**, *20*, 343. [CrossRef] [PubMed]
4. Iwaki, M.; Kanazawa, M.; Arakida, T.; Minakuchi, S. Mechanical Properties of a Polymethyl Methacrylate Block for CAD/CAM Dentures. *J. Oral. Sci.* **2020**, *62*, 420–422. [CrossRef] [PubMed]
5. Gad, M.M.; Abualsaud, R.; Al-Thobity, A.M.; Baba, N.Z.; Al-Harbi, F.A. Influence of Addition of Different Nanoparticles on the Surface Properties of Poly(methylmethacrylate) Denture Base Material. *J. Prosthodont.* **2020**, *29*, 422–428. [CrossRef]
6. Perea-Lowery, L.; Minja, I.K.; Lassila, L.; Ramakrishnaiah, R.; Vallittu, P.K. Assessment of CAD-CAM Polymers for Digitally Fabricated Complete Dentures. *J. Prosthet. Dent.* **2021**, *125*, 175–181. [CrossRef]
7. Ucar, Y.; Akova, T.; Aysan, I. Mechanical Properties of Polyamide Versus Different PMMA Denture Base Materials: Polyamide as Denture Base Material. *J. Prosthodont.* **2012**, *21*, 173–176. [CrossRef]
8. Lamfon, H.A.; Hamouda, I.M. Maxillary Denture Flange and Occlusal Discrepancies of Vertex ThermoSens in Comparison with Conventional Heat-Cured Denture Base Materials. *J. Biomed. Res.* **2019**, *33*, 139. [CrossRef]
9. Khan, A.A.; Fareed, M.A.; Alshehri, A.H.; Aldegheishem, A.; Alharthi, R.; Saadaldin, S.A.; Zafar, M.S. Mechanical Properties of the Modified Denture Base Materials and Polymerization Methods: A Systematic Review. *Int. J. Mol. Sci.* **2022**, *23*, 5737. [CrossRef]
10. Yunus, N.; Rashid, A.A.; Azmi, L.L.; Abu–Hassan, M.I. Some Flexural Properties of a Nylon Denture Base Polymer. *J. Oral Rehabil.* **2005**, *32*, 65–71. [CrossRef]
11. Song, S.Y.; Kim, K.S.; Lee, J.Y.; Shin, S.W. Physical Properties and Color Stability of Injection-Molded Thermoplastic Denture Base Resins. *J. Adv. Prosthodont.* **2019**, *11*, 32. [CrossRef]
12. Hada, T.; Kanazawa, M.; Iwaki, M.; Arakida, T.; Minakuchi, S. Effect of Printing Direction on Stress Distortion of Three-Dimensional Printed Dentures Using Stereolithography Technology. *J. Mech. Behav. Biomed. Mater.* **2020**, *110*, 103949. [CrossRef]

13. Kraemer Fernandez, P.; Unkovskiy, A.; Benkendorff, V.; Klink, A.; Spintzyk, S. Surface Characteristics of Milled and 3D Printed Denture Base Materials Following Polishing and Coating: An In-Vitro Study. *Materials* **2020**, *13*, 3305. [CrossRef]
14. Lee, S.; Hong, S.J.; Paek, J.; Pae, A.; Kwon, K.R.; Noh, K. Comparing Accuracy of Denture Bases Fabricated by Injection Molding, CAD/CAM Milling, and Rapid Prototyping Method. *J. Adv. Prosthodont.* **2019**, *11*, 55. [CrossRef]
15. Steinmassl, O.; Offermanns, V.; Stöckl, W.; Dumfahrt, H.; Grunert, I.; Steinmassl, P.A. In Vitro Analysis of the Fracture Resistance of CAD/CAM Denture Base Resins. *Materials* **2018**, *11*, 401. [CrossRef]
16. Wang, C.; Shi, Y.F.; Xie, P.J.; Wu, J.H. Accuracy of digital complete dentures: A systematic review of in vitro studies. *J. Prosthet. Dent.* **2021**, *125*, 249–256. [CrossRef]
17. Gad, M.M.; Fouda, S.M.; Abualsaud, R.; Alshahrani, F.A.; Al-Thobity, A.M.; Khan, S.Q.; Akhtar, S.; Ateeq, I.S.; Helal, M.A.; Al-Harbi, F.A. Strength and Surface Properties of a 3D-Printed Denture Base Polymer. *J. Prosthodont.* **2022**, *31*, 412–418. [CrossRef]
18. Meirowitz, A.; Rahmanov, A.; Shlomo, E.; Zelikman, H.; Dolev, E.; Sterer, N. Effect of Denture Base Fabrication Technique on Candida Albicans Adhesion In Vitro. *Materials* **2021**, *14*, 221. [CrossRef]
19. Janeva, N.M.; Kovacevska, G.; Elencevski, S.; Panchevska, S.; Mijoska, A.; Lazarevska, B. Advantages of CAD/CAM versus Conventional Complete Dentures—A Review. *Open Access Maced. J. Med. Sci.* **2018**, *6*, 1498–1502. [CrossRef]
20. Alp, G.; Murat, S.; Yilmaz, B. Comparison of Flexural Strength of Different CAD/CAM PMMA-Based Polymers: Comparison of Flexural Strength of Interim Resin Materials. *J. Prosthodont.* **2019**, *28*, e491–e495. [CrossRef]
21. Kim, B.J.; Yang, H.S.; Chun, M.G.; Park, Y.J. Shore Hardness and Tensile Bond Strength of Long-Term Soft Denture Lining Materials. *J. Prosthet. Dent.* **2014**, *112*, 1289–1297. [CrossRef] [PubMed]
22. Hussein, F.A. Advances in Soft Denture Liners: An Update. *J. Contemp. Dent. Pract.* **2015**, *16*, 314–318. [CrossRef] [PubMed]
23. Khanna, A.A. Comparative Evaluation of Shear Bond Strength Between Two Commercially Available Heat Cured Resilient Liners and Denture Base Resin with Different Surface Treatments. *J. Clin. Diagn. Res.* **2015**, *9*, 30–34. [CrossRef] [PubMed]
24. Palla, E.S.; Karaoglani, E.; Naka, O.; Anastassiadou, V. Soft Denture Liners' Effect on the Masticatory Function in Patients Wearing Complete Dentures: A Systematic Review. *J. Dent.* **2015**, *43*, 1403–1410. [CrossRef]
25. Pisani, M.X.; Malheiros-Segundo, A.D.L.; Balbino, K.L.; Souza, R.D.F.; Paranhos, H.D.F.O.; Lovato Da Silva, C.H. Oral Health Related Quality of Life of Edentulous Patients after Denture Relining with a Silicone-Based Soft Liner: Soft Liners and Quality of Life. *Gerodontology* **2012**, *29*, e474–e480. [CrossRef]
26. Krunic, N.; Kostic, M.; Petrovic, M.; Igic, M. Oral Health-Related Quality of Life of Edentulous Patients after Complete Dentures Relining. *Vojnosanit. Pregl.* **2015**, *72*, 307–311. [CrossRef]
27. Sônego, M.V.; Neto, C.L.M.M.; Dos Santos, D.M.; Moreno, A.L.D.M.; Bertoz, A.P.D.M.; Goiato, M.C. Quality of Life, Satisfaction, Occlusal Force, and Halitosis after Direct and Indirect Relining of Inferior Complete Dentures. *Eur. J. Dent.* **2022**, *16*, 215–222. [CrossRef]
28. Sarac, D.; Sarac, Y.S.; Basoglu, T.; Yapici, O.; Yuzbasioglu, E. The Evaluation of Microleakage and Bond Strength of a Silicone-Based Resilient Liner Following Denture Base Surface Pretreatment. *J. Prosthet. Dent.* **2006**, *95*, 143–151. [CrossRef]
29. Kulak-Ozkan, Y.; Sertgoz, A.; Gedik, H. Effect of Thermocycling on Tensile Bond Strength of Six Silicone-Based, Resilient Denture Liners. *J. Prosthet. Dent.* **2003**, *89*, 303–310. [CrossRef]
30. Emmer, T.J.; Emmer, T.J.; Vaidynathan, J.; Vaidynathan, T.K. Bond Strength of Permanent Soft Denture Liners Bonded to the Denture Base. *J. Prosthet. Dent.* **1995**, *74*, 595–601. [CrossRef]
31. Choi, J.E.; Ng, T.E.; Leong, C.K.Y.; Kim, H.; Li, P.; Waddell, J.N. Adhesive Evaluation of Three Types of Resilient Denture Liners Bonded to Heat-Polymerized, Autopolymerized, or CAD-CAM Acrylic Resin Denture Bases. *J. Prosthet. Dent.* **2018**, *120*, 699–705. [CrossRef]
32. Mutluay, M.M.; Ruyter, I.E. Evaluation of Bond Strength of Soft Relining Materials to Denture Base Polymers. *Dent. Mater.* **2007**, *23*, 1373–1381. [CrossRef]
33. Mese, A.; Guzel, K.G. Effect of Storage Duration on the Hardness and Tensile Bond Strength of Silicone- and Acrylic Resin-Based Resilient Denture Liners to a Processed Denture Base Acrylic Resin. *J. Prosthet. Dent.* **2008**, *99*, 153–159. [CrossRef]
34. *ISO 10139-2:2016*; Dentistry—Soft Lining Materials for Removable Dentures—Part 2: Materials for Long-Term Use. International Organisation for Standardization: Geneva, Switzerland, 2016.
35. *ISO 10365:2022*; Adhesives—Designation of Main Failure Patterns. International Organisation for Standardization: Geneva, Switzerland, 2022.
36. Awad, A.N.; Cho, S.H.; Kesterke, M.J.; Chen, J.H. Comparison of Tensile Bond Strength of Denture Reline Materials on Denture Bases Fabricated with CAD-CAM Technology. *J. Prosthet. Dent.* **2023**, *129*, 616–622. [CrossRef]
37. Wemken, G.; Burkhardt, F.; Spies, B.C.; Kleinvogel, L.; Adali, U.; Sterzenbach, G.; Beuer, F.; Wesemann, C. Bond Strength of Conventional, Subtractive, and Additive Manufactured Denture Bases to Soft and Hard Relining Materials. *Dent. Mater.* **2021**, *37*, 928–938. [CrossRef]
38. Azpiazu-Flores, F.X.; Schricker, S.R.; Seghi, R.R.; Johnston, W.M.; Leyva Del Rio, D. Adhesive strength of 3 long-term resilient liners to CAD-CAM denture base polymers and heat-polymerized polymethyl methacrylate with thermocycling. *J. Prosthet. Dent.* **2022**. [CrossRef]
39. Kim, J.H.; Choe, H.C.; Son, M.K. Evaluation of Adhesion of Reline Resins to the Thermoplastic Denture Base Resin for Non-Metal Clasp Denture. *Dent. Mater. J.* **2014**, *33*, 32–38. [CrossRef]
40. Vojdani, M.; Giti, R. Polyamide as a Denture Base Material: A Literature Review. *J. Dent.* **2015**, *16* (Suppl. S1), 1–9.

41. Hamanaka, I.; Shimizu, H.; Takahashi, Y. Bond Strength of a Chairside Autopolymerizing Reline Resin to Injection-Molded Thermoplastic Denture Base Resins. *J. Prosthodont. Res.* **2017**, *61*, 67–72. [CrossRef]
42. Koodaryan, R.; Hafezeqoran, A. Effect of Surface Treatment Methods on the Shear Bond Strength of Auto-Polymerized Resin to Thermoplastic Denture Base Polymer. *J. Adv. Prosthodont.* **2016**, *8*, 504. [CrossRef]
43. Kawano, F.; Dootz, E.R.; Koran, A., 3rd; Craig, R.G. Comparison of bond strength of six soft denture liners to denture base resin. *J. Prosthet. Dent.* **1992**, *68*, 368–371. [CrossRef] [PubMed]
44. Khan, Z.; Martin, J.; Collard, S. Adhesion characteristics of visible light-cured denture base material bonded to resilient lining materials. *J. Prosthet. Dent.* **1989**, *62*, 196–200. [CrossRef] [PubMed]
45. Bayati, O.H.; Yunus, N.; Ahmad, S.F. Tensile Bond Strengths of Silicone Soft Liners to Two Chemically Different Denture Base Resins. *Int. J. Adhes. Adhes.* **2012**, *34*, 32–37. [CrossRef]

Disclaimer/Publisher's Note: The statements, opinions and data contained in all publications are solely those of the individual author(s) and contributor(s) and not of MDPI and/or the editor(s). MDPI and/or the editor(s) disclaim responsibility for any injury to people or property resulting from any ideas, methods, instructions or products referred to in the content.

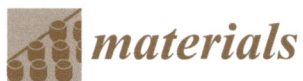

Article

Bioactive Glass-Enhanced Resins: A New Denture Base Material

Zbigniew Raszewski [1,*], Katarzyna Chojnacka [2], Marcin Mikulewicz [3] and Abdulaziz Alhotan [4]

1. SpofaDental, Markova 238, 506 01 Jicin, Czech Republic
2. Department of Advanced Material Technologies, Wroclaw University of Science and Technology, 50-370 Wroclaw, Poland; katarzyna.chojnacka@pwr.edu.pl
3. Department of Dentofacial Orthopedics and Orthodontics, Division of Facial Abnormalities, Medical University of Wroclaw, 50-367 Wroclaw, Poland; marcin.mikulewicz@umw.edu.wroc.pl
4. Department of Dental Health, College of Applied Medical Sciences, King Saud University, Riyadh P.O. Box 12372, Saudi Arabia; aalhotan@ksu.edu.sa
* Correspondence: zbigniew.raszewski@envistaco.com; Tel.: +420-702-208000

Abstract: Background: The creation of the denture base material with bioactive properties that releases ions and produces hydroxyapatite. Methods: Acrylic resins were modified by the addition of 20% of four types of bioactive glasses by mixing with powders. Samples were subjected to flexural strength (1, 60 days), sorption and solubility (7 days), and ion release at pH 4 and pH 7 for 42 days. Hydroxyapatite layer formation was measured using infrared. Results: Biomin F glass-containing samples release fluoride ions for a period of 42 days (pH = 4; Ca = 0.62 ± 0.09; P = 30.47 ± 4.35; Si = 22.9 ± 3.44; F = 3.1 ± 0.47 [mg/L]). The Biomin C (contained in the acrylic resin releases (pH = 4; Ca = 41.23 ± 6.19; P = 26.43 ± 3.96; Si = 33.63 ± 5.04 [mg/L]) ions for the same period of time. All samples have a flexural strength greater than 65 MPa after 60 days. Conclusion: The addition of partially silanized bioactive glasses allows for obtaining a material that releases ions over a longer period of time. Clinical significance: This type of material could be used as a denture base material, helping to preserve oral health by preventing the demineralization of the residual dentition through the release of appropriate ions that serve as substrates for hydroxyapatite formation.

Keywords: acrylic resin; mechanical properties; bioactive glass; ions releasing; hydroxyapatite

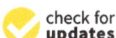

Citation: Raszewski, Z.; Chojnacka, K.; Mikulewicz, M.; Alhotan, A. Bioactive Glass-Enhanced Resins: A New Denture Base Material. *Materials* 2023, *16*, 4363. https://doi.org/10.3390/ma16124363

Academic Editors: Josip Kranjčić and Tina Poklepovic Pericic

Received: 16 May 2023
Revised: 9 June 2023
Accepted: 12 June 2023
Published: 13 June 2023

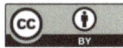

Copyright: © 2023 by the authors. Licensee MDPI, Basel, Switzerland. This article is an open access article distributed under the terms and conditions of the Creative Commons Attribution (CC BY) license (https://creativecommons.org/licenses/by/4.0/).

1. Introduction

The first stage of colonization by microorganisms is the adsorption of salivary membrane proteins by all accessible surfaces of the oral cavity and the acrylic surface of the prosthesis. On this surface, adhesion and growth of microorganisms occur. When microorganisms are appropriately accumulated, they form structures known as biofilms, which are highly organized microbial communities entangled in a three-dimensional matrix. This structure confers many benefits to colonizing species, such as antimicrobial and host defense, increased coaggregation and interaction properties [1]. However, biofilms formed on dentures are different in terms of bacterial colonization have higher content of *Streptococcus mutans*, *Streptococcus mitis*, and *Streptococcus oralis* compared to dental plaque. This can be observed as early as 24 h after placing the restorations in the oral cavity, and a mature biofilm forms after 72 h [2,3]. *S. aureus* and *C. albicans*, which are often found on the surface of dentures, can cause the transformation of homeostatic biofilm into a dysbiosis biofilm, which is already directly responsible for various types of diseases [4]. The literature states that more than 70% of difficult-to-treat and persistent infections are caused by microorganisms growing in biofilms [5].

Biofilm often accumulates on the surface of acrylic dentures during use (due to the absence of ionic charge), which leads to the formation of calculus over time. This problem may occur both in prostheses made using the traditional method, CAD CAM technology, or 3D printing [6]. It becomes an area where pathogenic bacteria multiply, which can cause various types of diseases within the body including demineralization of teeth, dental caries, gingivitis, periodontitis, periapical periodontitis, and peri-implantitis [7]. The process of colonization of acrylic restorations that are fixed on implants may lead to changes in the surface of the implant and the host tissues [8]. That is why it is desirable to create a material that will prevent the formation of biofilm on the surface of acrylic dentures. This is possible in three directions: antimicrobial agent release, contact-dependent strategies, and multifunctional strategies.

Application of an antimicrobial agent polyhexamethylene guanidine hydrochloride (PHMGH) inhibits biofilm formation on resinous materials against *S. mutans* [9]. Another way to obtain antibacterial properties is to use cationic resins at a concentration of 2.5–10% mass fraction of dimethylamino dodecyl methacrylate (DMADDM) which improves the antibacterial effect expressed in *S. mutans* and limits demineralization of the tested resin [9]. Greater effectiveness can be achieved when DMAHDM reacts with 2-methacryloyloxyethyl phosphorylcholine [10]. The same compound has also been shown to be effective as a reaction product with glass ionomer cement.

Another approach, known as contact-dependent strategies, involves creating a material with bactericidal properties by incorporating nanoparticles such as zinc oxide [11], zirconium dioxide, and silver nanoparticles [12,13], or silver vanadate (AgVO3) [14]. Nanomaterials, graphene oxide nanosheets, and carbon nanotubes were also successfully used, in which the mechanism of action is direct contact bacteria killing properties. This effect was achieved by applying a 2% supplement for 28 days [15]. The expansion of the concept of metals and the surface of acrylic plastic can also be modified by the addition of various types of metal salts with acrylic acid, zirconium methacrylate, tin methacrylate, and di-n-butyl methacrylate-tin [16]. The texture of the surface, as a result of material polishing, can reduce the adhesion of the microorganism and the formation of biofilm. This is due to changes in the surface of the denture and leads to an increase in the silicon atom concentration and a decrease in surface carbon [17]. Further modification of the surface can be achieved by interaction of plasma. Plasma-modified PMMA samples have 1.5–2.5 times lower microbial adhesion compared to unmodified samples, while their surface free energy increases up to 1.5 times due to the formation of additional polar oxygen-containing chemical groups induced by the plasma. The surface of the prosthesis subjected to plasma treatment showed good biocompatibility and less irritating effect compared to unmodified surfaces [18].

Another approach to modify the surface is use of different types of coatings (Shibata). studied the use of poly (2-methacryloyloxyethyl phosphorylcholine-co-n-butyl methacrylate), which drastically reduced the ability of cariogenic bacteria, such as *S. mutans* and *S. sobrinus*, to develop biofilms [19]. Finally, a further approach is to modify the surface to have a negative charge, which can be achieved with polyacrylic acid and poly itaconic acid, which have been tested as surface treatments on conventional denture base materials. Both acids demonstrated significant inhibition of *C. albicans* growth. The use of carboxyl groups by applying their coatings reduced the adhesion of *C. albicans* by 90%, which was tested by Acosta et al. [20]. However, using coatings has certain limitations, as the active layer can be removed under the influence of food or hygiene procedures (denture disinfectants, toothpaste, and toothbrush). Therefore, modifications of the entire material seem to be more promising. In the case of our team, bioactive glasses were added to traditional thermally polymerized PMMA resin [21,22]. We managed to obtain a material that was capable of releasing calcium, phosphorus, silicon, and ions for a period of 42 days. However, the amount of these ions was significantly reduced with time. The second problem was the reduction of mechanical properties (glasses were not chemically bonded with PMMA) [22]. To solve this problem, it was decided to use two variants of the same glass like in the previous study. One part has been silanized and the other has not been modified (50/50). The mixture of glasses improved in this way was added at a concentration of 20% to the heat curing denture base material. The thesis put forward at the beginning of this study is that by using modified glasses, the material will be able to release ions over a longer period of time in a more even manner. In addition, the use of the silanization process will improve the mechanical properties of the obtained material.

The paper's findings hold significant clinical implications, as the development of such denture base materials could improve patient outcomes by maintaining oral health and preserving residual dentition. The incorporation of partially silanized bioactive glasses may pave the way for further innovations in dental prosthetics and set the stage for future research aimed at optimizing and customizing these materials for individual patient needs.

2. Materials and Methods

Samples of acrylic resin polymerized hot curing method by the addition of bioactive glasses (totally 104 samples) were used for the tests. The same resin for making denture base (totally 30th sample) polymerized according to the manufacturer's recommendations was used as a reference sample. A detailed description of the sample's preparation is given below, and all performed tests are summarized in Figure 1.

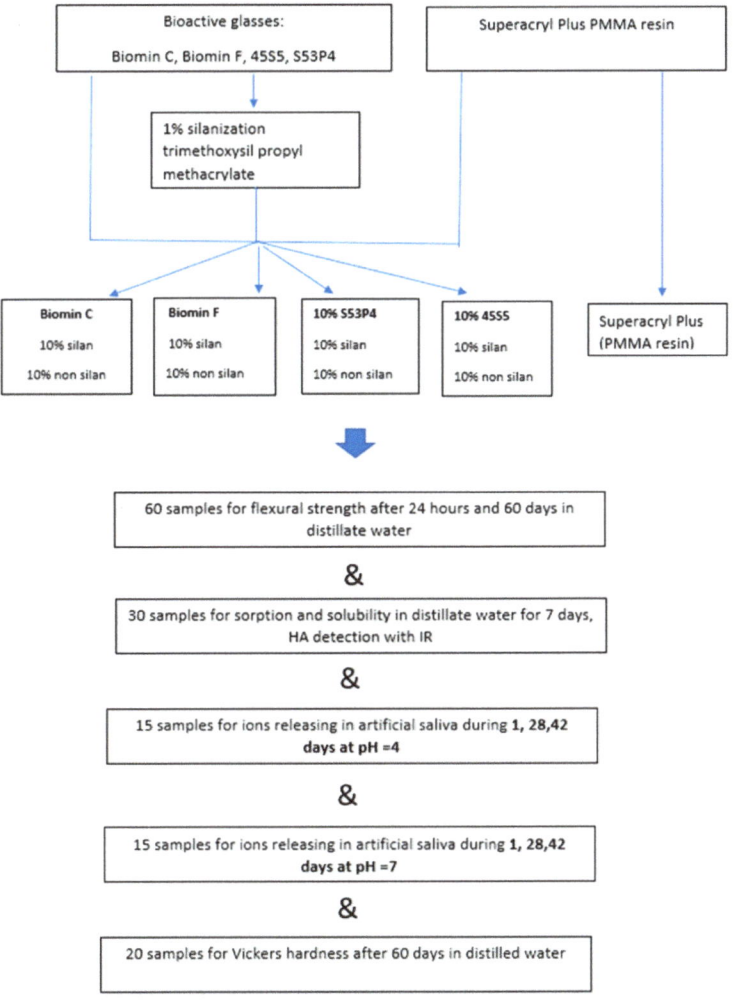

Figure 1. Scheme of sample preparation and testing in this work.

2.1. Silanization of Bioactive Glasses

Glasses used in our previous work (Biomin F, Biomin C, 53P4, and 45S5 (all samples were delivered by Cera Dynamic England, raw composition is presented in Table 1. For the silanization process, powder in the amount of 20 g was mixed with a solution of 90% ethyl alcohol containing 1% gamma trimethoxysil propyl methacrylate and 0.5% concentrated acetic acid (all raw materials from Sigma Aldrich, Praha, Czech Republic). The entire suspension was stirred with a magnetic stirrer for 60 min (Fisher Scientific, Praha, Czech Republic, 400 rpm). Then, it was washed with alcohol and water 3 times. The samples were dried at 105 °C for 24 h to complete the silanization process. The acrylic powders are then ground in a laboratory mortar and sieved through a 100-mesh sieve (Merck, Gernsheim, Germany).

Table 1. Raw composition of bioactive glasses, according to the bioactive glass manufacture Cera Dynamic.

	SiO_2	P_2O_5	CaO	Na_2O	CaF_2	$CaCl_2$
S53P4	53.8%	1.7%	21.8%	22.7%	0	0
Biomin F	36.0–40.0%	4–6%	28.0–30.0%	22.0–24.0%	1.5–3.0%	0
45S5	46.1%	2.6%	26.9%	24.4%	0	0
Biomin C	30.3–31.8%	5.0–5.3%	44.1–46.3%	0	0	16.7–20.6%

2.2. Preparation of a Sample of Resin Modified with Bioactive Glass

The acrylic powder Superacryl Plus (SpofaDental, Jicin, Czech Republic, batch number 567,823) in an amount of 80 g was mixed with 10 g of the appropriate nonsilanized glass and 10 g of silanized glass. To obtain a homogeneous mixture, the whole was placed in a porcelain ball mill (Izerska Porcelanka, Praha, Czech Republic), rotational speed 40 rpm. Number of balls 200 g, diameter 5 mm. The powders were then mixed with the Superacryl Plus liquid at a ratio of 2.4 g of powder to 1 g of monomer. The samples were placed in vessels for 10 min—dough time. When the dough was not sticky to the hand, it was placed in metal molds. For the determination of flexural strength, the samples had a length of 50 × 3 × 10 mm. For the testing of sorption, solubility and ion release, the material was placed in a mold with a diameter of 15 mm and a thickness of 2 mm.

The molds were placed in a manual laboratory press, under a load of 2000 kg, for a period of 10 min to press out excess dough. Resin samples were thermally polymerized in water, initially for 30 min at 60 °C and then for 60 min at 100 °C. After the curing process was completed, the polymerization frame was opened, and the samples were removed. Then, their edges were smoothed with sandpaper (120, Saint Gobain, Kolo, Poland).

2.3. Flexural Strength

Samples to test this parameter were placed in distilled water in sealed PE containers in a dryer at a temperature of 37 °C. The first six samples were subjected to a three-point fracture test after 24 h using a Shimadzu compressive strength instrument (AGS 10 kNG, Shimadzu, Kyoto, Japan), the width of the supports was 50 mm and the speed of the breaking head was 5 mm/min. The test ended with the fracture of the sample. For the first series of tests, 6 samples were used, and the next 6 samples were stored for 60 days in the same conditions. Distilled water was changed every 4 days. A second batch of samples was subjected to the same test after a period of 60 days. In total, 60 samples were made for the entire study. Pure polymethyl methacrylate (PMMA Superacryl Plus, SpofaDental, Jicin, Czech Republic batch 567,823) polymerized under the same conditions was used as reference material, and according to user instruction [20]. A detailed description of the tests and the amount of sample needed for testing are provided in ISO 20795-1: 2013 (EN) [23].

2.4. Sorption and Solubility

Sorption and solubility were analyzed according to ISO 20795-1: 2013 (EN), Dentistry—Denture base polymers [23]. Samples of the polymerized material (15X 2 mm, six of each composition, 30 totally) were placed in a desiccator and weighed every other day until a constant weight was obtained (M1). Then, they were placed in distilled water for 7 days. Once removed from the water, the discs were dried with a paper towel and reweighed on an analytical balance with an accuracy of 0.0001 g (Precioza 256, Turin, Italy), (M2). The samples were once again placed in a desiccator filled with molecular sieves (Sigma Aldrich, Poznan, Poland) and weighed until a constant mass of M3 was reached. Pure acrylic resin was used as a reference sample. The solubility and solubility of the materials were determined according to the following equations.

A—sorption, B—solubility.

These two parameters were calculated from the following Equations (1) and (2):

$$A = \frac{M2 - M1}{S} \quad (1)$$

$$B = \frac{M1 - M3}{S} \quad (2)$$

where M2 is the mass of the sample after 7 days in distillate water, M1 is the mass before immersion in water, and M3 is the mass drying of the material in the exicator after immersion in water. The S is the surface of the disc, measured by calibrated caliper [21].

2.5. Assessment of Ion Release of Glass and Acrylic Resins in Artificial Saliva

To assess the bioactive properties of the samples, we tested ions released into artificial saliva at pH 4 and 7 for 1, 28, and 42 days. The artificial saliva solution was prepared by dissolving sodium chloride (0.4 g) (NaCl, Sigma Aldrich, Poland), potassium chloride (1.21 g) (KCl, Sigma Aldrich, Poland), hydrated potassium dihydrogen phosphate (0.78 g) ($NaH_2PO_4 \cdot 2H_2O$, Sigma Aldrich, Poland), hydrated sodium sulfide (0.12 g) ($Na_2S \cdot 9H_2O$, Sigma Aldrich, Poland), and urea (1.0 g) (Sigma Aldrich, Poznan, Poland) in ultrapure water (1000.0 g) (Merck, Gernsheim, Germany). The prepared solution was transferred to two vessels and adjusted to pH 4 and 7 using hydrochloric acid (0.1 Mol) and sodium hydroxide (0.1 Mol), respectively (both from Merck, Gernsheim, Germany), as in previous of our study [22]. Fifteen samples were tested, including three of each type of glass and acrylic resin, as reference materials. The disks, 15 mm in diameter and 2 mm thick, were prepared according to a previously described method.

Sample extracts from artificial saliva were analyzed by inductively coupled plasma atomic emission spectrometry (ICP-AES) using an iCAP 6500 Duo optical spectrometer (Thermo Fisher Scientific, Waltham, MA, USA). The extraction process was completed after 1, 28, and 42 days, respectively. After the extraction process, the samples were acidified with trace pure nitric acid and made up to 20 mL. The blank and extraction samples were then used for multielement analysis.

To determine the fluoride ion concentration, the extract from the dental material was directly injected through a sterile 0.2-μm syringe filter before entering the chromatography column. The concentration of fluoride ions was measured using a Dionex ICS 1100 ion chromatograph (Thermo Fisher Scientific, Waltham, MA, USA). One-way ANOVA and the Tukey HSD test calculator on Astasta.com were used for statistical analysis, with a confidence level of $p < 0.05$.

2.6. Hydroxyapatite (HA) Formation

Pure acrylic resin samples and samples containing bioactive glasses, which were used for solubility and solubility tests, were subsequently used for surface testing using an IR spectrophotometer. The samples were placed on the window of this instrument, Nicolet I5S

(Thermoscientific, Prague, Czech Republic) and measured in the IR range of 4000–500 cm^{-1}. For each of the 5 sample groups, 3 measurements were made.

The scheme of the tests performed in this research is presented in Figure 1 in the form of a graphic abstract.

2.7. Vickers Hardness Measurement

To test the hardness of the material, 20 samples were used, which were obtained from the bending resistance test after 60 days of storage in distilled water. This parameter was assessed with a digital microhardness tester (FM-700, Future Tech Corp., Kawasaki, Japan). An indenter point in the form of a square-based pyramid was applied at a load of 300 g for 15 s at room temperature at 37 °C. Five indentations were made at different points along each specimen on the same surface side, with a minimum distance of 1 mm between any two indentations. The mean hardness value of each specimen group was then calculated. The Vickers microhardness (HVN) value was calculated using Equation (3)

$$HV = 1.854\left(\frac{F}{D2}\right) \qquad (3)$$

with F being the applied load (measured in kilograms-force) and $D2$ the area of the indentation (measured in square millimeters).

2.8. Statistical Analysis

The results were statistically analyzed using a one-way analysis of variance at a significance level of 0.05, as a reference using a sample of PMMA resin not modified with fillers. In addition, a post hoc analysis was performed by using Tukey's HSD test (using a free test calculator provided by Astatsa, San Jose, CA, USA).

3. Results

3.1. Flexural Strength

The results of flexural strength samples stored in distilled water for 24 h and 60 days are shown in Table 2.

Table 2. Flexural strength after storage in distilled water for 24 h and 60 Days Biomin F.

	Biomin F [MPa]	Biomin C [MPa]	53P4 [MPa]	45S5 [MPa]	Resin [MPa]
Flexural strength 24 h	78.13 ± 3.27 *	78.69 ± 5.72 *	80.75 ± 2.41	79.32 ± 2.24	86.5 ± 1.98
Flexural strength 60 days	70.74 ± 1.39 [®]	69.88 ± 1.73 [®]	69.88 ± 1.73 [®]	69.2 ± 2.10 [®]	79.30 ± 2.55 [®]

* Statistically significant values at confidence level $p < 0.05$. For samples modified with glass versus resin.
[®] Statistically significant values at confidence level $p < 0.01$. For samples modified with glass versus resin.

It should be noted, however, that all samples after storage in distilled water, both after 24 h and 60 days, have a flexural strength greater than 65 MPa. This means they meet the ISO 20795 Denture Base Polymers standard [22]. After storage in distilled water for 2 months, a decrease in flexural strength was observed from 11% (for Biomin C and Biomin F) to 18% (45S5, 53P4).

3.2. Sorption and Solublity

Another important material property is solubility and sorption, which indicate whether the material can extract ions from its composition (solubility) and to what extent water will penetrate into it (sorption). The results of this study after 7 days of storage in distilled water are presented in Table 3.

Table 3. Sorption and solubility of acrylic samples in distilled water for 7 days at 37 °C.

	Biomin F [μg/mm^3]	Biomin C [μg/mm^3]	53P4 [μg/mm^3]	45S5 [μg/mm^3]	Resin [μg/mm^3]
Sorption	16.10 ± 2.23	1.49 ± 3.06	19.15 ± 2.37 *	16.85 ± 3.04	14.05 ± 1.08
Solubility	0.85 ± 0.29	2.60 ± 0.88	1.20 ± 0.24	1.00 ± 0.18	1.10 ± 0.34

* Statistically significant at $p < 0.05$ for sample 53P4 vs. pure PMMA.

The highest solubility value was found for Biomin C—2.6 ± 0.88 μm/mm^3. For others, the solubility values were similar to that of pure PMMA (reference sample). The higher sorption was obtained for samples containing 20% 53P4 glass (19.15 ± 2.37 μg/mm^3).

3.3. Ions Releasing

Samples containing Biomin F after modification of half of the glass with silanes can release fluoride ions for a longer period of time (60 days). In a previous study, the secretion of this ion proceeded very rapidly during the first 24 h and then decreased to zero [22]. A gradual release was obtained for these two glasses also in the case of the release of calcium, phosphorus, and silicon ions over time, regardless of pH = 4 and pH = 7. Results from these tests are presented in Table 4.

Table 4. Ion release by samples of resins modified with bioactive glasses during 1, 28, and 42 days in acidic environment, pH = 4 and neutral pH = 7.

	Ca [mg/L]	P [mg/L]	Si [mg/L]	F [mg/L]
Blank				
pH 4 0	0	8.218 ± 1.23	0.00	0.00
pH 7 0	0	23.18 ± 3.48	0.00	0.00
Biomin F				
pH4 1 day	1.97 ± 0.3	33.12 ± 4.97	15.69 ± 2.35	3.0 ± 0.45
pH4 28 days	0.57 ± 0.09	30.91 ± 4.64	27,26 ± 4,09	3.05 ± 0.46
pH4 42 days	0.62 ± 0.09	30.47 ± 4.35	22.9 ± 3.44	3.1 ± 0.47
pH7 1 day	1.24 ± 0.19	35.40 ± 5.31	11.72 ± 1.76	2.93 ± 0.44
pH7 28 days	0.93 ± 0.14	32.56 ± 4.88	19.26 ± 2.89	3.29 ± 0.49
pH7 42 days	0.74 ± 0.11	31.58 ± 4.74	20.85 ± 3.13	3.09 ± 0.42
Biomin C				
pH4 1 day	16.49 ± 2.47	32.57 ± 4.88	18.28 ± 2.74	0.00
pH4 28 days	40.39 ± 6.06	20.38 ± 3.06	31.78 ± 4.77	0.00
pH4 42 days	41.23 ± 6.19	26.43 ± 3.96	33.63 ± 5.04	0.00
pH7 1 day	13.84 ± 2.08	33.17 ± 4.98	8.90 ± 1.33	0.00
pH7 28 days	26.90 ± 4.04	15.26 ± 2.29	25.32 ± 3.80	0.00
pH7 42 days	40.16 ± 6.02	17.50 ± 2.62	33.63 ± 5.04	0.00
45S53				
pH4 1 day	2.78 ± 0.42	35.44 ± 5.32	19.33 ± 2.9	0.00
pH4 28 days	3.35 ± 0.50	31.21 ± 4.68	74.12 ± 11.12	0.00
pH4 42 days	1.61 ± 0.24	27.24 ± 4.09	65.54 ± 9.83	0.00
pH7 1 day	1.07 ± 0.16	34.61 ± 0,5.19	17.60 ± 2.64	0.00
pH7 28 days	0.27 ± 0.04	30.49 ± 4.57	43.90 ± 6.59	0.00
pH7 42 days	1.04 ± 0.16	29.30 ± 4.40	53.16 ± 7.97	0.00
53P4				
pH4 1 day	2.73 ± 0.41	31.61 ± 4.74	23.20 ± 3.48	0.00
pH4 28 days	1.90 ± 0.29	25.83 ± 3.87	46.52 ± 6.99	0.00
pH4 42 days	1.14 ± 0.17	27.32 ± 4.10	49.23 ± 7.38	0.00
pH7 1 day	0.24 ± 0.03	32.72 ± 4.91	22.45 ± 3.37	0.00

Table 4. *Cont.*

	Ca	P	Si	F
	[mg/L]	[mg/L]	[mg/L]	[mg/L]
pH7 28 days	0.29 ± 0.04	28.83 ± 4.32	34.61 ± 5.19	0.00
pH7 42 days	0.28 ± 0.04	24.95 ± 3.72	45.30 ± 6.80	0.00
PMMA				
pH4 1 day	0.35 ± 0.05	23.94 ± 3.59	0.00	0.00
pH4 28 days	0.38 ± 0.06	26.22 ± 3.93	0.00	0.00
pH4 42 days	0.53 ± 0.08	22.51 ± 3.38	0.00	0.00
pH7 1 day	0.19 ± 0.03	19.80 ± 2.97	0.00	0.00
pH7 28 days	0.25 ± 0.04	30.95 ± 4.64	0.00	0.00
pH7 42 days	0.71 ± 0.11	29.38 ± 3.64	0.00	0.00

3.4. Vickers Hardness

The surface hardness test of the sample is shown in Table 5.

Table 5. Vickers hardness for a sample with 20% glass content stored for 60 days in distilled water.

		Vickers Hardness (HV)	SD
Biomin F	(A)	13.20	0.74
S53P4	(B)	15.36 [BE]	0.60
45S5	(C)	14.65 [CE]	0.55
Biomin C	(D)	14.31 [DE]	0.32
PMMA	(E)	12. 87	0.27

[BE, CE, DE]. Statistically significant values, relative to the pure PMMA (E) sample for the confidence level of confidence $p < 0.01$.

The addition of bioactive glasses in the amount of 20% (50/50 silanized/non) causes a slight 1–2 unit increase in the material's hardness.

3.5. Hydroxyapatite Formation

The formation of this layer of material on the pores after storage in distilled water at 37 °C after 7 days was examined by IR spectra (Figure 2).

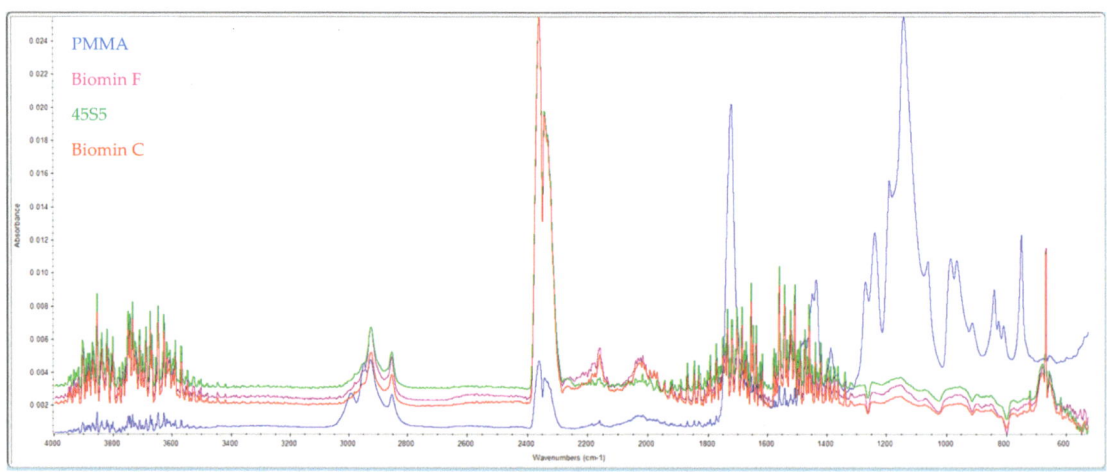

Figure 2. Shows the IR spectra of pure PMMA (blue) and samples with the addition of 53P4 (purple), 45S5 (green), and Biomin F (red) glasses after 7 days in distilled water.

High absorption in the range of 3500 cm^{-1} indicates the presence of OH$^-$ groups from hydroxyapatite. Furthermore, samples with bioactive glasses show absorption at 1460 cm^{-1} (CO_3^{2-}), 1041 cm^{-1} (corresponding to the PO_4^{3-} vibration), and 570 cm^{-1} (indicating the PO_4^{2-} group). Comparing these results with standard spectra from the library, it is evident that a layer of hydroxyapatite is formed on the surface of the samples stored in distilled water for 7 days.

4. Discussion

Modification of acrylic materials runs constantly and proceeds basically in two directions. The first is to increase their mechanical properties and the second is to increase their biological or bactericidal properties. Modifications that improve the mechanical properties are primarily additions of ZrO_2 nanomaterials [24,25], aluminum oxide [26], and cerium oxide [27].

Antibacterial properties can also be obtained by the addition of, e.g., $AgVO_3$ [14], mesoporous silica nanoparticles [28], zinc-modified phosphate-based glass microfiller [29], and ZnO [30].

Bioactive properties in the case of glasses can be classified as the possibility of releasing calcium, phosphorus, and fluoride ions, which can form a new layer of hydroxyapatite and have bactericidal properties or reduce adhesion to the surface of the material, e.g., in relation to *Candida albicans* (glass 45S5) [12].

The release of ions from various dental materials is a highly desirable property that can ensure their better biocompatibility. In this context, there are already a number of products on the market for filling crown and root canals, which release strontium ions and silicon, prereactive glass ionomer filler [31].

The thesis put forward at the beginning of this investigation has been partially confirmed. Materials such as Biomin C and S53P4 and 45S5 release silicon and phosphorus ions more uniformly, and fluoride ions through Biomin F. Mechanical properties have slightly deteriorated despite the use of 20% glass in the composition of the PMMA resin.

The release of calcium ions in Biomin F, 53P4, and 45S5 glasses is very fast. Different values are obtained for Biomin C, which releases these ions evenly over a long period of time, regardless of the pH of the solution. Similar results were obtained in our previous work [22]. Therefore, silanization does not affect the uniform release of calcium ions in Biomin F, 45S5, and S53P4 glasses. However, the Biomin C sample releases these ions in a uniform and more homogeneous manner when half of the silanized glass is inside.

The fluoride ions contained in Biomin F glass are released gradually and uniformly throughout the test period at pH = 4 and pH = 7. This is a difference from our previous work in which the same glasses added to acrylic were not silanized. Then, in a solution of pH = 4, all the fluoride was quickly washed out within 1 day. This is similar to the direct addition of fluorine compounds, e.g., NaF, to acrylic resin causes a very fast release of this ion within 1–7 days [32].

The influence of the silanization process (the pH of the solution) on the release of fluoride ions was described in the paper Nakornchai [33], for glass G018-090 and Piyananjaratsri [34].

In the case of Biomin F glass, which has been silanized in an acetic acid environment, after this step, a thin layer of polysalt matrix is formed on the surface of the fluor aluminosilicate glass. The matrix layer, which consisted of calcium and aluminum acetates and fluoride ions, was easily penetrated by water. Therefore, the leaching of fluoride ions from the surface of the so-modified matrix into the aqueous solution may be easier than the surface of the glass filler itself [32]. These authors have concluded that acrylic resin can release fluoride ions for 56 days for glasses [32] or 15 days for dopped ions to acrylic resins [33–35].

Low fluoride concentration ranged from 0.024–0.154 ppm/mL, reduced demineralization of the enamel surface [36]. In the case of Biomin F glass, the amount of fluorine ions released was 3 ppm/mL and remained at a constant level for a period of 42 days. Fluoride ions released in such quantities may have a bactericidal effect [36]. Therefore, we can assume for more tests in the future that this material will have properties that prevent demineralization of the enamel of the residual dentition, having direct contact with the denture base made with the addition of this type of glass.

Phosphorus ions are uniformly extracted in all test glasses at a constant level over a period of 42 days. Values of 20–30 mg/L are almost twice as high as those obtained in previous studies [22], which proves that the silanization process prolongs the period of releasing ions to artificial solutions.

The release of ions from the PMMA/glass material can be explained in three steps. At the beginning, the ions contained on the surface of the material pass into the solution. Next is washing out the residual monomer and other components with water from the resin. Some free spaces begin to form in the structure of the material, through which water can penetrate. It creates the possibility for ions migration by gradually hydrolyzing the glasses inside the resin, which explains why the materials are able to release these ions over a longer period of time. Since silanes are hydrophobic molecules, they significantly slow down this process [24,37]. This has been confirmed in these studies.

If the amount of unsilanized glass added is increased, a decrease in flexural strength can be observed [29]. For this reason, the measurable benefit of using half of the glass in the silanized form is the improvement of the mechanical properties of the new sample (Agarwal) [35]. They are lower than pure PMMA (reference sample), but at the same level as in previous studies, when the sample was filled with glass at 10%. At the moment, it is 20% concentration of glass in the acrylic resin [22]. The results of flexural strength of acrylic resins in the case of bioactive glasses tested in our case are in line with [32]. Silanized samples have better resistance to breakage even after 2 months of storage in distilled water. These values in the case of Japanese authors range from 72–76 MPa [32].

The amount of released ions will also be affected by the solubility of the material, i.e., the penetration of water into the resin. In the case of samples containing Biomin C, the largest amount of released calcium, phosphorus, and silicon ions was observed, which is accompanied by the highest solubility of this material among the tested samples.

The silanized glasses used in these studies reduced the solubility of the glasses in relation to the same PMMA/glass system from our previous work. The sorption has not changed. What can be concluded is that the process of silanization is an important process that increases the degree of cross-linking of the sample, which reduces their solubility (F) [38]. The important thing is that the flexural strength for all samples, even over a long period of 60 days, is greater than 65MPa. This means that all materials meet this requirement described in the ISO 20795-1:2013 Dentistry-denture base polymers standard [23].

Acrylic resins are relatively soft materials, which, under the influence of hygiene procedures or consumed food, may be subject to local abrasion. The polished surface at the beginning, after the manufacture of the prosthesis, is roughened, which is the precondition for colonization by microorganisms and the formation of a biofilm. Therefore, it is important that the material has the right hardness. In addition, a soft surface makes it easier to absorb dyes from food, which changes the color of the used restoration. Thus, the Vickers microhardness test is considered to be a valid method to evaluate rigid polymers [39].

The addition of bioactive glasses slightly increases the Vickers hardness from 12.87 ± 0.27 to 15.36 ± 0.60 HV. These are in line with the results obtained by a Farina [39], who obtained values of 15–17 HV for thermally polymerized materials. Higher hardness (18.57 HV) was obtained by Duymus for heat curing resin [40]. The differences may be due to the fact that other authors tested the material after polymerization. In this study, the samples were stored in water for 60 days. Water absorption causes a plasticizing effect and thus a decrease in the hardness of the material.

Immersion of acrylic samples containing bioactive glasses in the water causes that, under the influence of time, a layer of hydroxyapatite forms on their surface, which has been proved in these studies using IR spectroscopy. Hydroxyapatite can also form not only on the surface of the modified denture, but also on the residual dentition, which is in direct contact with the prothesis, which prevents demineralization of the enamel. In addition, the existence of this phenomenon has been confirmed by other authors in the case of composite materials [41,42].

However, the research conducted above has some limitations. In order for the material for the denture base to be created, further research on the analysis of the amount of hydroxyapatite produced, biological tests (cytotoxicity and others) and the study of the strength of the connection between the teeth and the denture plate and the content of residual monomers in the polymerized material are necessary, as the use of glasses can significantly affect all these parameters.

Future Perspectives

The results of this study demonstrate the potential of using partially silanized bioactive glasses in the development of acrylic resin materials for denture base applications. These materials exhibit promising ion release properties and mechanical strength, which could contribute to the prevention of demineralization and support the formation of hydroxyapatite in residual dentition. To fully comprehend the implications and possibilities of this technique, several issues need for more study and development. The long-term repercussions of the release of ions are a crucial factor to consider. Future research should prolong the observation time to explore the long-term ionization behavior, mechanical properties, hygiene and any possible effects on oral health. This study examined the ionization characteristics of materials over a 42-day period. Future research should examine these materials' cell toxicity and biocompatibility both in vitro and in vivo in order to confirm their safety for clinical usage. This will assist in determining whether the substance is safe for prolonged interaction with oral tissues and whether any negative responses are possible.

Another crucial aspect is the integration with dental prosthetics. Further research should focus on evaluating the bond strength between the teeth and the denture plate made from these modified acrylic resin materials. The success of dental prosthetics depends on the stability and durability of this connection, and it is essential to ensure that the addition of bioactive glasses does not compromise this aspect.

Future studies should explore the content of residual monomers in the polymerized material. The presence of residual monomers can affect the mechanical properties and biocompatibility of the denture base material, making this a crucial parameter to investigate.

The surface characteristics of these modified acrylic resins should also be investigated, with an emphasis on wettability, roughness, and the impact on the development of biofilms. This will give important information on how these materials could affect oral hygiene and the general health of the oral cavity.

Future investigations should also consider exploring the possibility of tailoring the material properties by adjusting the composition and percentage of bioactive glasses in the acrylic resin. This would allow for the development of customized denture base materials that cater to the specific needs of individual patients.

The use of this type of bioactive glass in further research can be extended to materials used in CAD CAM technology and 3D printing [6].

5. Conclusions

- The addition of bioactive glass Biomin F to the acrylic resin allows for a continuous release of fluoride ions over a period of 42 days.
- Samples containing Biomin C release a large amount of ion, phosphate, and silicate anions.
- The mechanical properties of acrylic resins that contain 20% of bioactive glasses (50/50 silanized or not) meet the flexural strength normative requirements for denture plate materials.
- On the surface of the sample, using the IR technique, it was possible to identify the formation of hydroxyapatite under the influence of storing the sample in distilled water.

Author Contributions: Z.R.: Contributed to conception, design, data acquisition and interpretation, performed all statistical analyses, drafted, and critically revised the manuscript. K.C.: Contributed to conception, design, data acquisition, and interpretation drafted and critically revised the manuscript. M.M.: Contributed to conception, design, and critically revised the manuscript. All authors gave their final approval and agreed to be accountable for all aspects of the work. A.A.: Contributed to conception, design, data acquisition, and interpretation. All authors have read and agreed to the published version of the manuscript.

Funding: This research received no external funding.

Institutional Review Board Statement: Not applicable.

Informed Consent Statement: Not applicable.

Data Availability Statement: Not applicable.

Acknowledgments: The authors would like to thank Xu Cao from James Kent Co., England for providing a sample of bioactive glass used in this research. The authors are also grateful to the Researchers Supporting Project number (RSPD2023R790), King Saud University, Saudi Arabia, Riyadh.

Conflicts of Interest: The authors declare no competing interest.

References

1. Bertolini, M.; Costa, R.C.; Barão, V.A.R.; Villar, C.C.; Retamal-Valdes, B.; Feres, M.; Silva Souza, J.G. Oral Microorganisms and Biofilms: New Insights to Defeat the Main Etiologic Factor of Oral Diseases. *Microorganisms* **2022**, *10*, 2413. [CrossRef] [PubMed]
2. Mazurek-Popczyk, J.; Nowicki, A.; Arkusz, K. Evaluation of biofilm formation on acrylic resins used to fabricate dental temporary restorations with the use of 3D printing technology. *BMC Oral Health* **2022**, *22*, 442. [CrossRef] [PubMed]
3. Nowakowska-Toporowska, A.; Malecka, K.; Raszewski, Z.; Wieckiewicz, W. Changes in hardness of addition-polymerizing silicone-resilient denture liners after storage in artificial saliva. *J. Prosthet. Dent.* **2019**, *121*, 317–321. [CrossRef] [PubMed]
4. Schnurr, E.; Paqué, P.N.; Attin, T.; Nanni, P.; Grossmann, J.; Holtfreter, S.; Bröker, B.M.; Kohler, C.; Diep, B.A.; Ribeiro, A.A. Staphylococcus aureus interferes with streptococci spatial distribution and with protein expression of species within a polymicrobial oral biofilm. *Antibiotics* **2021**, *10*, 116. [CrossRef]
5. Holban, A.M.; Farcasiu, C.; Andrei, O.C.; Grumezescu, A.M.; Farcasiu, A.T. Surface Modification to Modulate Microbial Biofilms-Applications in Dental Medicine. *Materials* **2021**, *14*, 6994. [CrossRef]
6. Grande, F.; Tesini, F.; Pozzan, M.C.; Zamperoli, E.M.; Carossa, M.; Catapano, S. Comparison of the Accuracy between Denture Bases Produced by Subtractive and Additive Manufacturing Methods: A Pilot Study. *Prosthesis* **2022**, *4*, 151–159. [CrossRef]
7. Abebe, G.M. Oral Biofilm and Its Impact on Oral Health, Psychological and Social Interaction. *Int. J. Oral Dent. Health* **2021**, *7*, 127. [CrossRef]
8. Collares, F.M.; Garcia, I.M.; Bohns, F.R.; Motta, A.; Melo, M.A.; Leitune, V.C.B. Guanidine hydrochloride polymer additive to undertake ultraconservative resin infiltrant against Streptococcus mutans. *Eur. Polym. J.* **2020**, *133*, 109746. [CrossRef]
9. Chen, H.; Zhang, B.; Weir, M.D.; Homayounfar, N.; Fay, G.G.; Martinho, F.; Lei, L.; Bai, Y.; Hu, T.; Xu, H.H.K. S. mutans gene-modification and antibacterial resin composite as dual strategy to suppress biofilm acid production and inhibit caries. *J. Dent.* **2020**, *93*, 103278. [CrossRef]
10. Wang, L.; Xie, X.; Qi, M.; Weir, M.D.; Reynolds, M.A.; Li, C.; Zhou, C.; Xu, H.H.K. Effects of single species versus multispecies periodontal biofilms on the antibacterial efficacy of a novel bioactive Class-V nanocomposite. *Dent. Mater.* **2019**, *35*, 847–861. [CrossRef]
11. Arun, D.; Adikari Mudiyanselage, D.; Gulam, M.R.; Liddell, M.; Monsur, H.N.M.; Sharma, D. Does the Addition of Zinc Oxide Nanoparticles Improve the Antibacterial Properties of Direct Dental Composite Resins? A Systematic Review. *Materials* **2021**, *14*, 40. [CrossRef] [PubMed]
12. Gad, M.M.; Abualsaud, R.; Rahoma, A.; Al-Thobity, A.M.; Akhtar, S.; Fouda, S.M. Double-layered acrylic resin denture base with nanoparticle additions: An in vitro study. *J. Prosthet. Dent.* **2020**, *123*, 386. [CrossRef] [PubMed]
13. Gad, M.M.; Al-Thobity, A.M.; Rahoma, A.; Abualsaud, R.; Al-Harbi, F.A.; Akhtar, S. Reinforcement of PMMA denture base material with a mixture of ZrO$_2$ nanoparticles and glass fibers. *Int. J. Dent.* **2019**, *2019*, 2489393. [CrossRef] [PubMed]
14. de Castro, D.T.; Vilela Teixeira, A.B.; Alves, O.L.; dos Reis, A.C. Cytotoxicity and Elemental Release of Dental Acrylic Resin Modified with Silver and Vanadium Based Antimicrobial Nanomater. *J. Health Sci.* **2021**, *23*, 12–17. [CrossRef]
15. Chen, J.; Peng, H.; Wang, X.; Shao, F.; Yuan, Z.; Han, H. Graphene oxide exhibits broad-spectrum antimicrobial activity against bacterial phytopathogens and fungal conidia by intertwining and membrane perturbation. *Nanoscale* **2014**, *6*, 1879–1889. [CrossRef]
16. Elwakiel, N.; El-Sayed, Y.; Elkafrawy, H. Synthesis, characterization of Ag+ and Sn2+ complexes and their applications to improve the biological and mechanical properties of denture base materials. *J. Mol. Struct.* **2020**, *1219*, 128521. [CrossRef]
17. Ionescu, A.; Wutscher, E.; Brambilla, E.; Schneider-Feyrer, S.; Giessibl, F.J.; Hahnel, S. Influence of surface properties of resin-based composites on in vitro Streptococcus mutans biofilm development. *Eur. J. Oral Sci.* **2012**, *120*, 458–465. [CrossRef]

18. Chang, Y.T.; Chen, G. Oral bacterial inactivation using a novel low-temperature atmospheric-pressure plasma device. *J. Dent. Sci.* **2016**, *11*, 65–71. [CrossRef]
19. Shibata, Y.; Yamashita, Y.; Tsuru, K.; Ishihara, K.; Fukazawa, K.; Ishikawa, K. Preventive effects of a phospholipid polymer coating on PMMA on biofilm formation by oral streptococci. *Appl. Surf. Sci.* **2016**, *390*, 602–607. [CrossRef]
20. Acosta, L.D.; Pérez-Camacho, O.; Acosta, R.; Escobar, D.M.; Gallardo, C.A.; Sánchez-Vargas, L.O. Reduction of Candida albicans biofilm formation by coating polymethyl methacrylate denture bases with a photopolymerized film. *J. Prosthet. Dent.* **2020**, *124*, 605–613. [CrossRef]
21. Raszewski, Z.; Nowakowska, D.; Wieckiewicz, W.; Nowakowska-Toporowska, A. Release and Recharge of Fluoride Ions from Acrylic Resin Modified with Bioactive Glass. *Polymers* **2021**, *13*, 1054. [CrossRef] [PubMed]
22. Raszewski, Z.; Chojnacka, K.; Mikulewicz, M. Preparation and characterization of acrylic resins with bioactive glasses. *Sci. Rep.* **2022**, *12*, 16624. [CrossRef] [PubMed]
23. ISO 20795-1: 2013 (EN); Dentistry—Denture base polymers (EN). International Organization for Standardization: Geneva, Switzerland, 2013.
24. Gad, M.M.; Abualsaud, R.; Alqarawi, F.K.; Emam, A.M.; Khan, S.Q.; Akhtar, S.; Mahrous, A.A.; Al-Harbi, F.A. Translucency of nanoparticle-reinforced PMMA denture base material: An in-vitro comparative study. *Dent Mater J.* **2021**, *40*, 972–978. [CrossRef] [PubMed]
25. Rasan, D.S.; Farhan, F.A. Effect of addition of polymerized polymethyl methacrylate (PMMA) and zirconia particles on impact strength, surface hardness, and roughness of heat cure PMMA: An in vitro study. *Dent. Hypotheses* **2022**, *14*, 36–38. [CrossRef]
26. Tamore, S.H.; Jyothi, K.S.; Muttagi, S.; Gaikwad, A.M. Flexural strength of surface-treated heat-polymerized acrylic resin after repair with aluminum oxide-reinforced autopolymerizing acrylic resin. *Contemp. Clin. Dent.* **2018**, *9*, S347–S353.
27. Jin, J.; Mangal, U.; Seo, J.Y.; Kim, J.Y.; Ryu, J.H.; Lee, Y.H.; Lugtu, C.; Hwang, G.; Cha, J.Y.; Lee, K.J.; et al. Cerium oxide nanozymes confer a cytoprotective and bio-friendly surface micro-environment to methacrylate based oro-facial prostheses. *Biomaterials* **2023**, *296*, 122063. [CrossRef]
28. Abualsaud, R.; Gad, M.M. Highlights on Drug and Ion Release and Recharge Capacity of Antimicrobial Removable Prostheses. *Eur. J. Dent.* **2022**. ahead of print. [CrossRef]
29. Lee, M.J.; Kim, M.J.; Mangal, U. Zinc-modified phosphate-based glass micro-filler improves Candida albicans resistance of auto-polymerized acrylic resin without altering mechanical performance. *Sci. Rep.* **2022**, *12*, 19456. [CrossRef]
30. Raj, I.; Mozetic, M.; Jayachandran, V.P.; Jose, J.; Thomas, S.; Kalarikkal, N. Fracture resistant, antibiofilm adherent, self-assembled PMMA/ZnO nanoformulations for biomedical applications: Physico-chemical and biological perspectives of nano reinforcement. *Nanotechnology* **2018**, *29*, 305704. [CrossRef]
31. Takahashi, Y.; Okamoto, M.; Komichi, S.; Imazato, S.; Nakatsuka, T.; Sakamoto, S.; Kimoto, K.; Hayashi, M. Application of a direct pulp capping cement containing S-PRG filler. *Clin. Oral Investig.* **2019**, *23*, 1723–1731. [CrossRef]
32. Sabir, D.B.; Omer, Z.Q. Evaluation of Fluoride release from orthodontic acrylic resin by using two different polymerizations techniques: An In-Vitro Study. *EDJ* **2019**, *2*, 149–158. [CrossRef]
33. Nakornchai, N.; Arksornnukit, M.; Kamonkhantikul, K.; Takahashi, H. The pH effect of solvent in silanization on fluoride released and mechanical properties of heat-cured acrylic resin containing fluoride-releasing filler. *Dent. Mater. J.* **2016**, *35*, 440–446. [CrossRef] [PubMed]
34. Piyananjaratsri, R.; Chaowicharat, E.; Saejok, K.; Susen, W.; Pankiew, A.; Srisuwan, A.; Jeamsaksiri, W.; Klunngien, N.; Hruanun, C.; Poyai, A. The effects of fluorine ion implantation on acrylic resin denture base. In Proceedings of the 2011 IEEE Nanotechnology Materials and Devices Conference, Jeju, Republic of Korea, 18–21 October 2011; pp. 577–580. [CrossRef]
35. Agarwal, B.; Singh, R.D.; Raghav, D.; Shekhar, A.; Yadav, P. Determination of Fluoride Release and Strength of a Fluoride Treated Heat Cured Acrylic Resin. *EAS J. Dent. Oral Med.* **2019**, *1*, 108–111.
36. Arksornnukit, M.; Takahashi, H.; Nishiyama, N. Effects of silane coupling agent amount on mechanical properties and hydrolytic durability of composite resin after hot water storage. *Dent. Mater. J.* **2004**, *23*, 31–36. [CrossRef] [PubMed]
37. Sepulveda, P.; Jones, J.R.; Hench, L.L. Characterization of melt-derived 45S5 and sol-gel-derived 58s bioactive glasses. *J. Biomed. Mater. Res.* **2001**, *58*, 734–740. [CrossRef]
38. Par, M.; Spanovic, N.; Bjelovucic, R.; Marovic, D.; Schmalz, G.; Gamulin, O.; Tarle, Z. Long-term water sorption and solubility of experimental bioactive composites based on amorphous calcium phosphate and bioactive glass. *Dent. Mater. J.* **2019**, *38*, 555–564. [CrossRef]
39. Farina, A.; Cecchin, D.; Soares, R.; Botelho, F.; Takahashi, J.; Mazzetto, M.; Marcelo, M. Evaluation of Vickers hardness of different types of acrylic denture base resins with and without glass fiber reinforcement. *Gerodontology* **2010**, *29*, e155–e160. [CrossRef]
40. Duymus, Z.; Ozdogan, A.; Ulu, H.; Ozbayram, O. Evaluation the Vickers Hardness of Denture Base Materials. *Open J. Stomatol.* **2016**, *6*, 114–119. [CrossRef]
41. Tiskaya, M.; Al-Eesa, N.A.; Wong, F.S.L.; Hill, R.G. Characterization of the bioactivity of two commercial composites. *Dent. Mat.* **2019**, *35*, 1757–1768. [CrossRef]
42. Al-Eesaa, N.A.; Johal, A.; Hill, R.G.; Wong, F.S.L. Fluoride-containing bioactive glass composite for orthodontic adhesives: Apatite formation properties. *Dent. Mater.* **2018**, *34*, 1127–1133. [CrossRef]

Disclaimer/Publisher's Note: The statements, opinions and data contained in all publications are solely those of the individual author(s) and contributor(s) and not of MDPI and/or the editor(s). MDPI and/or the editor(s) disclaim responsibility for any injury to people or property resulting from any ideas, methods, instructions or products referred to in the content.

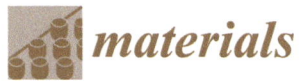 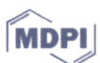

Article

Accuracy of Dental Models Fabricated Using Recycled Poly-Lactic Acid

Koudai Nagata [1], Keitaro Inaba [2], Katsuhiko Kimoto [3] and Hiromasa Kawana [1,*]

[1] Department of Oral and Maxillofacial Implantology, Kanagawa Dental University, 82 Inaoka-cho, Yokosuka 238-8580, Japan
[2] Department of Oral Microbiology, Kanagawa Dental University, 82 Inaoka-cho, Yokosuka 238-8580, Japan
[3] Department of Fixed Prosthodontics, Kanagawa Dental University, 82 Inaoka-cho, Yokosuka 238-8580, Japan
* Correspondence: kawana@kdu.ac.jp; Tel.: +81-468-88-8880

Abstract: Based on the hypothesis that the fabrication of dental models using fused deposition modeling and poly-lactic acid (PLA), followed by recycling and reusing, would reduce industrial waste, we aimed to compare the accuracies of virgin and recycled PLA models. The PLA models were recycled using a crusher and a filament-manufacturing machine. Virgin PLA was labeled R, and the first, second, and third recycles were labeled R1, R2, and R3, respectively. To determine the accuracies of the virgin and reused PLA models, identical provisional crowns were fitted, and marginal fits were obtained using micro-computed tomography. A marginal fit of 120 µm was deemed acceptable based on previous literature. The mesial, distal, buccal, and palatal centers were set at M, D, B, and P, respectively. The mean value of each measurement point was considered as the result. When comparing the accuracies of R and R1, R2, and R3, significant differences were noted between R and R3 at B, R and R2, R3 at P, and R and R3 at D ($p < 0.05$). No significant difference was observed at M. This study demonstrates that PLA can be recycled only once owing to accuracy limitations.

Keywords: material extrusion; 3D printer; poly-lactic acid; sustainable development goals; dental model; digital dentistry

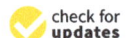

Citation: Nagata, K.; Inaba, K.; Kimoto, K.; Kawana, H. Accuracy of Dental Models Fabricated Using Recycled Poly-Lactic Acid. *Materials* **2023**, *16*, 2620. https://doi.org/10.3390/ma16072620

Academic Editors: Josip Kranjčić and Tina Poklepovic Pericic

Received: 13 February 2023
Revised: 23 March 2023
Accepted: 24 March 2023
Published: 25 March 2023

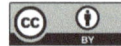

Copyright: © 2023 by the authors. Licensee MDPI, Basel, Switzerland. This article is an open access article distributed under the terms and conditions of the Creative Commons Attribution (CC BY) license (https:// creativecommons.org/licenses/by/ 4.0/).

1. Introduction

Over the past few years, dental materials and equipment have evolved remarkably, benefiting both dentists and patients by improving the quality of treatments and reducing treatment times. When creating prosthetics such as crowns and bridges, professionals commonly take impressions after the formation of the abutment tooth or after building the abutment, injecting plaster, and creating a dental model. Impression taking dates back to the 1800s when wax and plaster were the most commonly used materials. However, non-reversible hydrocolloid alginate impression materials extracted from seaweed and reacted with gypsum to form insoluble calcium alginate have been used since the 1900s owing to their low costs and ease of use. These materials still represent the mainstay of dental treatments [1–3]. However, the poor dimensional stability of alginate impression materials when used alone for abutment teeth and the difficulty in reproducing margins have led to the applications of union impressions using alginate and agar for abutment teeth [4]. In the late 1900s, a silicone impression material was developed with vinyl polysiloxane as a component. In silicone impression materials, vinyl polysiloxane and polysiloxane hydroxide are additionally polymerized using platinum chloride to create a cross-linked structure and induce hardening [5]. Basapogu et al. [6] reported that the dimensional accuracy of silicone impression materials had an error ranging from 0.6% to 0.2%; however, the dimensional accuracy was better than that of alginate impression materials. Rajendran et al. [7] also performed silicone impressions on implant abutments. The authors reported on the usefulness of silicone impression materials for implant treatments. However, owing to cost and operability issues, impressions using alginate and agar are more commonly used, whereas silicone impression materials are only seldom used [8]. Aroma injection, a paste-type allied alginate impression material, has been developed recently. Chen et al. [9] reported that this material was more consistent than silicone impressions, had a lower contact angle than silicone, was more fluid, and allowed for more seamless impression taking than agar. Plaster models have also been used for dental models since the 1800s. Currently, ordinary gypsum, primarily composed of beta hemihydrate gypsum; hard plaster, primarily composed of alpha hemihydrate gypsum; and ultrahard plaster, are used for various purposes [10,11]. It was also used to record intermaxillary relationships and dental models [12]. For prosthetic dentistry, Taggart introduced the casting method in 1907, which is considered the foundation of current prosthetic treatments [13]. Vojdani et al. [14] reported a marginal fit of 88 ± 11 μm and an internal gap of 77 ± 10 μm for metal crowns cast and fabricated from wax patterns, demonstrating an excellent fit accuracy. Yang et al. reported a good marginal fit for a single metal coping produced by lost wax casting: 93 μm for a Ni–Cr alloy and 52 μm for a noble alloy [15]. Reitemeier et al. [16] reported a 20-year survival rate of 79% in 95 patients with 190 cast single crowns. Thus, dentistry has benefited from advances in materials science. The fabrication of prostheses and models using intraoral scanners (IOSs), computer-aided design/computer-aided manufacturing (CAD/CAM) systems, and 3D printers is now feasible [17]. The first IOS is believed to be the one launched by CEREC in 1985. IOSs use confocal, holographic, and shape-from-motion methods to illuminate the surface of an object with a laser, acquire three-dimensional data, and convert the data into polygon information, a set of triangular surfaces. This facilitates the reduced use of plaster casts, less discomfort during impression taking, and digital data storage [18]. It also reduces the risk of errors owing to the absence of plaster expansion and deformation of impression materials in conventional workflows [19]. Di Fiore et al. [20] compared eight IOSs, that is, True Definition, Trios, CEREC Omnicam, 3Dprogress, CS3500, CS3600, Planmeca Emerald, and Dental Wings, with regard to the accuracy of abutments and reported results of 31 ± 8 μm, 32 ± 5 μm, 71 ± 55 μm, 107 ± 28 μm, 61 ± 14 μm, 101 ± 38 μm, 344 ± 121 μm, and 148 ± 64 μm, respectively. In addition, as dentists primarily provide oral care, they are at an increased risk of infection from bodily fluids, aerosols, and droplet infections, such as the currently prevalent COVID-19 [21]. Papi et al. [22] noted that in the traditional workflow, impression materials with blood or saliva and plaster could be sources of infections. Therefore, they reported that the digital workflow, which only requires sterilization of IOS tips, reduces the risk of infection. Furthermore, Joda et al. [23] compared treatment times between IOSs and conventional silicone-based impression taking. They reported that the average working time for a student group was 5 ± 2 min using an IOS and 12 ± 2 min using the conventional method, whereas dentists reported a duration of 5 ± 1 min using an IOS and 10 ± 1 min using the conventional method; both groups had shorter treatment times using IOSs. The widespread use of CAD/CAM has also improved the quality of ceramics and zirconia, allowing for greater precision and a shorter time for crafting dental prosthetics [24,25]. With the advent of digital technology, dental treatments are becoming increasingly effective. Albuha Al-Mussawi et al. [26] mentioned that virtual reality simulators and augmented reality (AR) technology could be applied to dentistry for dental training, education, and the fabrication of technological objects. Furthermore, Ariwa et al. [27] evaluated the accuracy of digital dental models, namely head-mounted displays (HMDs) and spatial reality displays (SRDs), as reflected in AR devices. They reported that the measurement errors ranged from 0.3 to 2 mm for the HMDs and from 0.02 to 0.6 mm for the SRDs, indicating that the error was significantly higher for the SRDs than for the HMDs. Digitalization in dentistry is expected to accelerate further.

From the perspective of environmental issues, sustainable development goals are attracting attention worldwide. In this study, we focused on one of the targets of Goal 12, "Ensure sustainable consumption and production patterns", which indicates that "by 2030, significantly reduce waste generation through prevention, reduction, recycling, and reuse". Wayman et al. [28] reported that 359 million metric tons (Mt) of plastics were produced in 2018, of which an estimated 14.5 Mt entered the ocean, causing potential harm to host organisms consuming them. Consequently, growing concerns have been raised regarding environmental issues, and attempts are being made worldwide to reduce plastics, for instance, by charging for plastic bags and eliminating plastic straws [29,30]. Research is underway to degrade polyethylene terephthalate and polypropylene food and beverage packaging waste to address the long-term persistence of plastics in the environment [31]. We believe that using IOSs will reduce impression material applications in the future. Plaster models are often replaced by resin models sculpted using stereolithography 3D printers (SLA) and digital light processing (DLP). This is because they are generally considered to exhibit reasonable accuracy. Ishida et al. [32] created a cylindrical pattern mimicking a full crown and compared the material extrusion (MEX) and SLA. They claimed that SLA was more accurate and that MEX had a high surface roughness. They also mentioned the importance of 3D printer performance, as dental 3D printers have better accuracy than private ones. Resin is not recyclable; therefore, resin models can cause industrial waste. However, thermoplastic materials such as those used in MEX are recyclable. Therefore, we used one of the MEXs, fused deposition modeling (FDM) and polylactic acid (PLA) filaments. MEX is applied in medical devices, building structures, automobiles, and aerospace owing to its high printing strength, a wide range of available materials, and low cost per part [33]. However, the use of MEX and PLA to create dental models has not yet been reported in the literature. In a previous study, we reported on the accuracy of fit for PLA, resin, and plaster models [34]: 118 ± 22 μm, 62 ± 16 μm, 50 ± 27 μm for buccal areas; 64 ± 32 μm, 48 ± 24 μm, 76 ± 11 μm for palatal areas; 62 ± 28 μm, 50 ± 17 μm, 78 ± 20 μm for mesial areas; and 86 ± 43 μm, 50 ± 12 μm, and 80 ± 39 μm for distal areas, respectively, suggesting the usefulness of PLA models. PLA is a plant-derived plastic material that is expected to reduce carbon dioxide emissions. It is biodegradable and can dissociate into water and carbon dioxide in a compost environment [35]. PLA filaments can be reused owing to their characteristics [36]. We consider that using MEX and PLA to fabricate dental models, followed by their reuse, would reduce industrial waste. However, assessing the corresponding accuracy for applications in clinical practice is essential.

This study aimed to compare the accuracies of recycled PLA and virgin PLA models.

2. Materials and Methods

A left upper first molar model (A55A-262, NISSIN, Tokyo, Japan) was attached to a jaw model (Prosthetic Restoration Jaw Model D16FE-500A(GSE)-QF, NISSIN, Tokyo, Japan) as the base model. Impressions of the base models were taken using an IOS (Trios 3®; 3 shape, Copenhagen, Denmark), and resin blocks (ASAHI PMMA DISK TEMP; ASAHI-ROENTGEN IND. CO., LTD., Kyoto, Japan) were machined using CAD/CAM (Exocad®; Exocad, Berlin, Germany) (Ceramill motion2®; Amann Girrbach, Wien, Austria) based on the stereolithography (STL) data recorded to fabricate provisional crowns. Based on the manufacturer's recommendations, the cement space was set to 0.11 mm, and the margin thickness was set to 0.06 mm. For the PLA model, impressions of the base models were taken using the IOS, and from the data obtained, PLA models were fabricated using 1.75 mm PLA filaments designed for Moment 3D printers (Moment Co., Ltd., Seoul, Republic of Korea) and MEX (Moment M350; Moment Co., Ltd., Seoul, Republic of Korea). Details regarding the filaments and MEX are summarized in Table 1.

In the recycling process, the PLA models were ground using a filament-grinding machine (SHR3D IT; 3devo B.V., Utrecht, The Netherlands), followed by filament production in a filament-making machine (COMPOSER; 3devo B.V). The manufactured filaments were used to fabricate the PLA models (Figure 1). The model made from virgin PLA was labeled R; PLA was recycled up to three times, and the first, second, and third PLA recycles were labeled as R1, R2, and R3, respectively. Five models for each type were fabricated, amounting to 20 in total. Following the manufacturer's recommendations, the temperature during MEX was set to 225 °C, the lamination pitch was set to 100 μm, and the temperature of the filament-manufacturing machine was set to 170–190 °C. No models were surface treated, and no other materials were added when the filaments were reused.

The marginal fits of the provisional crown and PLA model were used as accuracy measures. A PLA model with a provisional crown was placed perpendicular to the X-ray beam in a micro-computed tomography (CT) tube, and micro-CT (ScanXmate-L080T; Comscantecno Co., Ltd., Kanagawa, Japan) was used for imaging. The same provisional crown was placed on all the models. The occlusal surfaces of the provisional crown and adjacent teeth were fixed using utility wax (GC, Tokyo, Japan). The imaging conditions were as follows: 50 kV, 145 µA, voxel size of 34.5 µm, and magnification of 2.891×. After the images were recorded, the digital imaging and communications in medicine (DICOM) data were obtained for accuracy using a three-dimensional image analysis system volume analyzer (SYNAPSE VINCENT®, FUJIFILM, Tokyo, Japan). The measurement method included loading the DICOM data acquired by micro-CT into SYNAPSE VINCENT®, adjusting the contrast in the 3D viewer, selecting "linear measurement", and determining the marginal fits of the provisional crown and PLA model. In total, four measurement points were set as the mesial center (M), distal center (D), buccal center (B), and palatal center (P) (Figure 2). The average value of each measurement point was used as the result.

Table 1. Specifications of the filament and 3D printers used in this study.

	Specifications
PLA filament designed for Moment (Moment Co., Ltd., Seoul, Republic of Korea)	Material PLA: (>98%) Density: 1.25/cm Melting Point: 190 °C Recommended Print Temperature: 215–230 °C Thermal Distortion: 58 °C Water Absorption: 0.50% Molding shrinkage: 0.30
Moment M350 (Moment Co., Ltd., Seoul, Republic of Korea)	XYZ accuracy: XY: 12 µm, Z: 0.625 µm Laminating pitch: 0.05–0.3 mm Modeling size: 350 mm × 190 mm × 196 mm Nozzle: 0.4 mm

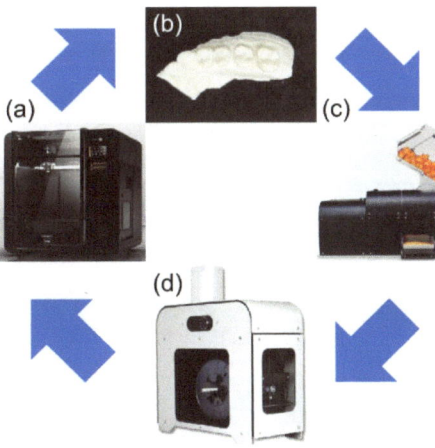

Figure 1. Process involved in poly-lactic acid (PLA) model recycling. (**a**) Moment M350 was used for MEX. (**b**) PLA models were prepared using 1.75 mm PLA filaments and MEX. (**c**) PLA models were ground using a filament-grinding machine (SHR3D IT). (**d**) After pulverization, filaments were produced again using a filament-manufacturing machine (COMPOSER).

The accuracy of the model was verified based on Dunnett's test using the bell curve in Excel (Social Survey Research Information Co., Ltd., Tokyo, Japan). Continuous data were expressed as mean ± standard deviation. Differences with a *p*-value < 0.05 were considered statistically significant.

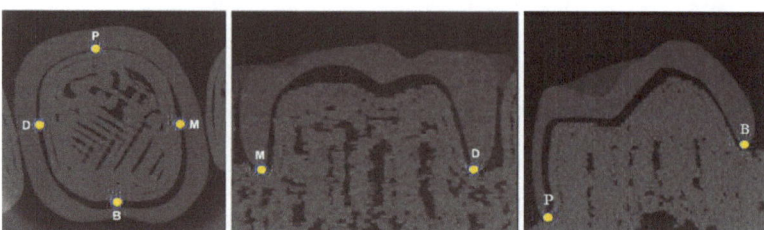

Figure 2. Provisional crown was placed on each model, and the marginal fit was measured using micro-computed tomography at the mesial center (M), distal center (D), buccal center (B), and palatal center (P) of the tooth.

3. Results

The results of this study are summarized in Table 2. For R, the accuracies at positions B, P, M, and D were 68 ± 16 µm, 66 ± 22 µm, 88 ± 13 µm, and 60 ± 31 µm, respectively. For R1, the accuracies at positions B, P, M, and D were 76 ± 34 µm, 86 ± 23 µm, 72 ± 27 µm, and 50 ± 12 µm, respectively. For R2, the accuracies at positions B, P, M, and D were 86 ± 36 µm, 216 ± 99 µm, 78 ± 44 µm, and 78 ± 48 µm, respectively. For R3, the accuracies at positions B, P, M, and D were 154 ± 94 µm, 336 ± 77 µm, 132 ± 49 µm, and 132 ± 41 µm, respectively; thus, the accuracies for R and R1 were lower than 120 µm, and those for R2 and R3 were greater than 120 µm at all measurement points if standard deviations were included.

Table 2. Marginal fit results for virgin PLA and reused PLA models at each measurement point (µm).

	B	P	M	D
R	68 ± 16	66 ± 22	88 ± 13	60 ± 31
R1	76 ± 34	86 ± 23	72 ± 27	50 ± 12
R2	86 ± 36	216 ± 99	78 ± 44	78 ± 48
R3	154 ± 94	336 ± 77	132 ± 49	132 ± 41

B—buccal center; P—palatal center; M—mesial center; D—distal center.

When comparing the accuracies of R with those of R1, R2, and R3, significant differences were noted between R and R3 at position B ($p < 0.05$), R and R2, R3 at position P ($p < 0.01$), and R and R3 at position D ($p < 0.01$) (Figure 3). A significant decrease was observed in the accuracy of R3.

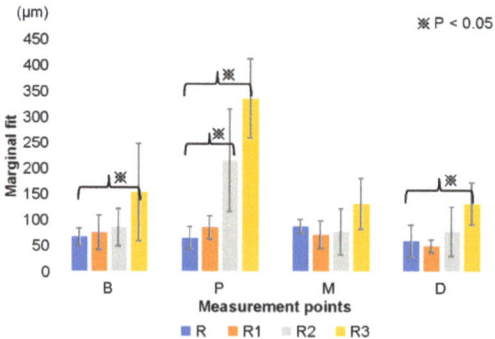

Figure 3. Mean and standard deviation of the marginal goodness of fit for each model and provisional crown were measured using SYNAPSE VINCENT®. The results for all models of R, R1, R2, and R3 are presented.

4. Discussion

With the widespread use of IOSs and CAD/CAM, the fabrication of prostheses without model creation is now feasible. However, models are still essential for margin, contact, and occlusal adjustments. Numerous reports indicate that the marginal fit discrepancy of CAD/CAM crowns should be less than 120 μm [37–39]. However, the results of this study, including standard deviations, exceed 120 μm at all measurement points for R2 and R3.

In MEX, the thermoplastic material is melted and extruded from a hot end to form a printed layer to produce the desired object [40,41]. Alsoufi et al. [42] reported that the shape error of PLA was within 3.00% on each side of a 40 mm (L) × 40 mm (W) × 15 mm (H) specimen, which is excellent accuracy for PLA fabricated by MEX. Only one PLA filament was used in this study. Cicala et al. [43] used MEX and three different commercial filaments to verify the accuracy using the same object. Two filaments that exhibited significant shear-thinning behavior and were correlated with mineral filler formulations printed well, but one had poor accuracy. Cicala et al. reported that differences in additives in the filament manufacturing process led to these accuracies. PLA is hydrolyzed during molding, which then degrades into low molecular weight oligomers. The oligomers further decompose into lactide and lactic acid, resulting in the loss of plastic properties. It has also been reported that when PLA is reused, the mechanical properties deteriorate because of hydrolysis and breakage of the reinforcing fibers [44,45]. Agüero et al. reported the following mechanical properties for reused PLA: impact strength (kJ·m^{-2}) of 58 ± 4 for virgin PLA, 56 ± 4 after one recycle, and 36 ± 5 after four recycles. The elongation at break (%) was 10 ± 0.04 for virgin PLA, 9 ± 0.3 after two recycles, and 7 ± 0.9 after four recycles. The authors reported that the material could be recycled up to six times, with a slight degradation in the mechanical properties after one and two cycles but a marked decrease from the fourth cycle [46]. Zhao et al. also reused PLA and reported that the viscosity at 160 °C was approximately 2000 Pa·s for virgin PLA, approximately 750 Pa·s after the first cycle, and approximately 100 Pa·s after the second cycle; moreover, they reported that the viscosity decreased with repeated reuse, and the molecular weight decreased with chain scission, resulting in the degradation of mechanical properties. Therefore, they reported that reuse after the second cycle was difficult [47].

Anderson et al. compared the mechanical properties of virgin PLA and one-time reused PLA. They reported an 11% decrease in the tensile strength, a 7% increase in the shear strength, and a 2% decrease in the hardness of the reused filament, with no differences in the average mechanical properties of one-time reused PLA compared to those of the virgin material. However, they reported an increase in the standard deviation and greater variability in the results for the recycled material [48]. These reports are similar to our results. We believe that the mechanical properties of PLA degrade, and their stability is impaired the more they are reused, resulting in a higher standard deviation. As dental models only tolerate minimal errors in micrometer units, reusing them after the second cycle may be difficult. However, research is underway to add other materials to PLA to compensate for the PLA weaknesses. Beltrán et al. added a chain extender and an organic peroxide to PLA and evaluated its mechanical properties. They discovered that both additives reacted with terminal carboxyl groups in the aged polymer, causing cross-linking, branching, and chain extension reactions. Notably, both additives failed to improve either the viscosity or the thermal stability of the heavily degraded PLA. However, they reported that they could improve the microhardness of the recycled material [49]. Patwa et al. reported that adding 1 wt% crystalline silk nanodisks to a PLA matrix increased the toughness by approximately 65%, elongation by approximately 40%, and tensile strength by approximately 10% [50]. López et al. reported that mixing virgin PLA with 30 wt% recycled PLA and adding an epoxy-based chain extender and microcrystalline cellulose as reinforcements improved the tensile strength by up to 88%, modulus by 127%, and Izod impact strength by 11% [51]. Other studies have focused on adding materials such as metals, carbon, and fibers to PLA to maintain and improve its mechanical properties [52,53]. Furthermore, some studies involve reusing PLA with other materials [54,55]. Thus, research on reusing PLA and adding additives to maintain or improve its mechanical properties is progressing worldwide. The decrease in accuracy after the second recycle in this study could be attributed to the fact that the mechanical properties of PLA are known to deteriorate when reused.

Although minimal progress has been achieved in maintaining the biodegradability and mechanical properties of PLA, we believe it is possible to increase the number of recycling times for PLA, with improvements in the future. To the best of our knowledge, this study is the first to consider the reuse of PLA in dentistry.

PLA is widely used in the medical field, and numerous reports on its good biocompatibility can be found in the literature [56–58].

Concerning the use of PLA in dentistry, Benli et al. compared the marginal gaps of PLA, polymethyl methacrylate, and polyetheretherketone as provisional crowns. The results for PLA, polymethyl methacrylate, and polyetheretherketone were 60.40 ± 2.85 μm, 61 ± 4 μm, and 56 ± 5 μm, respectively, demonstrating the usefulness of PLA crowns [59]. Molinello–Mourelle et al. reported similarly on the usefulness of provisional crowns fabricated using PLA [60]. Crenn et al. examined the mechanical properties of PLA to verify its feasibility for use as provisional crowns. The elastic modulus of PLA is $E = 3784 \pm 99$ MPa, that of nanoparticulate bisacryl resin is $E = 3977 \pm 878$ MPa, and that of acrylic resin is $E = 2382 \pm 226$ MPa. The flexural strength of PLA is $Rm = 116 \pm 2$ MPa, that of nanoparticulate bisacryl resin is $Rm = 86 \pm 6$ MPa, and that of acrylic resin is $Rm = 115 \pm 21$ MPa, indicating mechanical property problems compared to the other two materials [61]. Relatively fewer reports have been presented on the application of PLA in dentistry, and most reports focus on its applications in provisional crowns. However, the glass transition temperature of PLA is known to be 50–80 °C [62,63]. PLA improves crystallinity and increases heat resistance. Notably, methods adopted to improve crystallinity include plasticizing modification and adding nucleating agents [64,65]. Among these, plasticizing modification is the most effective approach to improve crystallinity. However, the approach is reported to lower the glass transition temperature [66] simultaneously. Xu et al. reported that adding ethylene butyl methacrylate glycidyl methacrylate terpolymer and talc as nucleating agents for PLA increased the heat deformation temperature from 58 °C to 139 °C. The glass transition temperature, however, remained almost unchanged [67]. Various other heat resistance analyses have been conducted. However, no straightforward method has been identified to improve the definite glass transition temperature [68,69]. Additionally, while improving heat resistance in the future, impurities added to achieve heat resistance must be ensured not to impair the biodegradability of PLA [70]. Placing PLA crowns in the oral cavity is challenging due to heat resistance issues. Instead, we consider them more effective when used as models.

PLA models are typically created using MEX. However, MEX is known to release volatile organic compounds (VOCs) during the molding process [71,72]. Ding et al. reported that the mass yields of VOCs emitted during MEX for PLA, acrylonitrile butadiene styrene, and polyvinyl alcohol were 0.03%, 0.21%, and 2%, respectively, at 220 °C [73]. Wojtyła et al. reported that the main VOC emitted from PLA was methyl methacrylate, which accounted for 44% of the total emissions. Thus, it is essential to keep the laboratory rooms unoccupied and ventilated during molding and restrict the use of several MEX processes simultaneously [74]. Notably, filaments left in an environment with 60–70% humidity for two weeks will degrade printing quality. Suharjanto et al. reported that filament storage using medium-density boards prevents and reduces air absorption of PLA filament and filament life, leading to the maintenance of the printing system. Note that the accuracy after modeling varies depending on the storage method [75].

In this study, we measured the marginal fit between the provisional crown and the model. However, it is necessary to measure the accuracy of the entire model in the future. Liu et al. examined the geometric accuracy of monkey tooth roots. After scanning the monkey's maxilla with cone-beam CT and segmentation of the incisor roots, titanium implants were fabricated using laser powder bed fusion (PBF), a metal composite fabrication method. The extracted teeth and 3D-printed implants were scanned with a micro-CT and compared with the original segmented STL data. Results were reported as 91 ± 5% for the segmented versus printed tooth and 67 ± 11% for segmented versus actual. They found that monkey denticles are small and difficult to segment with high precision and that irregular shapes, surfaces, and technical challenges make it difficult to delineate regions of interest and cause deviation errors [76]. In the future, measuring the overall accuracy of the base model and the PLA model after molding will be necessary. This study has some limitations: the mechanical properties of PLA could not be verified, and PLA could not be investigated with additives. They will be the topic of future research.

5. Conclusions

Sustainable development goals are attracting global attention in terms of environmental issues. Digital technology has led to improved accuracy in prosthetic treatment and shorter treatment times. However, SLA and DLP are widely employed in dentistry, and the resulting models are considered industrial waste. Therefore, we used MEX and PLA to reduce industrial waste in dentistry. Notably, PLA is a plant-derived plastic material that is expected to reduce carbon dioxide emissions. Further, biodegradable PLA filaments break down into water and carbon dioxide in a composting environment, and their properties allow them to be reused. This study examined the accuracy of MEX and PLA models in dentistry and the system for their reuse. The results show that PLA models made with MEX are within the acceptable range of 120 μm up to the first cycle and can be reused for up to one cycle. PLA may be considered the new material of choice in dentistry. The accuracy of MEX could be improved, and additives could be added to filaments to promote their reusability. This may reduce the industrial waste generated by dentistry.

Author Contributions: K.N.: data curation; formal analysis; investigation; methodology; roles/writing—original draft. K.I.: formal analysis; investigation; methodology; software. K.K.: conceptualization; methodology. H.K.: project administration; conceptualization. All authors have read and agreed to the published version of the manuscript.

Funding: This research received no external funding.

Institutional Review Board Statement: Not applicable.

Informed Consent Statement: Not applicable.

Data Availability Statement: The data presented in this study are available on request from the corresponding author. The data are not publicly available due to ethical issues.

Acknowledgments: We would like to express our deepest gratitude to 3D Printing Corporation for fabricating the PLA models for this study.

Conflicts of Interest: The authors declare no conflict of interest.

References

1. Hansson, O.; Eklund, J. A historical review of hydrocolloids and an investigation of the dimensional accuracy of the new alginates for crown and bridge impressions when using stock trays. *Swed. Dent. J.* **1984**, *8*, 81–95. [PubMed]
2. Cervino, G.; Fiorillo, L.; Herford, A.S.; Laino, L.; Troiano, G.; Amoroso, G.; Crimi, S.; Matarese, M.; D'Amico, C.; Nastro Siniscalchi, E.; et al. Alginate materials and dental impression technique: A current state of the art and application to dental practice. *Mar. Drugs* **2018**, *17*, 18. [CrossRef] [PubMed]
3. Papadiochos, I.; Papadiochou, S.; Emmanouil, I. The historical evolution of dental impression materials. *J. Hist. Dent.* **2017**, *65*, 79–89.
4. Johnson, G.H.; Craig, R.G. Accuracy and bond strength of combination agar/alginate hydrocolloid impression materials. *J. Prosthet. Dent.* **1986**, *55*, 1–6. [CrossRef] [PubMed]
5. Naumovski, B.; Kapushevska, B. Dimensional stability and accuracy of silicone—Based impression materials using different impression techniques—A literature review. *Prilozi* **2017**, *38*, 131–138. [CrossRef] [PubMed]
6. Basapogu, S.; Pilla, A.; Pathipaka, S. Dimensional accuracy of hydrophilic and hydrophobic VPS impression materials using different impression techniques—An invitro study. *J. Clin. Diagn. Res.* **2016**, *10*, ZC56–ZC59. [CrossRef]
7. Rajendran, R.; Chander, N.G.; Anitha, K.V.; Muthukumar, B. Dimensional accuracy of vinyl polyether and polyvinyl siloxane impression materials in direct implant impression technique for multiple dental implants. *Eur. Oral Res.* **2021**, *55*, 54–59. [CrossRef]

8. Hulme, C.; Yu, G.; Browne, C.; O'Dwyer, J.; Craddock, H.; Brown, S.; Gray, J.; Pavitt, S.; Fernandez, C.; Godfrey, M.; et al. Cost-effectiveness of silicone and alginate impressions for complete dentures. *J. Dent.* **2014**, *42*, 902–907. [CrossRef]
9. Chen, J.D.; Ma, A.B.; Sun, L.; Hong, G. The physical properties of new paste type alginate impression materials. In Proceedings of the 2021 IADR/AADR/CADR General Session (Virtual Experience), Virtual, 21–24 July 2021. Final Presentation ID: 0552.
10. Buckingum, T.L. The force of expansion of plaster of Paris. *Dent. Cosmos* **1959**, *1*, 238–240.
11. Mori, T.; Mcaloon, J.; Aghajani, F. Gypsum-bonded investment and dental precision casting (I) two investments. *Dent. Mater. J.* **2003**, *22*, 412–420. [CrossRef]
12. Urstein, M.; Fitzig, S.; Moskona, D.; Cardash, H.S. A clinical evaluation of materials used in registering interjaw relationships. *J. Prosthet. Dent.* **1991**, *65*, 372–377. [CrossRef] [PubMed]
13. Donaldson, J.A. The use of gold in dentistry: An historical overview. *J. Hist. Dent.* **2012**, *60*, 134–147.
14. Vojdani, M.; Torabi, K.; Farjood, E.; Khaledi, A. Comparison the marginal and internal fit of metal copings cast from wax patterns fabricated by CAD/CAM and conventional wax up techniques. *J. Dent.* **2013**, *14*, 118–129.
15. Yang, J.; Li, H. Accuracy of CAD-CAM milling versus conventional lost-wax casting for single metal copings: A systematic review and meta-analysis. *J. Prosthet. Dent.* **2022**, *S0022-3913*, 00344-4. [CrossRef] [PubMed]
16. Reitemeier, B.; Hänsel, K.; Range, U.; Walter, M.H. Prospective study on metal ceramic crowns in private practice settings: 20-year results. *Clin. Oral Investig.* **2019**, *23*, 1823–1828. [CrossRef] [PubMed]
17. Lo Russo, L.; Caradonna, G.; Biancardino, M.; De Lillo, A.; Troiano, G.; Guida, L. Digital versus conventional workflow for the fabrication of multiunit fixed prostheses: A systematic review and meta-analysis of vertical marginal fit in controlled in vitro studies. *J. Prosthet. Dent.* **2019**, *122*, 435–440. [CrossRef] [PubMed]
18. Kihara, H.; Hatakeyama, W.; Komine, F.; Takafuji, K.; Takahashi, T.; Yokota, J.; Oriso, K.; Kondo, H. Accuracy and practicality of intraoral scanner in dentistry: A literature review. *J. Prosthodont. Res.* **2020**, *64*, 109–113. [CrossRef]
19. Chochlidakis, K.M.; Papaspyridakos, P.; Geminiani, A.; Chen, C.J.; Feng, I.J.; Ercoli, C. Digital versus conventional impressions for fixed prosthodontics: A systematic review and meta-analysis. *J. Prosthet. Dent.* **2016**, *116*, 184–190.e12. [CrossRef]
20. Di Fiore, A.; Meneghello, R.; Graiff, L.; Savio, G.; Vigolo, P.; Monaco, C.; Stellini, E. Full arch digital scanning systems performances for implant-supported fixed dental prostheses: A comparative study of 8 intraoral scanners. *J. Prosthodont. Res.* **2019**, *63*, 396–403. [CrossRef]
21. Izzetti, R.; Nisi, M.; Gabriele, M.; Graziani, F. COVID-19 transmission in dental practice: Brief review of preventive measures in Italy. *J. Dent. Res.* **2020**, *99*, 1030–1038. [CrossRef]
22. Papi, P.; Di Murro, B.; Penna, D.; Pompa, G. Digital prosthetic workflow during COVID-19 pandemic to limit infection risk in dental practice. *Oral Dis.* **2021**, *27* (Suppl. S3), 723–726. [CrossRef] [PubMed]
23. Joda, T.; Lenherr, P.; Dedem, P.; Kovaltschuk, I.; Bragger, U.; Zitzmann, N.U. Time efficiency, difficulty, and operator's preference comparing digital and conventional implant impressions: A randomized controlled trial. *Clin. Oral Implant. Res.* **2017**, *28*, 1318–1323. [CrossRef] [PubMed]
24. Davidowitz, G.; Kotick, P.G. The use of CAD/CAM in dentistry. *Dent. Clin. N. Am.* **2011**, *55*, 559–570. [CrossRef] [PubMed]
25. Spitznagel, F.A.; Boldt, J.; Gierthmuehlen, P.C. CAD/CAM ceramic restorative materials for natural teeth. *J. Dent. Res.* **2018**, *97*, 1082–1091. [CrossRef] [PubMed]
26. Albuha Al-Mussawi, R.M.; Farid, F. Computer-based technologies in dentistry: Types and applications. *J. Dent.* **2016**, *13*, 215–222.
27. Ariwa, M.; Itamiya, T.; Koizumi, S.; Yamaguchi, T. Comparison of the observation errors of augmented and spatial reality systems. *Appl. Sci.* **2021**, *11*, 12076. [CrossRef]
28. Wayman, C.; Niemann, H. The fate of plastic in the ocean environment—A minireview. *Environ. Sci. Process. Impacts* **2021**, *23*, 198–212. [CrossRef]
29. Seo, Y.; Kudo, F. Charging plastic bags: Perceptions from Japan. *PLoS Sustain. Transform.* **2022**, *1*, e0000011. [CrossRef]
30. Jonsson, A.; Andersson, K.; Stelick, A.; Dando, R. An evaluation of alternative biodegradable and reusable drinking straws as alternatives to single-use plastic. *J. Food Sci.* **2021**, *86*, 3219–3227. [CrossRef]
31. Blanco, I. Lifetime prediction of food and beverage packaging wastes. *J. Therm. Anal. Calorim.* **2016**, *125*, 809–816. [CrossRef]
32. Ishida, Y.; Miura, D.; Miyasaka, T.; Shinya, A. Dimensional accuracy of dental casting patterns fabricated using consumer 3D printers. *Polymers* **2020**, *12*, 2244. [CrossRef] [PubMed]
33. Arrigo, R.; Frache, A. FDM printability of PLA based-materials: The key role of the rheological behavior. *Polymers* **2022**, *14*, 1754. [CrossRef] [PubMed]
34. Nagata, K.; Muromachi, K.; Kouzai, Y.; Inaba, K.; Inoue, E.; Fuchigami, K.; Nihei, T.; Atsumi, M.; Kimoto, K.; Kawana, H. Fit accuracy of resin crown on a dental model fabricated using fused deposition modeling 3D printing and a polylactic acid filament. *J. Prosthodont. Res.* **2023**, *67*, 144–149. [CrossRef] [PubMed]
35. Singhvi, M.S.; Zinjarde, S.S.; Gokhale, D.V. Polylactic acid: Synthesis and biomedical applications. *J. Appl. Microbiol.* **2019**, *127*, 1612–1626. [CrossRef] [PubMed]
36. Mikula, K.; Skrzypczak, D.; Izydorczyk, G.; Warchoł, J.; Moustakas, K.; Chojnacka, K.; Witek-Krowiak, A. 3D printing filament as a second life of waste plastics-a review. *Environ. Sci. Pollut. Res. Int.* **2021**, *28*, 12321–12333. [CrossRef] [PubMed]
37. Shembesh, M.; Ali, A.; Finkelman, M.; Weber, H.P.; Zandparsa, R. An in vitro comparison of the marginal adaptation accuracy of CAD/CAM restorations using different impression systems. *J. Prosthodont.* **2017**, *26*, 581–586. [CrossRef] [PubMed]

38. Ryu, J.E.; Kim, Y.L.; Kong, H.J.; Chang, H.S.; Jung, J.H. Marginal and internal fit of 3D printed provisional crowns according to build directions. *J. Adv. Prosthodont.* **2020**, *12*, 225–232. [CrossRef]
39. Dolev, E.; Bitterman, Y.; Meirowitz, A. Comparison of marginal fit between CAD-CAM and hot-press lithium disilicate crowns. *J. Prosthet. Dent.* **2019**, *121*, 124–128. [CrossRef]
40. Teng, P.S.P.; Leong, K.F.; Kong, P.W.; Er, B.H.; Chew, Z.Y.; Tan, P.S.; Tee, C.H. A methodology to design and fabricate a smart brace using low-cost additive manufacturing. *Virtual Phys. Prototyp.* **2022**, *17*, 932–947. [CrossRef]
41. Wickramasinghe, S.; Do, T.; Tran, P. Flexural behavior of 3D printed bio-inspired interlocking suture structures. *Mater. Sci. Addit. Manuf.* **2022**, *1*, 9. [CrossRef]
42. Alsoufi, M.S.; Elsayed, A.E. Surface roughness quality and dimensional accuracy—A comprehensive analysis of 100% infill printed parts fabricated by a personal/desktop cost-effective FDM 3D printer. *Mater. Sci. Appl.* **2018**, *9*, 11–40. [CrossRef]
43. Cicala, G.; Giordano, D.; Tosto, C.; Filippone, G.; Recca, A.; Blanco, I. Polylactide (PLA) filaments a biobased solution for additive manufacturing: Correlating rheology and thermomechanical properties with printing quality. *Materials* **2018**, *11*, 1191. [CrossRef] [PubMed]
44. Palsikowski, P.A.; Kuchnier, C.N.; Pinheiro, I.F.; Morales, A.R. Biodegradation in soil of PLA/PBAT blends compatibilized with chain extender. *J. Polym. Environ.* **2018**, *26*, 330–341. [CrossRef]
45. Beltrán, F.R.; Arrieta, M.P.; Moreno, E.; Gaspar, G.; Muneta, L.M.; Carrasco-Gallego, R.; Yáñez, S.; Hidalgo-Carvajal, D.; de la Orden, M.U.; Martínez Urreaga, J. Evaluation of the technical viability of distributed mechanical recycling of PLA 3D printing wastes. *Polymers* **2021**, *13*, 1247. [CrossRef]
46. Agüero, A.; Morcillo, M.D.C.; Quiles-Carrillo, L.; Balart, R.; Boronat, T.; Lascano, D.; Torres-Giner, S.; Fenollar, O. Study of the influence of the reprocessing cycles on the final properties of polylactide pieces obtained by injection molding. *Polymers* **2019**, *11*, 1908. [CrossRef] [PubMed]
47. Zhao, P.; Rao, C.; Gu, F.; Sharmin, N.; Fu, J. Close-looped recycling of polylactic acid used in 3D printing: An experimental investigation and life cycle assessment. *J. Clean. Prod.* **2018**, *197*, 1046–1055. [CrossRef]
48. Anderson, I. Mechanical properties of specimens 3D printed with virgin and recycled polylactic acid. *3D Print Addit Manuf.* **2017**, *4*, 110–115. [CrossRef]
49. Beltrán, F.R.; Infante, C.; de la Orden, M.U.; Martínez Urreaga, J.M. Mechanical recycling of poly(lactic acid): Evaluation of a chain extender and a peroxide as additives for upgrading the recycled plastic. *J. Clean. Prod.* **2019**, *219*, 46–56. [CrossRef]
50. Patwa, R.; Kumar, A.; Katiyar, V. Effect of silk nano-disc dispersion on mechanical, thermal, and barrier properties of poly(lactic acid) based bionanocomposites. *J. Appl. Polym. Sci.* **2018**, *135*, 46671. [CrossRef]
51. Cisneros-López, E.O.; Pal, A.K.; Rodriguez, A.U.; Wu, F.; Misra, M.; Mielewski, D.F.; Kiziltas, A.; Mohanty, A.K. Recycled poly(lactic acid)–based 3D printed sustainable biocomposites: A comparative study with injection molding. *Mater. Today Sustain.* **2020**, *7–8*, 100027. [CrossRef]
52. Coppola, B.; Cappetti, N.; Di Maio, L.; Scarfato, P.; Incarnato, L. 3D printing of PLA/clay nanocomposites: Influence of printing temperature on printed samples properties. *Materials* **2018**, *11*, 1947. [CrossRef] [PubMed]
53. Bardot, M.; Schulz, M.D. Biodegradable poly(lactic acid) nanocomposites for fused deposition modeling 3D printing. *Nanomaterials* **2020**, *10*, 2567. [CrossRef] [PubMed]
54. Gomes, T.E.; Cadete, M.S.; Dias-de-Oliveira, J.; Neto, V. Controlling the properties of parts 3D printed from recycled thermoplastics: A review of current practices. *Polym. Degrad. Stab.* **2022**, *196*, 109850. [CrossRef]
55. Lagazzo, A.; Moliner, C.; Bosio, B.; Botter, R.; Arato, E. Evaluation of the mechanical and thermal properties decay of PHBV/sisal and PLA/sisal biocomposites at different recycle steps. *Polymers* **2019**, *11*, 1477. [CrossRef]
56. Gai, M.; Li, W.; Frueh, J.; Sukhorukov, G.B. Polylactic acid sealed polyelectrolyte complex microcontainers for controlled encapsulation and NIR-laser based release of cargo. *Colloids Surf. B Biointerfaces* **2019**, *173*, 521–528. [CrossRef]
57. Li, Z.; Wu, T.; Chen, Y.; Gao, X.; Ye, J.; Jin, Y.; Chen, B. Oriented homo-epitaxial crystallization of polylactic acid displaying a biomimetic structure and improved blood compatibility. *J. Biomed. Mater. Res. A* **2022**, *110*, 684–695. [CrossRef]
58. Ahuja, R.; Kumari, N.; Srivastava, A.; Bhati, P.; Vashisth, P.; Yadav, P.K.; Jacob, T.; Narang, R.; Bhatnagar, N. Biocompatibility analysis of PLA based candidate materials for cardiovascular stents in a rat subcutaneous implant model. *Acta Histochem.* **2020**, *122*, 151615. [CrossRef]
59. Benli, M.; Eker-Gümüş, B.; Kahraman, Y.; Huck, O.; Özcan, M. Can polylactic acid be a CAD/CAM material for provisional crown restorations in terms of fit and fracture strength? *Dent. Mater. J.* **2021**, *40*, 772–780. [CrossRef]
60. Molinero-Mourelle, P.; Canals, S.; Gómez-Polo, M.; Solá-Ruiz, M.F.; Del Río Highsmith, J.; Viñuela, A.C. Polylactic acid as a material for three-dimensional printing of provisional restorations. *Int. J. Prosthodont.* **2018**, *31*, 349–350. [CrossRef]
61. Crenn, M.J.; Rohman, G.; Fromentin, O.; Benoit, A. Polylactic acid as a biocompatible polymer for three-dimensional printing of interim prosthesis: Mechanical characterization. *Dent. Mater. J.* **2022**, *41*, 110–116. [CrossRef]
62. Plavec, R.; Horváth, V.; Hlaváčiková, S.; Omaníková, L.; Repiská, M.; Medlenová, E.; Feranc, J.; Kruželák, J.; Přikryl, R.; Figalla, S.; et al. Influence of multiple thermomechanical processing of 3D filaments based on polylactic acid and polyhydroxybutyrate on their rheological and utility properties. *Polymers* **2022**, *14*, 1947. [CrossRef] [PubMed]
63. Menčík, P.; Přikryl, R.; Stehnová, I.; Melčová, V.; Kontárová, S.; Figalla, S.; Alexy, P.; Bočkaj, J. Effect of selected commercial plasticizers on mechanical, thermal, and morphological properties of poly(3-hydroxybutyrate)/poly(lactic acid)/plasticizer biodegradable blends for three-dimensional (3D) print. *Materials* **2018**, *11*, 1893. [CrossRef] [PubMed]

64. Greco, A.; Ferrari, F. Thermal behavior of PLA plasticized by commercial and cardanol-derived plasticizers and the effect on the mechanical properties. *J. Therm. Anal. Calorim.* **2021**, *146*, 131–141. [CrossRef]
65. Li, Y.; Mi, J.; Fu, H.; Zhou, H.; Wang, X. Nanocellular foaming behaviors of chain-extended poly(lactic acid) induced by isothermal crystallization. *ACS Omega* **2019**, *4*, 12512–12523. [CrossRef]
66. Yang, Y.; Xiong, Z.; Zhang, L.; Tang, Z.; Zhang, R.; Zhu, J. Isosorbide dioctoate as a "green" plasticizer for poly(lactic acid). *Mater. Des.* **2016**, *91*, 262–268. [CrossRef]
67. Xu, P.; Tian, H.; Han, L.; Yang, H.; Bian, J.; Pan, H.; Zhang, H. Improved heat resistance in poly (lactic acid)/ethylene butyl methacrylate glycidyl methacrylate terpolymer blends by controlling highly filled talc particles. *J. Ther. Anal. Calorim.* **2022**, *147*, 5719–5732. [CrossRef]
68. Barczewski, M.; Mysiukiewicz, O.; Hejna, A.; Biskup, R.; Szulc, J.; Michałowski, S.; Piasecki, A.; Kloziński, A. The effect of surface treatment with isocyanate and aromatic carbodiimide of thermally expanded vermiculite used as a functional filler for polylactide-based composites. *Polymers* **2021**, *13*, 890. [CrossRef]
69. Andrzejewski, J.; Skórczewska, K.; Kloziński, A. Improving the toughness and thermal resistance of polyoxymethylene/poly(lactic acid) blends: Evaluation of structure-properties correlation for reactive processing. *Polymers* **2020**, *12*, 307. [CrossRef]
70. Zhao, X.; Liu, J.; Li, J.; Liang, X.; Zhou, W.; Peng, S. Strategies and techniques for improving heat resistance and mechanical performances of poly(lactic acid) (PLA) biodegradable materials. *Int. J. Biol. Macromol.* **2022**, *218*, 115–134. [CrossRef]
71. Chan, F.L.; Hon, C.Y.; Tarlo, S.M.; Rajaram, N.; House, R. Emissions and health risks from the use of 3D printers in an occupational setting. *J. Toxicol. Environ. Health A* **2020**, *83*, 279–287. [CrossRef]
72. Dobrzyńska, E.; Kondej, D.; Kowalska, J.; Szewczyńska, M. State of the art in additive manufacturing and its possible chemical and particle hazards-review. *Indoor Air* **2021**, *31*, 1733–1758. [CrossRef] [PubMed]
73. Ding, S.; Ng, B.F.; Shang, X.; Liu, H.; Lu, X.; Wan, M.P. The characteristics and formation mechanisms of emissions from thermal decomposition of 3D printer polymer filaments. *Sci. Total Environ.* **2019**, *692*, 984–994. [CrossRef] [PubMed]
74. Wojtyła, S.; Klama, P.; Baran, T. Is 3D printing safe? Analysis of the thermal treatment of thermoplastics: ABS, PLA, PET, and nylon. *J. Occup. Environ. Hyg.* **2017**, *14*, D80–D85. [CrossRef] [PubMed]
75. Suharjanto, G.; Adi, J.P. Design and manufacture of polylacticacid (PLA) filament storage for 3-dimensional printing with composite material. *IOP Conf. Ser. Earth Environ. Sci.* **2022**, *998*, 012028. [CrossRef]
76. Liu, Y.; Sing, S.L.; Lim, R.X.E.; Yeong, W.Y.; Goh, B.T. Preliminary Investigation on the Geometric Accuracy of 3D Printed Dental Implant Using a Monkey Maxilla Incisor Model. *Int. J. Bioprint.* **2022**, *8*, 476. [CrossRef]

Disclaimer/Publisher's Note: The statements, opinions and data contained in all publications are solely those of the individual author(s) and contributor(s) and not of MDPI and/or the editor(s). MDPI and/or the editor(s) disclaim responsibility for any injury to people or property resulting from any ideas, methods, instructions or products referred to in the content.

Color Stability of Various Orthodontic Clear Aligner Systems after Submersion in Different Staining Beverages

Nicolae Daniel Olteanu [1], Ionut Taraboanta [1], Tinela Panaite [1], Carina Balcos [1], Sorana Nicoleta Rosu [1,*], Raluca Maria Vieriu [1], Stefania Dinu [2] and Irina Nicoleta Zetu [1]

[1] Department of Oral and Maxillofacial Surgery, Faculty of Dental Medicine "Grigore T. Popa", University of Medicine and Pharmacy from Iasi, Str. Universitatii 16, 700115 Iasi, Romania; daniel.olteanu@umfiasi.ro (N.D.O.); ionut-taraboanta@umfiasi.ro (I.T.); tinela-panaite@umfiasi.ro (T.P.); carina.balcos@umfiasi.ro (C.B.); raluca-maria.vieriu@umfiasi.ro (R.M.V.); irina.zetu@umfiasi.ro (I.N.Z.)

[2] Department of Pedodontics, Faculty of Dental Medicine, "Victor Babes", University of Medicine and Pharmacy Timisoara, No. 9, Revolutiei Bv., 300041 Timisoara, Romania; dinu.stefania@umft.ro

* Correspondence: soranarosu@gmail.com; Tel.: +40-757-070-891

Abstract: This study aimed to compare the color changes in two different orthodontic clear aligner systems after submersion in various beverages for 14 days. The tested aligner systems were Taglus Premium made of polyethylene terephthalate glycol (the TAG group) and CA® Prodin+ made of a transparent copolyester and a thermoplastic elastomer (the PRO group). A total of 56 samples were firstly divided into two groups according to the tested system, TAG and PRO. Each group was subsequently divided in four subgroups according to immersion solution: A—artificial saliva, B—cola, C—coffee, D—red wine. Color measurements were performed on Days 1, 7 and 14 using a portable colorimeter and the CIE L*a*b* system. The obtained results showed significant color changes in both materials when exposed to coffee and red wine ($p > 0.05$). Samples in the PRO group showed a greater susceptibility to discoloration (higher ΔE values) when compared to the TAG group after submersion in cola ($p = 0.025$), coffee ($p = 0.005$) and red wine ($p = 0.041$) solutions. Statistical analysis revealed that all of the color parameters ΔL*, Δa*, Δb* and ΔE of both tested materials were affected by submersion in coffee solution for 14 days. In conclusion, the CA® Pro+ aligner system is more prone to staining compared to the Taglus material after submersion for 14 days in cola, coffee and red wine solutions. Submersion for 14 days in coffee solution alters all of the color parameters (ΔL, Δa, Δb and ΔE) of both tested aligner materials.

Keywords: clear aligner; polyethylene terephthalate glycol; thermoplastic elastomer; color stability; staining beverages

1. Introduction

Currently, patients seeking orthodontic treatment demand not only high-quality results, but also a comfortable and aesthetic treatment experience [1]. The patients' preference for esthetic dental treatments has led to the development of various orthodontic appliances that are as inconspicuous as possible and readily accepted by patients due to their clinical, esthetical and social comfort.

The recent improvements in computer-aided manufacturing/design (CAD/CAM) and the development of new dental materials have allowed the appearance of revolutionary orthodontic treatments [2]. These materials are composed of thermoplastic resin polymers such as polyvinyl chloride, polyethylene terephthalate, polyethylene terephthalate glycol and thermoplastic polyurethane [1,2].

The ideal orthodontic appliance has been described by Proffit et al.; therefore, it must be esthetic, lightweight, should not interfere with occlusion or hygiene, should not affect oral tissues, should be capable of withstanding masticatory forces, allow controlled forces to be applied between treatment sessions and provide good anchorage control [3]. The concept of transparent aligners was first introduced in 1946 as a tooth positioner manufactured by thermoplastic molding technology and used to generate minor tooth movements during the final stages of orthodontic treatment [4].

Although the initial main purpose of orthodontic therapy based on clear aligners was to address low and moderate dento-alveolar incongruence and to close small spaces, the technique has continuously evolved through the development of new materials used in the manufacture of aligners, dental attachments and special auxiliary systems, which now allow the approach of a wide range of malocclusions [1,4].

The color stability of aligners is crucial, as any discoloration may significantly affect their aesthetic value. Previous studies on thermoformed aligners have examined their resistance to staining in detail, attributing color stability to both material properties and manufacturing process [5,6]. Other research has shown that thermoformed aligners maintain their color when exposed to staining beverages such as coffee, tea and wine, due to the surface characteristics and chemical composition of the polyurethane [7].

However, through prolonged contact with acidic beverages, these materials might undergo surface wear, making them susceptible to discoloration. Also, an important role is played by the water absorption capacity of the materials, which leads to a hydrolytic degradation of the polymers, affecting the mechanical and aesthetic properties [8]. Moreover, the beverage temperature may cause the thermal expansion or contraction of these materials, increasing their susceptibility to deterioration and discoloration over time [9].

The current orthodontic therapy applied to both children and adults benefits from minimally invasive approaches as well as esthetic appliances, according to patients' requirements. Patients' current demands for a healthy smile have led to the development of new types of orthodontic appliances, such as invisible ones. In the last decade, orthodontic aligners have become more thin, transparent and comfortable to patients and at the same time, efficient in the therapy of several dento-maxillary anomalies [10].

In spite of their increasing popularity, investigations to assess the staining susceptibility of aligner materials are scarce [11]. Through this study, we propose to address this gap by following the behavior of aligners after a prolonged exposure to different coloring solutions. The study results will be likely to provide valuable insight on the durability and longevity of aligner materials under real-life conditions and offer guidance to clinicians and patients in taking decisions on the material selection and care of aligners.

The aim of this in vitro study was to compare the colorimetric changes in two materials used as transparent aligners after immersion for 14 days in different staining beverages (cola, coffee and red wine). Color measurements were performed after Days 1, 7 and 14. The null hypothesis of the study stated that no differences in the color of each of the two materials would be observed after submersion for 1, 7 and 14 days in red wine, cola and coffee solutions.

2. Materials and Methods

The study was conducted in accordance with the Declaration of Helsinki and the rules imposed by the Ethics Committee of "Grigore T. Popa" University of Medicine and Pharmacy of Iasi, Romania (Agreement No. 66/2021).

2.1. Sample Preparation

The sample size was calculated using G*Power software version 3.1. developed at the Heinrich-Heine University of Düsseldorf, Germany. An effect size of 0.5, an alpha value of 0.05 and a power of 0.8 were used. The obtained results indicated a minimum number of 34 samples to be used in the study.

A total of 56 samples were used to perform this study. The samples were divided into 2 groups corresponding to the material from which they were made. Each group was then divided into 4 subgroups corresponding to the immersion solution. The distribution of the samples into groups and subgroups is shown in Figure 1.

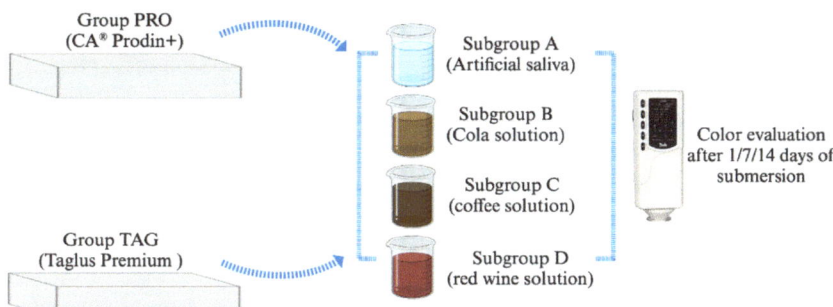

Figure 1. Study design and distribution of samples in groups and subgroups.

The samples in the TAG group (n = 28) made of the Taglus Premium system (Taglus Company, Mumbai, India) contained polyethylene terephthalate glycol, while samples in the PRO group (n = 28) made of the CA® Prodin+ system (SCHEU-DENTAL GmbH, Iserlohn, Germany) contained a transparent copolyester and a thermoplastic elastomer. The samples were realized by a thermoforming process using BIOSTAR® (SCHEU-DENTAL GmbH, Iserlohn, Germany) with a 3D-printed mold obtained with a SprintRay 3D printer (SprintRay GmbH, Weiterstadt, Germany), thus resulting rectangular samples of 10 mm length/10 mm width/0.75 mm height. The samples were then kept in distilled water at 37 °C for 24 h in a Biobase incubator (Biobase BJPXH30II, Biodusty, Jinan, China).

2.2. Submersion in Coloring Solutions

The samples were then submersed in the following coloring solutions: Subgroup A—AFNOR artificial saliva (Biochemazone™, Leduc, AB, Canada) considered as a control subgroup; and three study subgroups: Subgroup B—Pepsi Cola, (PepsiCo. Inc., New York, NY, USA), Subgroup C—coffee Nescafe Brasero (Nestle, Vevey, Switzerland) and Subgroup D—dry red wine, 13.5% alcohol by volume, Negru de Purcari 2015 (Purcari Winery, Purcari, Republic of Moldova). AFNOR artificial saliva was composed of NaCI 6.7 g/L, KCl 1.2 g/L, $NaHCO_3$ 1.5 g/L, NaH_2PO_4 H_2O 0.26 g/L, KSCN 0.33 g/L and urea 1.35 g/L. Instant coffee was prepared by dissolving 3.6 g of coffee in 300 mL hot distilled water and filtered after 10 min. Samples were immersed in solution for 14 days and stored in an incubator at 37 °C. The coloring solutions were changed every 24 h. The pH values of the tested solutions were the following: artificial saliva—7.4; cola solution—2.71; coffee solution—5.33; red wine solution—3.85. The pH value was evaluated every 24 h using a portable pH meter (Thermo Scientific Eutech pH 5+, Vernon Hills, IL, USA).

2.3. Color Evaluation

The CIE L*a*b* system was used to determine the color variation in each study sample using a Precision Colorimeter NR10QC spectrophotometer (3NH Technology Co., Ltd., Shenzhen, China) with manual calibration and a 0.3 mm focused light beam.

Measurements were performed after 1, 7 and 14 days of submersion in the staining solutions. Subsequently, the samples were washed of residual dyes with distilled water and dried with the water–air spray from the dental unit. For color determination, samples were placed on a white sheet of paper to avoid color absorption. L*, a* and b* values were determined by a single operator and repeated three times for each sample. The mean of the three measurements was the value assigned to the sample. The color variation was calculated using the following formula:

$\Delta E = [(\Delta L^*)^2 + (\Delta a^*)^2 + (\Delta b^*)^2]^{\frac{1}{2}}$ $\frac{1}{2}$ (11), where ΔE values represent the total color deviation, ΔL^* is the brightness deviation, Δa^* is the red–green axis deviation and Δb^* is the yellow–blue axis deviation. The values were calculated according to the following formulas [12,13]:

$$\Delta a^* = a^*T - a^*R \text{ (where T is the test solution; R the control solution—artificial saliva)}$$

$$\Delta b^* = b^*T - b^*R$$

$$\Delta L^* = L^*T - L^*R$$

2.4. Statistical Analysis

The obtained data were statistically analyzed using IBM SPSS software version 29.0.0. (IBM SPSS Inc., Chicago, IL, USA). The normality of data distribution was assessed using the Shapiro–Wilk test and the homogeneity of variances was verified with Levene's test, while the differences between the groups and subgroups were analyzed using ANOVA one-way and Tukey post-hoc tests, independent samples t tests and the Kruskal–Wallis test. The significance level was set at 0.05.

3. Results

In Figure 2, the mean values and standard deviations of the ΔL^* parameter within each study stage for the TAG and PRO groups are presented. It can be observed that in the TAG group, on Day 1 the highest value was recorded for the samples submersed in red wine solution (-1.28 ± 0.97), on Day 7 for the samples submersed in coffee solution (-1.52 ± 0.68) and on Day 14 also for the samples submersed in coffee (-2.73 ± 1.50). For the PRO group, on Day 1 the highest negative value was recorded for the samples submersed in red wine solution (-2.71 ± 1.26), on Day 7 for the samples submersed in red wine (-3.48 ± 1.82) and on Day 14 for the samples submersed in coffee (-4.52 ± 1.37).

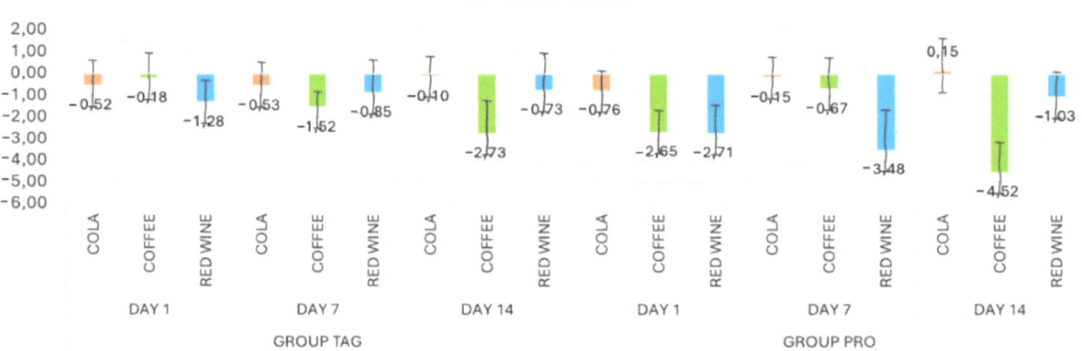

Figure 2. Mean values and standard deviations of the ΔL^* parameter within each study stage for the TAG and PRO groups.

Statistical analysis of the data within the TAG group shows that between the values obtained on Day 1 of submersion in coffee solution vs. Day 14 of submersion in the same solution, there were statistically significant differences in the parameter L* ($p = 0.002$). Within the PRO group, significant differences were recorded between the samples submersed in coffee solution for Day 1 vs. Day 7 ($p = 0.023$), Day 1 vs. Day 14 ($p = 0.033$) and Day 7 vs. Day 14 ($p < 0.00$), respectively, and between the samples submersed in red wine solution: Day 7 vs. Day 14 ($p = 0.004$).

In Figure 3, the mean values and standard deviations of the Δa^* parameter within each subgroup of both the TAG and PRO groups are presented. Within the TAG group, on Day 1 the highest value was recorded for the samples submersed in red wine solution (0.21 ± 0.25), on Day 7 for the samples submersed in wine (0.89 ± 0.22) and on Day 14 also for the samples submersed in red wine (1.54 ± 0.19). As for the PRO group, on Day 1 the highest value was recorded for the samples submersed in red wine solution (0.61 ± 0.51), on Day 7 also for the samples submersed in wine (1.67 ± 0.28) and on Day 14 for the samples submersed in coffee (0.96 ± 0.38).

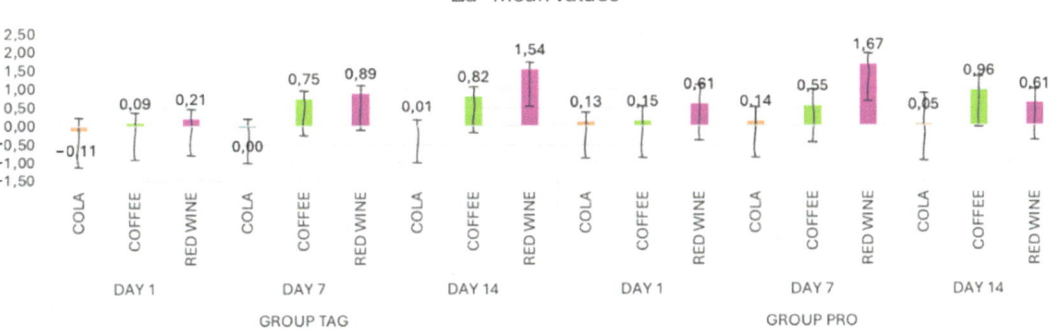

Figure 3. Mean values and standard deviations of the Δa* parameter within each study stage for the TAG and PRO groups.

Statistical analysis of the data within the TAG group shows that there were significant differences within the samples submersed in coffee between Day 1 vs. Day 7 ($p < 0.001$) and Day 1 vs. Day 14 ($p < 0.001$), and between the samples submersed in wine: Day 1 vs. Day 7 ($p = 0.029$) and Day 1 vs. Day 14 ($p < 0.001$). In the PRO group, significant differences were recorded between the values obtained on Day 1 vs. Day 14 for the samples submersed in coffee solution ($p = 0.016$).

When analyzing the mean values of the Δb* parameter (Figure 4) for the TAG group, it can be observed that on Day 1 the highest mean value was recorded for the samples submersed in coffee (0.86 ± 0.28), on Day 7 for the samples submersed in coffee (2.38 ± 0.23) and on Day 14 also for the samples submersed in coffee (4.01 ± 0.34). For the PRO group, on Day 1 the highest value was recorded for the samples submersed in wine (0.56 ± 0.07), on Day 7 for the samples submersed in coffee (0.98 ± 0.98) and on Day 14 for the samples submersed in coffee (0.67 ± 0.41).

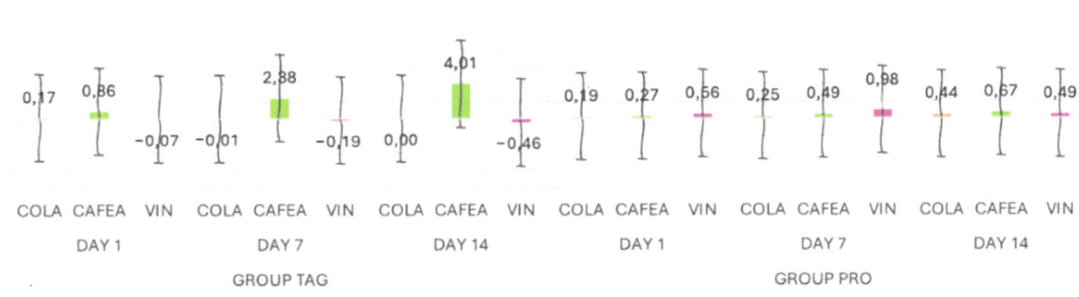

Figure 4. Mean values and standard deviations of the Δb* parameter within each study stage for the TAG and PRO groups.

The results of the statistical tests show that within the TAG group there were significant differences between the samples submersed in coffee on Day 1 vs. Day 7 ($p < 0.001$) and

Day 1 vs. Day 14 ($p < 0.001$). For the PRO group, statistically significant differences were obtained between Day 1 vs. Day 14 ($p = 0.00$) for the samples submersed in coffee solution.

In Table 1, the mean values and standard deviations of the ΔE values within each study stage for TAG group are presented. It can be noted that on Day 1 the highest value was recorded for the samples submersed in coffee (1.43 ± 0.83), on Day 7 for the samples submersed in wine (2.96 ± 0.52) and on Day 14 for the samples submersed in coffee (5.06 ± 0.87).

Table 1. Mean values, standard deviations of ΔE and statistically significant differences between groups.

	Day 1			Day 7			Day 14		
	Cola	Coffee	Red Wine	Cola	Coffee	Red Wine	Cola	Coffee	Red Wine
TAG Group	−0.52 ± 1.12	−0.18 ± 1.12	−1.28 ± 0.97	−0.53 ± 1.03	−1.52 ± 0.68	−0.85 ± 1.48	−0.10 ± 0.90	−2.73 ± 1.50	−0.73 ± 0.89
PRO Group	−0.76 ± 0.89	−2.65 ± 0.97	−2.71 ± 1.26	−0.15 ± 0.92	−0.67 ± 1.41	−3.48 ± 1.82	0.15 ± 1.48	−4.52 ± 1.37	−1.03 ± 1.11
p values	**	* 0.003	* 0.015	**	**	* 0.004	* 0.025	* 0.005	* 0.041

* Statistically significant differences. ** Statistically non-significant differences.

Within the PRO group, the highest ΔE value on Day 1 was recorded for the samples submersed in wine (2.91 ± 1.11), on Day 7 for the samples submersed in wine (4.03 ± 1.49) and on Day 14 for the samples submersed in coffee (6.86 ± 0.66).

In Figure 5, box-plot graph is used to illustrate the distribution of the ΔE values of each group and subgroup by the end of each test day. The results of the statistical tests showed significant differences within the TAG group between the samples submersed in coffee on Day 1 vs. Day 7 ($p < 0.001$), Day 1 vs. Day 14 ($p < 0.001$) and Day 7 vs. Day 14 ($p < 0.001$). For the PRO group, statistically significant differences were obtained between the samples submersed in coffee solution between the values recorded on Day 1 vs. Day 14 ($p < 0.001$) and Day 7 vs. Day 14 ($p < 0.001$), and between the samples submersed in wine solution: Day 7 vs. Day 14 ($p = 0.002$).

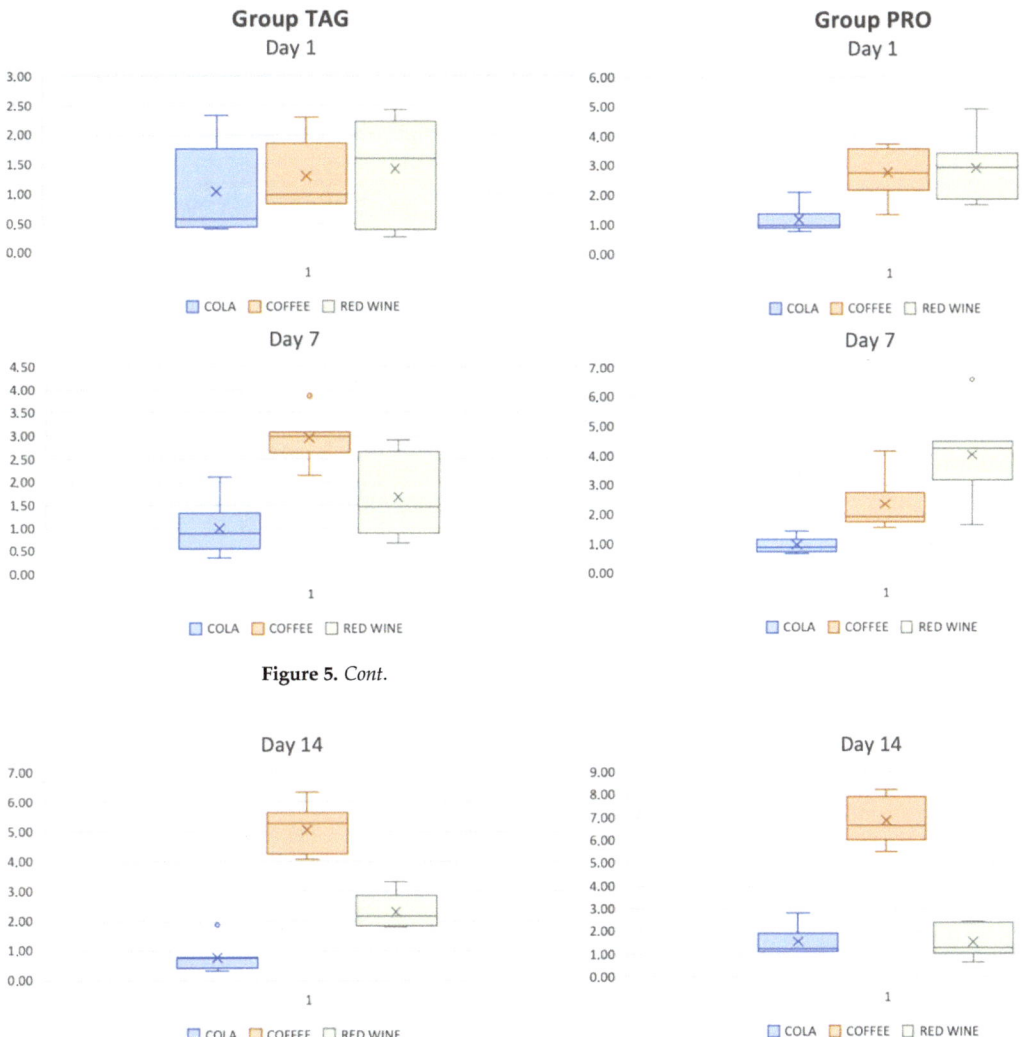

Figure 5. Box-plot representation of the distribution of ΔE values of each group and subgroup on each test day.

Comparative statistical analysis of the ΔE values of the two tested materials showed differences between the values recorded for the samples submersed for 1 day in coffee solution ($p = 0.003$) and in wine ($p = 0.015$), and for those submersed for 7 days in wine solution ($p = 0.004$) and for the samples submersed for 14 days in cola solution ($p = 0.025$), coffee ($p = 0.005$) and wine ($p = 0.041$).

4. Discussion

This in vitro study is of significant applicability in clinical practice, as orthodontic therapy with aligners is increasingly used due to their esthetic and clinical advantages [14]. Most of the currently used aligners are thermoplastic polymers, polyurethanes and polyesters, such as those based on polyethylene terephthalate glycol [15].

Aligners are made of amorphous polymers such as polyurethane, polycarbonate and polyethylene terephthalate glycol that benefit from a highly transparent appearance, all three types of materials being widely used in dentistry, especially in orthodontics, due to their superior mechanical and aesthetic properties [9].

Polyurethane has excellent mechanical properties such as elasticity, flexibility, chemical resistance and ease of processing. These properties make it ideal for use in various dental appliances such as bruxism mouth guards, prosthodontic bases and other orthodontic appliances requiring flexibility and durability [16].

Polycarbonate is widely used in orthodontic appliances such as esthetic brackets and clear aligners because of its excellent optical, physical and chemical characteristics. Polycarbonate is preferred in dentistry because of its transparency, making it esthetically attractive to patients, as well as its impact resistance, thus ensuring durability in use [17].

Polyethylene terephthalate glycol (PET-G) is an amorphous co-polymer of PET that does not crystallize and is a relatively hard material with good mechanical properties, wear resistance and dimensional stability. In dentistry, it is commonly used to produce transparent aligners due to its resistance to deformation and ability to maintain a precise shape in the long term [16,18]. Although they are biocompatible materials, they still have some disadvantages related to dimensional instability, low resistance to wear and chewing forces, but also a change in esthetic properties determined by the absorption of water and of food colorants [6]. The polyethylene terephthalate glycol aligners are maintained in the oral cavity for a period of about 14 days, after which the clinical situation is assessed, and they are replaced with others until the final result is obtained. During this period, the food and drinks consumed by patients may lead to a loss of transparency. This phenomenon is explained by an increase in water absorption that may lead to the adsorption of food pigments [6,16].

In a study conducted in 2016 in which aligners made of different materials were tested and immersed for 14 days in coffee, black tea and red wine solutions, a higher color change was obtained in polyurethane aligners compared to polycarbonate or polyethylene terephthalate glycol. The authors explained the results by stating that the polyurethane material adsorbs pigments from colored beverages more than the other materials, because its water absorption capacity is higher and thus entrains the pigments in coffee and tea in particular. The roughness of the materials submersed in the three tested solutions was also analyzed in that study, and the authors observed that the same polyurethane material exhibited a rougher surface; thus, the surface condition of the materials may play an important role in enhancing the coloration [6].

Also, the pigmentation of the aligners may be influenced by the acidity of the food or drink ingested by the patients, the frequency of their consumption and the time they are kept in contact with the staining factors [19]. Our study consisted of the colorimetric evaluation after 1, 7 and 14 days of two new generation materials, composed of polyethylene terephthalate glycol and thermoplastic copolyesters and elastoplastic, which were immersed in different colored beverages (coffee, red wine and cola). The manufacturers of the polyurethane aligners recommend that patients not consume colored food or beverages while wearing the appliances.

The Taglus Premium material showed more pronounced changes in mean ΔL^* values in samples submersed in red wine solution (-1.28 ± 0.97), followed by cola (-0.52 ± 1.12) and coffee (-0.18 ± 1.12). In contrast, in the CA® Pro+ material, the changes in transparency after one day were higher for samples soaked in wine (-2.71 ± 1.26), followed by coffee (-2.65 ± 0.97) and cola (-0.76 ± 0.89).

Polyethylene terephthalate glycol materials did not show significant changes in transparency after one day of contact with staining solutions, due to their stable chemical composition and resistance to wear and chemical degradation in the oral environment [20]. The higher colorimetric values obtained for the CA® Pro+ material can be explained by its water absorption capacity of 0.13% over 24 h, at a constant temperature of 23 °C. However, the samples evaluated by us were kept during the tests in an incubator at 37 °C, simulating the normal temperature in the oral cavity. The ΔE parameter, which represents the total color deviation, recorded the highest value on Day 1 for the samples submersed in coffee solution (1.43 ± 0.83), on Day 7 for the samples submersed in wine (2.96 ± 0.52) and on Day 14 for those submersed in coffee (1.24 ± 0.83). Our obtained results showed that the CA® Pro+ material is more prone to staining compared to Taglus Premium after submersion for 1 day in coffee solution, while in red wine solution it showed significant changes for the whole tested period. Submersion for 14 days in coffee solution alters all of the color parameters (ΔL*, Δa*, Δb* and ΔE*) of both tested materials.

These results agree with another in vitro study which showed that polymers presented changes in transparency after 7 days of soaking in colored beverages [14]. The results of other studies have shown that thermomolding affects the transparency of the thicker material, decreasing it and increasing the water absorption properties, but may also alter the surface hardness. Thus, previous research also suggests that the thermomolding process decreases the thickness of the aligners compared to the initial size of the thermoplastic foil [21]. Specific conditions in the oral cavity, related to the salivary environment such as salivary enzymes, pH, temperature and the bacterial environment may negatively affect aligner transparency maintenance throughout the treatment.

Polyurethanes are susceptible to degradation over time through exposure to light, heat, moisture and enzymes. They can also exhibit oxidative degradation and absorb water if used for longer periods of time, leading to changes in physical and aesthetic properties [22]. The same conclusion as ours was reached by other studies that examined polyethylene terephthalate glycol or copolyester-based materials, stating that these materials compared to polyurethanes do not markedly change their transparency after submersion in staining beverages [11,23].

Three-dimensionally printed thermoplastic materials used as aligners can have acrylonitrile-butadiene-styrene, epoxy resins, polylactic acid, polyamide, glass-filled polyamide, silver, steel, titanium, photopolymers, wax and polycarbonate in their composition. Their choice is based on their excellent characteristics, which are essential for obtaining the desired clinical results and perfect adaptation to the teeth [9]. Their production process may influence the final thickness of the aligners, negatively affecting them if they are created by 3D printing, although this process is time-saving and produces stronger and more elastic aligners compared to conventionally thermoformed ones [17,24]. Other authors have stated that the variations in thickness do not affect the clinical efficiency and the thermoforming process does not alter the active or passive configurations of these appliances [25,26].

The colorimetric variation in the aligners tested in our study can be explained by the fact that the tested dry red wine contained a variety of pigments, the most relevant of which are anthocyanins and tannins. Anthocyanins are the main pigments that confer red wine with its distinctive color. Anthocyanins are flavonoids and can range in color from red to blue, depending on the wine's pH. Tannins, on the other hand, contribute to the structure and color of red wine. They play a role in wine color stability by interacting with anthocyanins and form polymerized pigments that are responsible for a more stable and deeper color of red wine as it ages. Other pigments are flavonols, such as quercetin and kaempferol, which although less abundant, contribute to the color and antioxidant characteristics of the wine. Overall, the combination of these pigments and their complex interactions confer an unique color and chromatic stability to dry red wine [13,27].

Coffee contains slow-release low-polarity yellow pigments that penetrate organic substrates. Therefore, significant changes were observed in both groups for the samples submersed in coffee for 1 day, these results being in agreement with other studies [6,19].

The other tested staining solution was Pepsi Cola that contains caramel as the main colorant. This is an artificial pigment obtained by heating sugar and is often used in carbonated drinks to confer the characteristic brown color. The pigment-impregnating capacity of the solutions in the study is also determined by their pH value. The increased acidity of the solutions may lead to surface changes in the tested materials by producing chemical and physical alterations of the surface through acid wear [20,28,29]. Both pigments and the pH of the solutions play a major role in the color changes in the materials used for alignment [30]. The pigments in coffee, tannins in red wine, or caramel in cola drinks adhere easily to the surface of clear aligners producing visible color changes. On the other hand, an acidic environment may increase the susceptibility to staining due to altered properties and an enhanced surface roughness of the material that attracts the retention of colorants. Thus, pigments color the surfaces whereas the presence of an acidic pH enhances the coloring effect [30,31].

The results of our in vitro study demonstrated that the inappropriate use of aligners during mealtimes can lead to a loss of transparency, as colorants in food and beverages can affect the color stability of thermoplastic materials [20,32]. Thus, orthodontists should advise patients who are concerned about esthetics to be aware of the possibility of visible changes in the color of aligners during use, these changes being closely related to their diet, hygiene habits and the fact that they have to remove these devices from their oral cavity during meals [12,19,33–35].

The results of the study reject the null hypothesis that there are no statistically significant differences between the two study materials submersed in the coloring solutions during the evaluation period. The limitations of the conducted study were that we evaluated only two materials from the same category of transparent aligners, namely polyethylene terephthalate glycol, at the same thickness of 0.75 mm and we did not use models on the teeth, which by their shape may influence the results of the physical and chemical tests.

However, to justify the conclusions of the study, further in vitro and in vivo studies are needed using other evaluation methods, such as scaling electron microscopy, microhardness and wear resistance analysis of these materials after immersion in colored solutions, to validate the results obtained.

For greater clinical relevance, future in vitro studies should be able to reproduce oral environmental conditions, such as temperature and pH variations, enzymatic and microbial activity and the mechanics of masticatory movements.

5. Conclusions

The CA® Pro+ aligner system is more prone to staining compared to the Taglus material after submersion for 14 days in cola, coffee and red wine solutions.

Submersion for 14 days in coffee solution alters all of the color parameters (ΔL, Δa, Δb and ΔE) of the CA® Pro+ and Taglus Premium aligner systems.

Immersion for 1, 7 or 14 days in red wine solution induced differences in the color stability of the two tested materials.

In order to obtain optimal esthetic results during the treatment period, which is usually 14 days, patients must follow the orthodontists' instructions regarding diet, the consumption of coloring beverages and oral hygiene.

Author Contributions: Conceptualization, N.D.O., R.M.V. and I.N.Z.; methodology, T.P. and C.B.; software, I.T.; validation, I.T., N.D.O. and I.N.Z.; formal analysis, S.N.R.; investigation, N.D.O. and I.T.; resources, N.D.O. and I.N.Z.; data curation, I.T. and C.B.; writing—original draft preparation, N.D.O. and I.T.; writing—review and editing, I.N.Z., S.D., R.M.V., T.P. and C.B.; visualization, S.N.R. and S.D.; supervision, I.N.Z.; project administration, N.D.O.; funding acquisition, N.D.O. All authors have read and agreed to the published version of the manuscript.

Funding: This research received no external funding.

Institutional Review Board Statement: Not applicable.

Informed Consent Statement: Not applicable.

Data Availability Statement: The data presented in this study are available from the corresponding author upon reasonable request.

Conflicts of Interest: The authors declare no conflicts of interest.

References

1. Tsai, M.H.; Chen, S.S.H.; Chen, Y.J.; Yao, J.C.C. Treatment Efficacy of Invisalign: Literature Review Update. *Taiwan. J. Orthod.* **2020**, *32*, 1. [CrossRef]

2. Alassiry, A.M. Orthodontic Retainers: A Contemporary Overview. *J. Contemp. Dent. Pract.* **2019**, *20*, 857–862. [PubMed]
3. Proffit, W.R. *Contemporary Orthodontics*; Elsevier: Toronto, ON, Canada, 2013.
4. Graber, T.M. *Orthodontics: Current Principles and Techniques in Clear Aligner Treatment*; Paquette, D., Colville, C., Wheeler, T., Eds.; Mosby: St. Louis, MO, USA, 2012; Volume 1.
5. Lai, Y.L.; Lui, H.F.; Lee, S.Y. In vitro color stability, stain resistance, and water sorption of four removable gingival flange materials. *J. Prosthet. Dent.* **2003**, *90*, 293–300. [CrossRef] [PubMed]
6. Liu, C.L.; Sun, W.T.; Liao, W.; Lu, W.X.; Li, Q.W.; Jeong, Y.; Liu, J.; Zhao, Z.-H. Colour stabilities of three types of orthodontic clear aligners exposed to staining agents. *Int. J. Oral Sci.* **2016**, *8*, 246–253. [CrossRef] [PubMed]
7. Timm, L.H.; Rößler, R.; Baxmann, M. Comparison of Clear Aligner Treatment in First-Treatment and Re-Treatment Patients: A Retrospective Cohort Study. *Appl. Sci.* **2023**, *13*, 4303. [CrossRef]
8. Alharbi, N.; Alharbi, A.; Osman, R. Stain Susceptibility of 3D-Printed Nanohybrid Composite Restorative Material and the Efficacy of Different Stain Removal Techniques: An In Vitro Study. *Materials* **2021**, *14*, 5621. [CrossRef] [PubMed]
9. Tartaglia, G.M.; Mapelli, A.; Maspero, C.; Santaniello, T.; Serafin, M.; Farronato, M.; Caprioglio, A. Direct 3D Printing of Clear Orthodontic Aligners: Current State and Future Possibilities. *Materials* **2021**, *14*, 1799. [CrossRef] [PubMed]
10. Venkatasubramanian, P.; Jerome, M.S.; Ragunanthanan, L.; Maheshwari, U.; Vijayalakshmi, D. Color stability of aligner materials on exposure to indigenous food products: An in-vitro study. *J. Dent. Res. Dent. Clin. Dent. Prospect.* **2022**, *16*, 221–228. [CrossRef] [PubMed]
11. Al-Angari, S.S.; Eckert, G.J.; Sabrah, A.H.A. Color stability, Roughness, and Microhardness of Enamel and Composites Submitted to Staining/Bleaching Cycles. *Saudi Dent. J.* **2021**, *33*, 215–221. [CrossRef]
12. Assaf, C.; Abou Samra, P.; Nahas, P. Discoloration of Resin Composites Induced by Coffee and Tomato Sauce and Subjected to Surface Polishing: An In Vitro Study. *Med. Sci. Monit. Basic Res.* **2020**, *26*, e923279-1–e923279-7. [CrossRef] [PubMed]
13. Pérez, M.d.M.; Saleh, A.; Yebra, A.; Pulgar, R. Study of the Variation between CIELAB.DELTA.E* and CIEDE2000 Color-differences of Resin Composites. *Dent. Mater. J.* **2007**, *26*, 21–28. [CrossRef]
14. Daniele, V.; Macera, L.; Taglieri, G.; Spera, L.; Marzo, G.; Quinzi, V. Color Stability, Chemico-Physical and Optical Features of the Most Common PETG and PU Based Orthodontic Aligners for Clear Aligner Therapy. *Polymers* **2021**, *14*, 14. [CrossRef] [PubMed]
15. Zhang, N.; Bai, Y.; Ding, X.; Zhang, Y. Preparation and characterization of thermoplastic materials for invisible orthodontics. *Dent. Mater. J.* **2011**, *30*, 954–959. [CrossRef] [PubMed]
16. Lombardo, L.; Martines, E.; Mazzanti, V.; Arreghini, A.; Mollica, F.; Siciliani, G. Stress relaxation properties of four orthodontic aligner materials: A 24-hour in vitro study. *Angle Orthod.* **2016**, *87*, 11–18. [CrossRef] [PubMed]
17. Jindal, P.; Worcester, F.; Siena, F.L.; Forbes, C.; Juneja, M.; Breedon, P. Mechanical behaviour of 3D printed vs thermoformed clear dental aligner materials under non-linear compressive loading using FEM. *J. Mech. Behav. Biomed. Mater.* **2020**, *112*, 104045. [CrossRef] [PubMed]
18. Hamanaka, I.; Iwamoto, M.; Lassila, L.; Vallittu, P.; Shimizu, H.; Takahashi, Y. Influence of water sorption on mechanical properties of injection-molded thermoplastic denture base resins. *Acta Odontol. Scand.* **2014**, *72*, 859–865. [CrossRef] [PubMed]
19. Oliveira, C.B.d.; Maia, L.G.M.; Santos-Pinto, A.; Gandini Júnior, L.G. In vitro study of color stability of polycrystalline and monocrystalline ceramic brackets. *Dent. Press. J. Orthod.* **2014**, *19*, 114–121. [CrossRef] [PubMed]
20. Bernard, G.; Rompré, P.; Tavares, J.R.; Montpetit, A. Colorimetric and spectrophotometric measurements of orthodontic thermoplastic aligners exposed to various staining sources and cleaning methods. *Head Face Med.* **2020**, *16*, 2. [CrossRef] [PubMed]
21. Ryu, J.H.; Kwon, J.S.; Jiang, H.B.; Cha, J.Y.; Kim, K.M. Effects of thermoforming on the physical and mechanical properties of thermoplastic materials for transparent orthodontic aligners. *Korean J. Orthod.* **2018**, *48*, 316. [CrossRef] [PubMed]
22. Agarwal, M.; Wible, E.; Ramir, T.; Altun, S.; Viana, G.; Evans, C.; Lukic, H.; Megremis, S.; Atsawasuwan, P. Long-term effects of seven cleaning methods on light transmittance, surface roughness, and flexural modulus of polyurethane retainer material. *Angle Orthod.* **2018**, *88*, 355–362. [CrossRef] [PubMed]
23. Aldweesh, A.H.; Al-Maflehi, N.S.; AlGhizzi, M.; AlShayea, E.; Albarakati, S.F. Comparison of mechanical properties and color stability of various vacuum-formed orthodontic retainers: An in vitro study. *Saudi Dent. J.* **2023**, *35*, 953–959. [CrossRef] [PubMed]
24. Edelmann, A.; English, J.D.; Chen, S.J.; Kasper, F.K. Analysis of the thickness of 3-dimensional-printed orthodontic aligners. *Am. J. Orthod. Dentofac. Orthop.* **2020**, *158*, e91–e98. [CrossRef] [PubMed]
25. Yadav, R.; Saini, S.; Sonwal, S.; Meena, A.; Huh, Y.S.; Brambilla, E.; Ionescu, A.C. Optimization and ranking of dental restorative composites by ENTROPY-VIKOR and VIKOR-MATLAB. *Polym. Adv. Technol.* **2024**, *35*, e6526. [CrossRef]
26. Iliadi, A.; Koletsi, D.; Eliades, T. Forces and moments generated by aligner-type appliances for orthodontic tooth movement: A systematic review and meta-analysis. *Orthod. Craniofac. Res.* **2019**, *22*, 248–258. [CrossRef] [PubMed]
27. Taraboanta, I.; Pancu, G.; Ghiorghe, C.A.; Topoliceanu, C.; Nica, I.; Gamen, A.C.; Iovan, A.; Andrian, S. Evaluation of some exogenous colorants effects on resin based materials used in incipient caries lesions therapy. *Mater. Plast.* **2019**, *56*, 629–634. [CrossRef]
28. Papadopoulou, A.K.; Cantele, A.; Polychronis, G.; Zinelis, S.; Eliades, T. Changes in Roughness and Mechanical Properties of Invisalign® Appliances after One- and Two-Weeks Use. *Materials* **2019**, *12*, 2406. [CrossRef] [PubMed]
29. Kim, S.H.; Lee, Y.K. Measurement of discolouration of orthodontic elastomeric modules with a digital camera. *Eur. J. Orthod.* **2009**, *31*, 556–562. [CrossRef] [PubMed]

30. Villalta, P.; Lu, H.; Okte, Z.; Garcia-Godoy, F.; Powers, J.M. Effects of staining and bleaching on color change of dental composite resins. *J. Prosthet. Dent.* **2006**, *95*, 137–142. [CrossRef] [PubMed]
31. Imirzalioglu, P.; Karanca, B.; Yilmaz, B. The effect of surface treatments on the color of composite resins. *J. Esthet. Restor. Dent.* **2012**, *24*, 373–379.
32. Memè, L.; Notarstefano, V.; Sampalmieri, F.; Orilisi, G.; Quinzi, V. ATR-FTIR Analysis of Orthodontic Invisalign® Aligners Subjected to Various In Vitro Aging Treatments. *Materials* **2021**, *14*, 818. [CrossRef] [PubMed]
33. Saini, S.; Yadav, R.; Sonwal, S.; Meena, A.; Huh, Y.S.; Brambilla, E.; Ionescu, A.C. Tribological, mechanical, and thermal properties of nano tricalcium phosphate and silver particulates reinforced Bis-GMA/TEGDMA dental resin composites. *Tribol. Int.* **2024**, *199*, 110010. [CrossRef]
34. Mitchell, D.C.; Knight, C.A.; Hockenberry, J.; Teplansky, R.; Hartman, T.J. Beverage caffeine intakes in the U.S. *Food Chem. Toxicol.* **2014**, *63*, 136–142. [CrossRef] [PubMed]
35. Charavet, C.; Gourdain, Z.; Graveline, L.; Lupi, L. Cleaning and Disinfection Protocols for Clear Orthodontic Aligners: A Systematic Review. *Healthcare* **2022**, *10*, 340. [CrossRef] [PubMed]

Disclaimer/Publisher's Note: The statements, opinions and data contained in all publications are solely those of the individual author(s) and contributor(s) and not of MDPI and/or the editor(s). MDPI and/or the editor(s) disclaim responsibility for any injury to people or property resulting from any ideas, methods, instructions or products referred to in the content.

Stress Distribution within the Peri-Implant Bone for Different Implant Materials Obtained by Digital Image Correlation

Ragai Edward Matta [1,*], Lara Berger [1], Moritz Loehlein [1], Linus Leven [1], Juergen Taxis [2], Manfred Wichmann [1] and Constantin Motel [1]

1. Dental Clinic 2-Dental Prosthodontics, University Hospital Erlangen, Glueckstrasse 11, 91054 Erlangen, Germany; lara.berger@uk-erlangen.de (L.B.); msl98@gmx.de (M.L.); linus_leven@yahoo.de (L.L.); claudia.ehrhardt@uk-erlangen.de (M.W.); constantin.motel@uk-erlangen.de (C.M.)
2. Clinic for Oro- and Maxillofacial Surgery, University hospital Regensburg, Franz-Josef-Strauß-Allee 11, 93053 Regensburg, Germany; juergen.taxis@ukr.de
* Correspondence: ragai.matta@uk-erlagen.de

Abstract: Stress distribution and its magnitude during loading heavily influence the osseointegration of dental implants. Currently, no high-resolution, three-dimensional method of directly measuring these biomechanical processes in the peri-implant bone is available. The aim of this study was to measure the influence of different implant materials on stress distribution in the peri-implant bone. Using the three-dimensional ARAMIS camera system, surface strain in the peri-implant bone area was compared under simulated masticatory forces of 300 N in axial and non-axial directions for titanium implants and zirconia implants. The investigated titanium implants led to a more homogeneous stress distribution than the investigated zirconia implants. Non-axial forces led to greater surface strain on the peri-implant bone than axial forces. Thus, the implant material, implant system, and direction of force could have a significant influence on biomechanical processes and osseointegration within the peri-implant bone.

Keywords: dental implants; implant biomechanics; peri-implant stress distribution; implant materials; implant loading; optical measurement

1. Introduction

The replacement of missing teeth with osseointegrated dental implants has been an established dental procedure since the late 1960s [1]. With the ever-increasing interest and innovations in the field of treatment planning and implementation, research in the field of biological–mechanical relationships is progressing [2]. The mechanical tension that acts at the junction of dental implants and peri-implant bone can lead to micromovements of the dental implants and is considered to influence osseointegration [3–5]. This aspect belongs to the broad field of dental biomechanics, the understanding and influence of which are of great importance for the long-term success of dental implants [6]. The transmission of force from implant to bone and, thus, the mechanical stress at the implant–bone junction depend on the direction of the applied force (axial vs. non-axial), the length and diameter of the implant, the design of the junction, and the quality of the bone [7–10]. Several different implant materials are currently being scientifically investigated or already in clinical use. The most common are titanium and zirconium oxide ceramic (zirconia) [11]. Titanium is the gold standard, as it is by far the best-studied implant material since its first use in the late 1960s [1,12,13]. Its advantages are excellent biocompatibility and well-studied and predictable osseointegration [14–16]. In addition, due to the very widespread use of dental titanium implants in dental practice, many different implant systems are available, which can be flexibly selected according to the patient's situation [17]. The disadvantages include limited esthetics, particularly in the case of a high smile line with exposed implant shoulders, such as in the case of soft tissue loss or a very thin mucosa through which titanium implants can show [18]. Furthermore, the modulus of elasticity of titanium (~110 GPa) is significantly higher than that of cortical bone, which has a modulus of elasticity of ~13 GPa [19,20]. Over the last 15 years, zirconia has become established as an implant material [21]. This material also offers very good biocompatibility, and the absence of a microgap in one-piece zirconia implants is also seen as an advantage, in conjunction with reduced biofilm [22]. With the exception of very thin mucosal layers, Jung et al. found no color difference in the area of the gingival margin after implantation of zirconia implants in the porcine jaw [18]. In contrast, exposed portions of zirconia implants can lead to esthetically unsatisfactory results due to the appearance of an unnatural coloration in the event of mucosal recession [23]. Another disadvantage for a long time was that zirconia dental implants were mostly manufactured in one piece (i.e., the implant–abutment complex consisted of a single workpiece). This means that the possibility to individualize implant therapy was low. In a regular case, it was only possible to choose from differently configured, prefabricated implant–abutment complexes [24,25]. Two-piece implant systems made of zirconia are now also available [26]. Another disadvantage of zirconia implants is their extremely high modulus of elasticity (~210 GPa) relative to the modulus of elasticity of bone [27]. Therefore, this implant material could lead to high stress peaks in the peri-implant bone [28]. In addition, zirconia implants were established in the dental field only a few years ago and are not as well studied as titanium implants. Little is currently known about the influence of different implant materials on the stress distribution in the peri-implant area under masticatory loading. Studies simulated the stress distribution in this area using the finite element method in a three-dimensional computer model, but this procedure is subjected to the limitation of the mathematical simplification of virtual test models [29]. The direct, three-dimensional measurement of stress distribution on the peri-implant bone under simulated masticatory force application was established for the first time by this working group. Surface changes during measurement by the ARAMIS system from Carl Zeiss GOM Metrology GmbH (Braunschweig, Germany) under masticatory loading correspond to the accuracy of strain gauges [30]. The aim of the present study was to investigate the influence of different implant materials, specifically, titanium and zirconia, on stress distribution in the porcine jaw. For this purpose, zirconia implants and titanium implants were loaded axially with masticatory forces of 300 N at an angle of 30° and the deformation of the bone surface was detected using the ARAMIS system. As null hypotheses, we assumed that the implant material and the masticatory force direction had no influence on stress distribution in the peri-implant bone under masticatory loading.

2. Materials and Methods

Five pieces of bone were prepared from the dorsal ramus region of five pig mandibles and embedded in plaster (Fujirock®, super hard stone type 4, GC Europe N.V., Leuwen, Belgium). It was necessary to keep the sample size as small as possible, as the porcine mandibles available for scientific use were limited. The relatively small sample size of 5 specimens allowed for a meaningful statistical evaluation in this context. Due to the nature of porcine bone, there were individual differences in the shape of the bone pieces, which were approximately 8 cm wide and 6 cm high. The drill studs for the two implants examined in each piece of bone (titanium: bone-level implant, diameter 4.1 mm, length 10 mm; zirconia: ceramic implant monotype, diameter 4.1 mm RD, length 10 mm; Straumann GmbH, Freiburg, Germany) were prepared according to the supplier's instructions. Regarding the bone dimension around the implant after insertion, it varied individually. Typically, approximately 1 mm of bone remained buccally and orally around the implant site. These variations reflect the natural variability in the bone structure. The bone surface was then sprayed with an acrylic resin-based varnish (Sparvar color spray, Spray-Color GmbH, Merzenich, Germany) and a graphite varnish (CRC Industries Deutschland GmbH, Iffezheim, Germany) to create a stochastic contrast pattern. For both implant types examined, five implants were inserted individually into one bone block each and loaded by a compression testing machine (inspekt mini, Hegewald & Peschke Mess- und Prüftechnik GmbH, Nossen, Germany) with a 300 N force in two different directions (0°, "axial" and 30°, "non-axial"). The sample size of five implants per implant type was chosen deliberately. This number allowed statistical comparisons to be made with confidence, as it met the requirement for meaningful statistical analysis. For the titanium implants, insertion posts were inserted and screwed into place to support the masticatory load. The zirconia implants were a one-piece implant system. In the 0° test series, the force was applied in the direction of the longitudinal axis of the implant. In the 30° test series, the force was applied with an inclination of 30° with respect to the longitudinal axis of the implant (Figure 1a,b). The strain on the surface of the bone caused by the load on the implants was measured using the ARAMIS 3D optical camera system (Carl Zeiss GOM Metrology GmbH, Braunschweig, Germany), a non-contact optical three-dimensional deformation measurement system that is able to analyze movements and deformations through digital image correlation [31]. The displacement was calculated by assigning gray value distributions in the deformed image to gray value distributions in the undeformed reference image. The ARAMIS system was positioned orthogonally to the course of the examined bone. The calibration and distance between the peri-implant measurement area and the lenses of the ARAMIS system corresponded to the manufacturer's specifications. The ARAMIS Professional software Version 2020 (Carl Zeiss GOM Metrology GmbH, Braunschweig, Germany) was used to examine the technical strain in the X and Y directions, as well as the main deformation. In the study, the X-axis corresponded to the mesio-distal orientation, whereby the left side in the test arrangement was defined as mesial. Accordingly, the force was applied in the 30° test series from a distal direction. The Y-axis corresponded to the corono-apical dimension. Figure 1c,d show the visual surface representation using the ARAMIS system without force application and, therefore, without deformation (plain blue region of interest in Figure 1d). An exemplary visual evaluation with force application of 300 N is presented in Figure 1e,f.

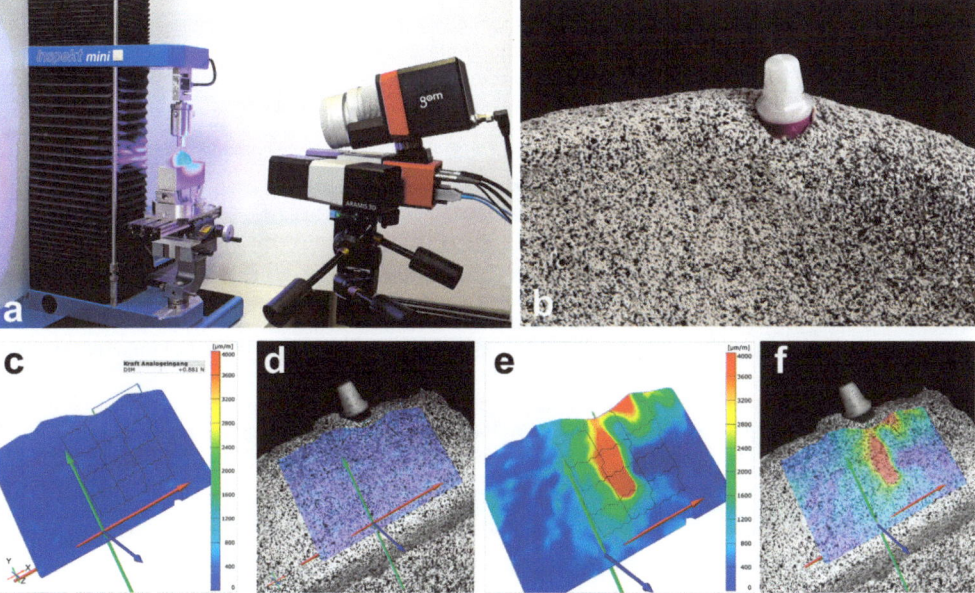

Figure 1. Overview of the experimental setup and presentation of the computer-aided evaluation in the study presented. (**a**) Experimental setup with the prepared bone, inserted implant, universal power machine on the left and ARAMIS camera system on the right (consisting of two cameras and

a blue light lamp); (**b**) macrograph of the bone preparation with an inserted zirconia implant and a stochastic contrast pattern; (**c**,**d**) exemplary representation of the ARAMIS Professional software without force application (test setup with force direction of 30°); (**e**,**f**) exemplary representation of the ARAMIS Professional software with force application of 300 N (test setup with force direction of 30°, changes in shape in green, yellow, and red).

The numerical evaluation was carried out in the form of absolute measured values using raw data tables from the ARAMIS Professional software, which were transferred to Excel (Microsoft Corporation, Redmond, WA, USA). To differentiate the strain distribution, the peri-implant bone was divided into a total of 12 equally sized areas, which were arranged in four three-part rows. The dimensions resulted from the macro design of the implant. The width of each area was the same as the individual implant diameter, while the length of the area was one-third of the implant's individual length. One row of measurement areas was added at the implant's apex. The described arrangement led to four measurement areas on the left (a,d,g,j), right (c,f,i,l), and in a projection (b,e,h,k) of the implants examined. The measurement areas b, e, and h reflect the projection of the implant on the surface of the bone. The areas j,k,l represent the area at the implant's apex. To enable statistical comparisons between the implant types, the deflection values were averaged within the specified measurement areas. The mean values are presented descriptively for the two implant types, separated by force and loading direction, and were compared non-parametrically between the implant types using single-factor analysis of variance (ANOVA) for statistical analysis. In addition, the percentage distribution of the fields with the highest deflection in terms of an averaged normalized relative deflection per field is presented graphically for both implant types and both force directions in relation to each individual implant position.

3. Results

The comparison of surface deformation of the peri-implant bone under axial loading showed a significantly greater main deformation when a force of 300 N was applied on the zirconia implant; the same applied to the deformation in the X and Y directions (more precisely). The titanium implant showed an average main deformation of 198.38 μm/m, a deformation of 336.02 μm/m in the X-axis, and a deformation of 320.90 μm/m in the Y-axis. The main deformation of the peri-implant bone with the zirconia implant amounted to 898.95 μm/m. The deformation in the X-axis was 471.83 μm/m, and that in the Y-axis 654.69 μm/m. The overall descriptive statistics are shown in Table 1. Figure 2 shows the data in the form of a box–whisker plot. When loading was applied at an angle of 30° to the longitudinal axis of the implant, a significantly greater change in the main shape was observed in the area of the peri-implant bone with the zirconia implant. There were also significantly greater changes in shape in the X and Y directions. In this case, the titanium implant was associated with in a main deformation of 720.77 μm/m, with a deformation of 501.09 μm/m in the X-axis and 475.05 μm/m in the Y-axis. For the zirconia implant, the main deformation was 1601.46 μm/m, with a deformation of 906.31 μm/m in the X-axis and 1095.38 μm/m in the Y-axis. The descriptive statistics regarding the force application at an angle of 30° can also be found in Table 1, and the graphical representation in Figure 2. Table 2 provides the p-values from the non-parametric analyses of variance.

To illustrate the results, Figures 3–5 show the percentage shape change in relation to the peri-implant measurement areas for the axial and non-axial examinations, respectively. This is the percentage of the average change in shape over the individual test series in relation to the largest change in shape within the test series. For example, a change in shape of 0.9 means that an average change in shape of 90% was calculated in the specified measurement area, measured against the highest individually measured change in shape within the test series. The largest deformation of the main shape was found in the axial direction for both implant materials; in the case of the titanium implant, this was concentrated apically to the implant (measurement area k), while for the zirconia implant, it was concentrated in the area of the apical third in relation to the implant axis (measurement area h). For the change in shape in the X and Y directions, relatively symmetrical results were obtained for the axial load in relation to the implant axis. On the X-axis (mesio-distal direction), the greatest changes in shape were calculated in the cervical third for the titanium implant and in the apical third for the zirconia implant, in the projection of the implant in each case. On the Y-axis (apical–cervical direction), the largest changes in shape were calculated further apically for both implant materials. Even in the test series with a force application at an angle of 30°, the largest deformation changes, including those on the X- and Y-axes, were found in the projection of the longitudinal axis of the implant. Overall, when loading at an angle of 30°, an asymmetrical distribution of the size of the deformation changes was observed in the individual observations. Larger changes in shape could be calculated on the mesial side of the peri-implant bone, opposite to the load.

Table 1. Descriptive statistics of the mean surface shape changes in the investigated dimensions regarding both implant materials [1].

Material	Angulation	Main Change in Shape		Change in Shape in X-axis		Change in Shape in Y-axis	
		Mean	SD	Mean	SD	Mean	SD
Titanium	0°	198.38	155.57	336.02	139.62	320.9	270.41
	30°	720.77	594.95	501.09	383.49	475.05	287.1
Zirconium	0°	898.95	373.53	471.83	47.25	654.69	271.02
	30°	1601.46	661.08	906.31	499.68	1095.38	216.24

[1] All measured values are in μm/m.

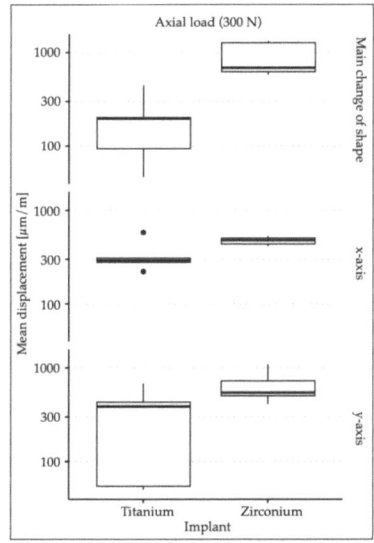 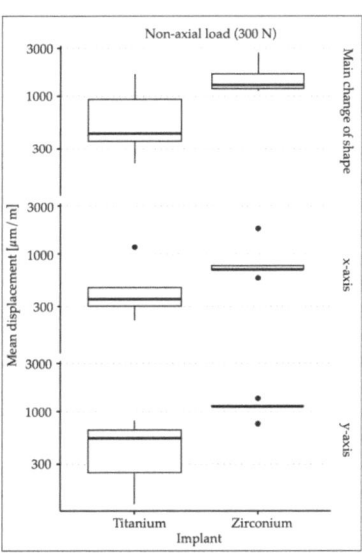

Figure 2. Box–whisker plots of the surface shape changes in the three investigated dimensions with axial and non-axial force application for both implant materials.

Table 2. p-values regarding the differences between the two implant materials in relation to the mean surface shape changes in the three dimensions investigated (calculation by ANOVA).

Angulation	Dimension	p-Value
0°	main change in shape	0.009
	X-axis	0.1172
	Y-axis	0.0758

Table 2. *Cont.*

Angulation	Dimension	*p*-Value
30°	main change in shape	0.0472
	X-axis	0.0758
	Y-axis	0.0163

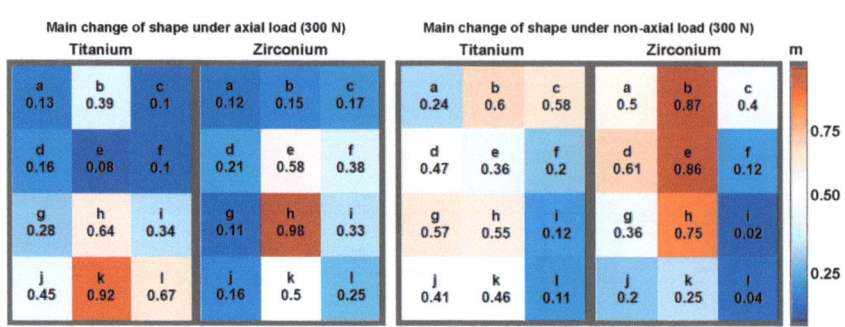

Figure 3. Relative representation of the main change in shape according to the measurement areas with axial and non-axial loading for both implant materials.

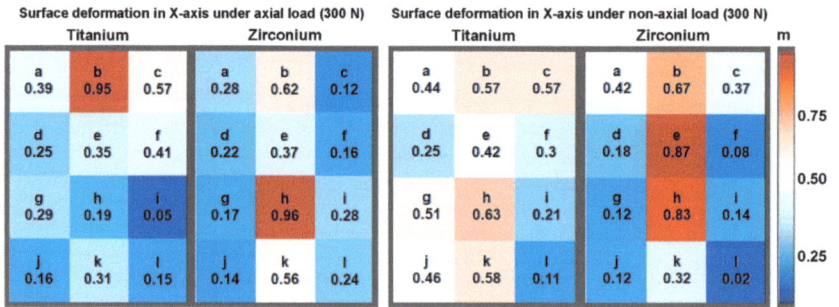

Figure 4. Relative representation of the surface deformation in the X-axis according to the measurement areas under axial and non-axial loading for both implant materials.

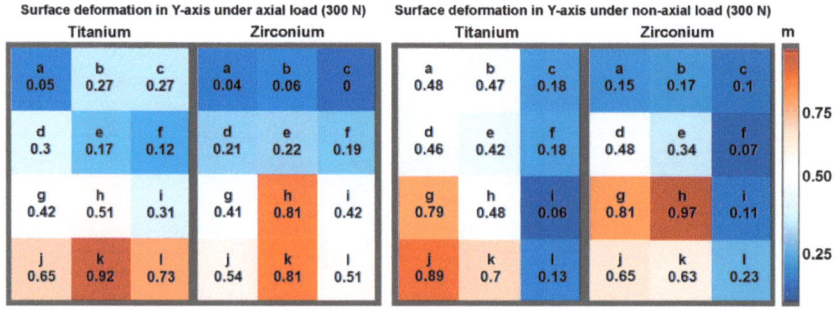

Figure 5. Relative representation of the surface deformation in the Y-axis according to the measurement areas under axial and non-axial loading for both implant materials.

4. Discussion

The 3D optical image correlation used in the present study to detect changes in the shape of superficial bone due to stress induction is already well established in dentistry [32–34]. The transfer of this technology to the measurement of peri-implant bone during masticatory force application was presented as part of a pilot study in 2021 [30]. Good repeatability and measurement stability can be attributed to the method. The present study is the first to use this technology to investigate peri-implant stress under masticatory force application as a function of the implant material. Very few studies investigated stress propagation in bone using the finite element method [11]. A finite element method-based study showed that implant materials with a lower modulus of elasticity cause greater stress within the cortical bone under a chewing force application of 100 N compared to those with a higher modulus of elasticity. A chewing force simulation on one-piece implants made of titanium, zirconia, and various PEEK materials was investigated. In contrast, a study by Haseeb et al. comparing carbon-fiber-reinforced PEEK implants with conventional pure-titanium implants showed a comparable stress distribution in the peri-implant bone [11,35]. When considering these two studies, a particular limitation of the finite element method becomes clear. It is a simulative research method that is dependent on the parameter definitions and therefore makes it fundamentally difficult to compare different studies [36]. In this context, the data collected in the present study showed contradictory results. With regard to the main shape change, significantly greater superficial changes in the shape of the peri-implant bone were found with the zirconia implant. Notably, the measurement method used in this study, as a direct, optical procedure, differs fundamentally from the simulative method of the finite element method. In addition, different masticatory forces were considered. At this point, it should be noted that the present data were collected using an avital bone preparation. This means that osseointegration could not take place, and the results, therefore, represent a situation of primary stability or immediate loading. The results related to the axial force application revealed an overall symmetrical distribution around the examined implants. The different localization of the largest deformation changes depending on the implant material was striking. In the case of the zirconia implant, the largest changes in shape were found in the apical third of the projection of the implant, in relation to both the main change in shape and the X- and Y-axes. In contrast, in the case of the titanium implant, a more heterogeneous distribution of the largest shape changes was observed in the three dimensions. This indicated an overall greater local concentration of stress in the area of the peri-implant bone with the zirconia implant than with the titanium implant. Conversely, the results indicated a more even distribution of stress in the peri-implant bone in the case of the titanium implant. This was reflected in the comparatively smaller changes in shape in the case of the titanium implant and could have a positive effect on osseointegration. The stronger concentration of stress in implants with a comparatively higher modulus of elasticity ("stress isolation") was recently demonstrated by Masoomi et al. in a finite element analysis [37]. In this context, this shows a very good comparability of finite element analysis and digital image correlation. In particular, further investigation of the geometry of the implants and their effect on stress distribution in the surrounding bone will be clinically relevant in the future. The results of the analysis of force application at an angle of 30° suggested that the strain in the dimensions examined was closer to the projection of the implant in the peri-implant bone with the zirconia implant than with the titanium implant. For both implant materials, greater elongation was observed in all dimensions on the side contralateral to the force application compared to the ipsilateral side. In contrast, more eccentric strain distributions were observed for the titanium implant. These were comparable to the those obtained with axial force application, more homogeneous over the measurement area of the peri-implant bone, and less pronounced overall. In principle, the greater modulus of elasticity of the zirconia implants could lead to a more direct transfer of masticatory forces into the peri-implant bone, which may be reflected in a greater surface deformation. However, despite the significant differences in deformation, the overall differences were small. Incidentally, the zirconia implant was a one-piece implant system. In contrast, the titanium implant consisted of a screw-retained implant–abutment complex, which represents a combination of implant and abutment. This im-plant–abutment connection could potentially lead to reduced stress distribution into the peri-implant bone. This could have come into play, particularly with a masticatory force application at a 30° angle. A greater difference in the change in shape between the titanium and the zirconia implants was found for each of the three investigated changes in shape when force was applied at a 30° angle than when an axial chewing force was applied. To the best of our knowledge, no directly comparative data are available regarding stress distribution in the peri-implant bone with single-piece implants and implant–abutment systems. In this context, Tribst et al. were able to demonstrate that a semi-rigid implant–abutment connection can lead to a lower stress propagation in the peri-implant bone compared to a rigid connection, which fundamentally supports the results of the present study [38]. The overall greater and asymmetrical stress transmission into the peri-implant bone with non-axial masticatory force transmission could also argue against the immediate or early loading of implants in the anterior region, as it was already shown that non-axial forces can lead to greater deflections even with relatively low loading [39]. Such micromovements can lead to the formation of fibrous tissue between the implant and the bone in implants that are not yet fully osseointegrated and thus to implant loss [40–42].

For the clinical application of dental implants, it is imperative to meticulously examine the strategies by which peri-implant stress can be mitigated during the period prior to osseointegration. This phase is characterized solely by the attainment of primary stability, which critically impacts the subsequent healing processes. Peri-implant bone's stress distribution plays a pivotal role in the bone's healing trajectory. When the loading exceeds the mechanical tolerance of the peri-implant bone, pathological outcomes such as cartilagogenesis or fibrous tissue formation may ensue, highlighting the detrimental effects of excessive mechanical loading during the initial healing phase [43,44]. This study posits that a uniform stress distribution within the peri-implant bone may confer therapeutic benefits. Consequently, it is evident that comprehensive investigations into the specific patterns of peri-implant stress distribution and its influence on bone integrity are essential. These studies are crucial for formulating precise clinical guidelines concerning the immediate loading of dental implants, thereby optimizing treatment outcomes.

The design of the present study is subject to various limitations. First, an in vitro procedure was used that cannot fully reflect the actual conditions in the oral cavity. In addition, the standardization of chewing force initiation, which was necessary for experimental reasons, limits the possibility of generalizing the results of the present study. Furthermore, the methodology used only detects superficial changes in shape and does not allow for any direct transfer to processes within the bone. Overall, the results presented should be supplemented by further investigations.

5. Conclusions

In the present study, the implant material and implant system significantly influenced the deformation of the superficial peri-implant bone under masticatory force application. Zirconia caused locally more concentrated stress propagation into the peri-implant bone, with relatively small overall strain. In addition, non-axial forces led to greater peri-implant stress than axial masticatory forces, and the strain was greater on the contralateral side of the force direction than on the ipsilateral side. In connection with physiological bone remodeling, which loads on dental implants may have positive or negative influences on the physiological processes of bone metabolism remains to be investigated.

Author Contributions: Conceptualization, R.E.M. and C.M.; methodology, M.L. and L.L.; software, R.E.M. and C.M.; validation, R.E.M. and C.M.; formal analysis, R.E.M.; investigation, L.B. and J.T.; resources, M.W.; data curation, R.E.M. and M.L.; writing—original draft preparation, R.E.M.; writing—review and editing, C.M. and M.W.; visualization, L.B. and J.T.; supervision, R.E.M.; project administration, R.E.M.; funding acquisition, R.E.M. All authors have read and agreed to the published version of the manuscript.

Funding: This research received no external funding.

Data Availability Statement: The underlying data can be requested via the correspondence address.

Acknowledgments: The study was supported by the company Straumann GmbH, Freiburg, Germany. The company provided the implants used. In this context, the authors would particularly like to thank Karin Paulmeier, Armin Vollmer, and Thomas Kreuzwieser for their support. Parts of the results of the present study will be used in Linus Leven's doctoral thesis.

Conflicts of Interest: The authors declare no conflicts of interest. The funders had no role in the design of the study; in the collection, analyses, or interpretation of the data; in the writing of the manuscript; or in the decision to publish the results.

References

1. Branemark, P.I.; Adell, R.; Breine, U.; Hansson, B.O.; Lindstrom, J.; Ohlsson, A. Intra-osseous anchorage of dental prostheses. I. Experimental studies. *Scand. J. Plast. Reconstr. Surg.* **1969**, *3*, 81–100. [CrossRef] [PubMed]
2. Assif, D.; Marshak, B.; Horowitz, A. Analysis of load transfer and stress distribution by an implant-supported fixed partial denture. *J. Prosthet. Dent.* **1996**, *75*, 285–291. [CrossRef] [PubMed]
3. Frost, H.M. Wolff's Law and bone's structural adaptations to mechanical usage: An overview for clinicians. *Angle Orthod.* **1994**, *64*, 175–188. [CrossRef] [PubMed]
4. Wiskott, H.W.; Belser, U.C. Lack of integration of smooth titanium surfaces: A working hypothesis based on strains generated in the surrounding bone. *Clin. Oral Implants Res.* **1999**, *10*, 429–444. [CrossRef] [PubMed]
5. Frost, H.M. A 2003 update of bone physiology and Wolff's Law for clinicians. *Angle Orthod.* **2004**, *74*, 3–15. [CrossRef] [PubMed]
6. Cehreli, M.C.; Iplikcioglu, H.; Bilir, O.G. The influence of the location of load transfer on strains around implants supporting four unit cement-retained fixed prostheses: In vitro evaluation of axial versus off-set loading. *J. Oral Rehabil.* **2002**, *29*, 394–400. [CrossRef]
7. Lee, J.H.; Frias, V.; Lee, K.W.; Wright, R.F. Effect of implant size and shape on implant success rates: A literature review. *J. Prosthet. Dent.* **2005**, *94*, 377–381. [CrossRef]
8. Nishioka, R.S.; Nishioka, L.N.; Abreu, C.W.; de Vasconcellos, L.G.; Balducci, I. Machined and plastic copings in three-element prostheses with different types of implant-abutment joints: A strain gauge comparative analysis. *J. Appl. Oral Sci.* **2010**, *18*, 225–230. [CrossRef]
9. de Vasconcellos, L.G.; Nishioka, R.S.; de Vasconcellos, L.M.; Balducci, I.; Kojima, A.N. Microstrain around dental implants supporting fixed partial prostheses under axial and non-axial loading conditions, in vitro strain gauge analysis. *J. Craniofacial Surg.* **2013**, *24*, e546–e551. [CrossRef]
10. Kheiralla, L.S.; Younis, J.F. Peri-implant biomechanical responses to standard, short-wide, and mini implants supporting single crowns under axial and off-axial loading (an in vitro study). *J. Oral Implantol.* **2014**, *40*, 42–52. [CrossRef]
11. Fabris, D.; Moura, J.P.A.; Fredel, M.C.; Souza, J.C.M.; Silva, F.S.; Henriques, B. Biomechanical analyses of one-piece dental implants composed of titanium, zirconia, PEEK, CFR-PEEK, or GFR-PEEK: Stresses, strains, and bone remodeling prediction by the finite element method. *J. Biomed. Mater. Res. B Appl. Biomater.* **2022**, *110*, 79–88. [CrossRef] [PubMed]
12. Osman, R.B.; Swain, M.V. A Critical Review of Dental Implant Materials with an Emphasis on Titanium versus Zirconia. *Materials* **2015**, *8*, 932–958. [CrossRef] [PubMed]
13. Khaohoen, A.; Sornsuwan, T.; Chaijareenont, P.; Poovarodom, P.; Rungsiyakull, C.; Rungsiyakull, P. Biomaterials and Clinical Application of Dental Implants in Relation to Bone Density-A Narrative Review. *J. Clin. Med.* **2023**, *12*, 6924. [CrossRef] [PubMed]
14. Albrektsson, T.; Jacobsson, M. Bone-metal interface in osseointegration. *J. Prosthet. Dent.* **1987**, *57*, 597–607. [CrossRef] [PubMed]
15. Palmquist, A.; Omar, O.M.; Esposito, M.; Lausmaa, J.; Thomsen, P. Titanium oral implants: Surface characteristics, interface biology and clinical outcome. *J. R. Soc. Interface* **2010**, *7* (Suppl. S5), S515–S527. [CrossRef]
16. Hoque, M.E.; Showva, N.N.; Ahmed, M.; Rashid, A.B.; Sadique, S.E.; El-Bialy, T.; Xu, H. Titanium and titanium alloys in dentistry: Current trends, recent developments, and future prospects. *Heliyon* **2022**, *8*, e11300. [CrossRef]
17. Binon, P.P. Implants and components: Entering the new millennium. *Int. J. Oral Maxillofac. Implants* **2000**, *15*, 76–94. [PubMed]
18. Jung, R.E.; Sailer, I.; Hammerle, C.H.; Attin, T.; Schmidlin, P. In vitro color changes of soft tissues caused by restorative materials. *Int. J. Periodontics Restor. Dent.* **2007**, *27*, 251–257.
19. Sevimay, M.; Turhan, F.; Kilicarslan, M.A.; Eskitascioglu, G. Three-dimensional finite element analysis of the effect of different bone quality on stress distribution in an implant-supported crown. *J. Prosthet. Dent.* **2005**, *93*, 227–234. [CrossRef]

20. Manzano, G.; Herrero, L.R.; Montero, J. Comparison of clinical performance of zirconia implants and titanium implants in animal models: A systematic review. *Int. J. Oral Maxillofac. Implants* **2014**, *29*, 311–320. [CrossRef]
21. Wenz, H.J.; Bartsch, J.; Wolfart, S.; Kern, M. Osseointegration and clinical success of zirconia dental implants: A systematic review. *Int. J. Prosthodont.* **2008**, *21*, 27–36. [PubMed]
22. Roehling, S.; Astasov-Frauenhoffer, M.; Hauser-Gerspach, I.; Braissant, O.; Woelfler, H.; Waltimo, T.; Kniha, H.; Gahlert, M. In Vitro Biofilm Formation on Titanium and Zirconia Implant Surfaces. *J. Periodontol.* **2017**, *88*, 298–307. [CrossRef] [PubMed]
23. Happe, A.; Schulte-Mattler, V.; Strassert, C.; Naumann, M.; Stimmelmayr, M.; Zoller, J.E.; Rothamel, D. In vitro color changes of soft tissues caused by dyed fluorescent zirconia and nondyed, nonfluorescent zirconia in thin mucosa. *Int. J. Periodontics Restor. Dent.* **2013**, *33*, e1–e8. [CrossRef] [PubMed]
24. Kohal, R.J.; Knauf, M.; Larsson, B.; Sahlin, H.; Butz, F. One-piece zirconia oral implants: One-year results from a prospective cohort study. 1. Single tooth replacement. *J. Clin. Periodontol.* **2012**, *39*, 590–597. [CrossRef] [PubMed]
25. Jung, R.E.; Grohmann, P.; Sailer, I.; Steinhart, Y.N.; Feher, A.; Hammerle, C.; Strub, J.R.; Kohal, R. Evaluation of a one-piece ceramic implant used for single-tooth replacement and three-unit fixed partial dentures: A prospective cohort clinical trial. *Clin. Oral Implants Res.* **2016**, *27*, 751–761. [CrossRef] [PubMed]
26. Kohal, R.J.; Finke, H.C.; Klaus, G. Stability of prototype two-piece zirconia and titanium implants after artificial aging: An in vitro pilot study. *Clin. Implant Dent. Relat. Res.* **2009**, *11*, 323–329. [CrossRef] [PubMed]
27. Sannino, G.; Gloria, F.; Ottria, L.; Barlattani, A. Influence of finish line in the distribution of stress trough an all ceramic implant-supported crown.: A 3D Finite Element Analysis. *Oral Implantol.* **2009**, *2*, 14–27.
28. Lopez, C.A.V.; Vasco, M.A.A.; Ruales, E.; Bedoya, K.A.; Benfatti, C.M.; Bezzon, O.L.; Deliberador, T.M. Three-Dimensional Finite Element Analysis of Stress Distribution in Zirconia and Titanium Dental Implants. *J. Oral Implantol.* **2018**, *44*, 409–415. [CrossRef] [PubMed]
29. Brenner, S.C. *The Mathematical Theory of Finite Element Methods*, 3rd ed.; Springer: New York, NY, USA, 2008; p. 96.
30. Matta, R.E.; Riegger, K.; Trägler, H.; Adler, W.; Eitner, S.; Wichmann, M.; Motel, C. Establishment of a New Biomechanical Measurement Method for Surface Deformation of Bone by Force Application via Dental Implants—A Pilot Study. *Appl. Sci.* **2021**, *11*, 7568. [CrossRef]
31. Bakalarz, M.M.; Tworzewski, P.P. Application of Digital Image Correlation to Evaluate Strain, Stiffness and Ductility of Full-Scale LVL Beams Strengthened by CFRP. *Materials* **2023**, *16*, 1309. [CrossRef]
32. Goellner, M.; Berthold, C.; Holst, S.; Wichmann, M.; Schmitt, J. Correlations between photogrammetric measurements of tooth mobility and the Periotest method. *Acta Odontol. Scand.* **2012**, *70*, 27–35. [CrossRef] [PubMed]
33. Lezaja, M.; Veljovic, D.; Manojlovic, D.; Milosevic, M.; Mitrovic, N.; Janackovic, D.; Miletic, V. Bond strength of restorative materials to hydroxyapatite inserts and dimensional changes of insert-containing restorations during polymerization. *Dent. Mater.* **2015**, *31*, 171–181. [CrossRef] [PubMed]
34. Miletic, V.; Peric, D.; Milosevic, M.; Manojlovic, D.; Mitrovic, N. Local deformation fields and marginal integrity of sculptable bulk-fill, low-shrinkage and conventional composites. *Dent. Mater.* **2016**, *32*, 1441–1451. [CrossRef] [PubMed]
35. Haseeb, S.A.; Vinaya, K.C.; Vijaykumar, N.; Sree Durga, B.A.; Kumar, A.S.; Sruthi, M.K. Finite element evaluation to compare stress pattern in bone surrounding implant with carbon fiber-reinforced poly-ether-ether-ketone and commercially pure titanium implants. *Natl. J. Maxillofac. Surg.* **2022**, *13*, 243–247. [CrossRef] [PubMed]
36. Wight, C.M.; Schemitsch, E.H. In vitro testing for hip head-neck taper tribocorrosion: A review of experimental methods. *Proc. Inst. Mech. Eng. Part H* **2022**, *236*, 9544119221074582. [CrossRef]
37. Masoomi, F.; Mahboub, F. Stress distribution pattern in all-on-four maxillary restorations supported by porous tantalum and solid titanium implants using three-dimensional finite element analysis. *Eur. J. Transl. Myol.* **2024**, *34*. [CrossRef] [PubMed]
38. Tribst, J.P.M.; Dal Piva, A.M.O.; Ozcan, M.; Borges, A.L.S.; Bottino, M.A. Influence of Ceramic Materials on Biomechanical Behavior of Implant Supported Fixed Prosthesis with Hybrid Abutment. *Eur. J. Prosthodont. Restor. Dent.* **2019**, *27*, 76–82. [CrossRef] [PubMed]
39. Boldt, J.; Knapp, W.; Proff, P.; Rottner, K.; Richter, E.J. Measurement of tooth and implant mobility under physiological loading conditions. *Ann. Anat.* **2012**, *194*, 185–189. [CrossRef] [PubMed]
40. Pilliar, R.M.; Lee, J.M.; Maniatopoulos, C. Observations on the effect of movement on bone ingrowth into porous-surfaced implants. *Clin. Orthop. Relat. Res.* **1986**, *208*, 108–113. [CrossRef]
41. Brunski, J.B. Biomechanical factors affecting the bone-dental implant interface. *Clin. Mater.* **1992**, *10*, 153–201. [CrossRef]
42. Kao, H.C.; Gung, Y.W.; Chung, T.F.; Hsu, M.L. The influence of abutment angulation on micromotion level for immediately loaded dental implants: A 3-D finite element analysis. *Int. J. Oral Maxillofac. Implants* **2008**, *23*, 623–630. [PubMed]
43. Sakka, S.; Baroudi, K.; Nassani, M.Z. Factors associated with early and late failure of dental implants. *J. Investig. Clin. Dent.* **2012**, *3*, 258–261. [CrossRef] [PubMed]
44. Duyck, J.; Vandamme, K. The effect of loading on peri-implant bone: A critical review of the literature. *J. Oral Rehabil.* **2014**, *41*, 783–794. [CrossRef] [PubMed]

Disclaimer/Publisher's Note: The statements, opinions and data contained in all publications are solely those of the individual author(s) and contributor(s) and not of MDPI and/or the editor(s). MDPI and/or the editor(s) disclaim responsibility for any injury to people or property resulting from any ideas, methods, instructions or products referred to in the content.

Article

Comparative Verification of the Accuracy of Implant Models Made of PLA, Resin, and Silicone

Kana Wakamori [1,†], Koudai Nagata [1,†], Toshifumi Nakashizu [2], Hayato Tsuruoka [1], Mihoko Atsumi [1] and Hiromasa Kawana [1,*]

1. Department of Oral and Maxillofacial Implantology, Kanagawa Dental University, 82 Inaoka-cho, Yokosuka 238-8580, Japan
2. Division of the Dental Practice Support, Kanagawa Dental University, 82 Inaoka-cho, Yokosuka 238-8580, Japan
* Correspondence: kawana@kdu.ac.jp; Tel.: +81-468-88-8880
† These authors contributed equally to this work.

Abstract: Polylactic acid (PLA) has gained considerable attention as an alternative to petroleum-based materials due to environmental concerns. We fabricated implant models with fused filament fabrication (FFF) 3D printers using PLA, and the accuracies of these PLA models were compared with those of plaster models made from silicone impressions and resin models made with digital light processing (DLP). A base model was obtained from an impact-training model. The scan body was mounted on the plaster, resin, and PLA models obtained from the base model, and the obtained information was converted to stereolithography (STL) data by the 3D scanner. The base model was then used as a reference, and its data were superimposed onto the STL data of each model using Geomagic control. The horizontal and vertical accuracies of PLA models, as calculated using the Tukey–Kramer method, were 97.2 ± 48.4 and 115.5 ± 15.1 µm, respectively, which suggests that the PLA model is the least accurate among the three models. In both cases, significant differences were found between PLA and gypsum and between the PLA and resin models. However, considering that the misfit of screw-retained implant frames should be ≤150 µm, PLA can be effectively used for fabricating implant models.

Keywords: 3D printing; fused filament fabrication (FFF); digital light processing (DLP); polylactic acid (PLA); dental implant

1. Introduction

The history of dental implants in current use can be traced back to the first clinical use of root-shaped titanium implants in 1965, which are still in use today. The bonding mode between bone and titanium is called osseointegration [1]. Various surface treatments, including blasting, etching, sandblasting, and anodizing, are used to ensure osseointegration [2–4]. Oates et al. reported that implant stability can be accelerated by two weeks if implants are sandblasted and surface-treated with acid etching [5]. In a 20-year follow-up study of 631 patients and 1472 implant bodies, Cheng et al. reported a 94% implant survival rate [6]. Various surface treatment techniques have accelerated implant stability and established the long-term prognosis of implant therapy [7]. In recent years, digital technology has been widely used in implant treatment. The concepts of top-down treatment and static and dynamic navigation in surgery have become widespread, allowing for safe and esthetic implant treatment for patients [8–10]. In implant prosthetic treatment, intraoral scanners (IOSs) and computer-aided design/computer-aided manufacturing (CAD/CAM) have been applied to single-tooth and multiple-tooth defect cases. This has enabled the digitization of almost all processes, leading to improved accuracy of prosthetics, shorter treatment times, and reduced fabrication times of technical work [11–13].

The Sustainable Development Goals, adopted at the 2015 United Nations Summit, are currently attracting attention from the environmental perspective. In particular, Goal 12, "ensure sustainable patterns of consumption and production", targets waste reduction [14]. According to the WHO, biomedical waste (BMW) is one of the most important categories of waste, posing significant potential risks to people and the environment. BMW is defined as "the generation of waste in medical institutions, medical research facilities, laboratories, and private practices". The global growth of the medical and dental sectors and the increase in disposable products have resulted in the generation of large amounts of medical and dental waste [15]. A survey on dental waste in Greece [16] reported that 141 kg of waste was collected from 20 dental clinics with a total patient population of 2542, with 8% of the total weight being household waste and 92% hazardous waste. Koolivand et al. also reported that in Urmia, Iran, general dental offices accounted for 58.94 kg of waste per day, specialized dental clinics for 17.92 kg/day, dental clinics for 10.22 kg/day, household waste for 35.46%, potentially infectious waste for 32.24%, and toxic waste for 11.83%, while chemical and pharmaceutical wastes accounted for 5.56% of the total [17]. According to the Survey Report on Industrial Waste Discharge and Disposal by Sector reported by Japan's Ministry of the Environment in 2021, the amount of industrial waste discharged by the medical industry accounted for 438 (thousand tons) in 2021. Our dental hospital in Japan also generates approximately 2660 kg of industrial waste per year. Therefore, the reduction, management, and reuse of dental waste is a challenge that healthcare professionals face [18]. Papi et al. discussed how impression materials and plaster casts with blood or saliva on them can be a source of infection [19]. Frahdian et al. stated that alginate impressions are one of the reasons for the increase in dental waste [20]. Silicone impression material, alginate, and plaster are considered industrial waste in the field of dentistry in Japan. Plaster is commonly used to fabricate dental models, but plaster models are gradually being replaced by resin models sculpted by light-based 3D printers due to the widespread use of IOSs and 3D printers in dentistry [21,22]. This is because the light-based 3D printer method is considered to have better accuracy. Ishida et al. [23] fabricated dental patterns and verified their accuracy using consumer 3D printers such as a fused filament fabrication (FFF) device, a stereolithography (SLA) device, and two types of dental 3D printers (a Multijet device and an SLA device). As a result, the surface roughness of the civilian consumer FFF devices is significantly larger than that of the SLA devices, and the accuracy of the SLA devices is better than that of the civilian FFF devices. Kim et al. [24] measured the accuracy of models fabricated using SLA, digital light processing (DLP), FFF, and PolyJet. Overall tooth measurements were 88 ± 14 µm for SLA, 76 ± 14 µm for DLP, 99 ± 14 µm for FFF, and 68 ± 9 µm for PolyJet, indicating that 3D printing technology is applicable to dental models. SLA uses a UV laser to form the liquid resin. DLP uses a projector to project an image of one layer onto the entire surface of the build platform and cures the entire layer on a "surface" rather than curing it at "dots" as with the SLA devices [25]. In dentistry, SLA and DLP are used to produce orthodontic devices and surgical guides for implant surgery due to their accuracy [26,27]. However, light-based 3D printers can only use resin, and light-mediated resin cannot be broken down since it is a polymer. Therefore, resin models cannot be reused and they do not help reduce industrial waste [28]. That is why we turned our attention to FFF. In the FFF manufacturing process, raw material is melted to form an object called a filament. This material is pulled by a drive wheel through filaments placed on a roll and heated by a temperature-controlled nozzle head to produce a semi-liquid material that is precisely extruded and guided layer by layer to produce the desired object [29]. FFF uses various filaments, such as polylactic acid (PLA), acrylonitrile butadiene styrene, and polyethylene terephthalate [30].

Since PLA is present in the filament used for FFF, we believe that PLA could be reused after the model is fabricated and remolded, thereby reducing industrial waste. PLA is characterized by decomposition into water and carbon dioxide under composting conditions of high temperature, high humidity, and the presence of microorganisms [31,32]. PLA is widely used in medical practice, and its biocompatibility has been widely reported [33–35]. However, there have been few reports on the use of FFF or PLA in dentistry. Benli et al. [36] and Molinero-Mourelle et al. [37] reported the superiority of PLA as a provisional crown. Crenn et al. [38] compared the mechanical properties of PLA to those of conventional resins and reported that PLA has mechanical properties similar to those of conventional resins with low porosity and could be used for provisional crowns. However, Park et al. [39] reported that three-unit provisional crowns fabricated from SLA and DLP had superior bending strength, and it was difficult to fabricate three-unit provisional crowns from FFF. Results may vary depending on the nature of the 3D printer and the filament. The glass transition temperature of PLA is as low as 60 °C. Methods to increase the heat resistance of PLA have been studied, but no clear method has been found that does not impair the biodegradability of PLA [40,41]. Therefore, it is currently difficult to use PLA as a crown, and practically, it is more useful for making dental models.

Regarding FFF, Muta et al. [42] compared plaster models and polyvinyl alcohol (PVA) models made with FFF and reported the usefulness of FFF and PVA. Wang and Su [43] compared the accuracy of edentulous trays fabricated using DLP and FFF with that of conventional manual edentulous trays and found the digitally fabricated trays to have higher precision. Research on filament reuse has also been conducted. Lagazzo et al. [44] reported the effectiveness of PLA and poly (3-hydroxybutyrate-co-3-hydroxyvalerate)-based biocomposites for composite material recycling. Vidakis et al. also reported that PA12 polymers can be reused up to three times [45]. Anderson et al. [46] compared the mechanical properties of virgin PLA and one-time-recycled PLA and reported a 10.9% decrease in tensile strength, 6.8% increase in shear strength, and 2.4% decrease in the hardness of the reused filaments. While there are many reports on the reuse of PLA, no clear process for reuse has been defined. Majgaonkar et al. [47] believe that it is important to have a sustainable strategy for recycling PLA waste due to current environmental concerns, although recycling PLA will degrade its mechanical properties. They also considered recycling strategies that involve the alcoholysis of post-consumer PLA into lactic acid esters. We believe that the use of an IOS and PLA to fabricate and reuse implant models would lead to dental care with reduced waste [48]. However, to the best of our knowledge, there are no reports documenting the accuracy of implant models using FFF or PLA. In our previous study, we compared dental models made of PLA with those made of resin and plaster, and reported that the PLA models were equally accurate [49]. Therefore, in this study, we aimed to compare the accuracy of implant plaster models made from silicon impression material and plaster, implant resin models made with DLP, and implant PLA models made with FDM.

2. Materials and Methods

Straumann® $\phi 4.1 \times 10$ implants (bone-level tapered implant, Basel, Switzerland) were placed on a jaw model for implant training ([D18D-KP.80]; NISSIN, Tokyo, Japan), Switzerland) and were used as the base model. Next, the scan body (S-WAVE, SHOFU INC, Tokyo, Japan) was mounted and scanned with a 3D scanner (Ceramill Map® 400; Amann Girrbach, Vienna, Austria) to acquire stereolithography (STL) data of the mother model. The process of making each model and obtaining STL data is described below. The models are shown in Figure 1. This study was conducted in compliance with SQUIRE guidelines.

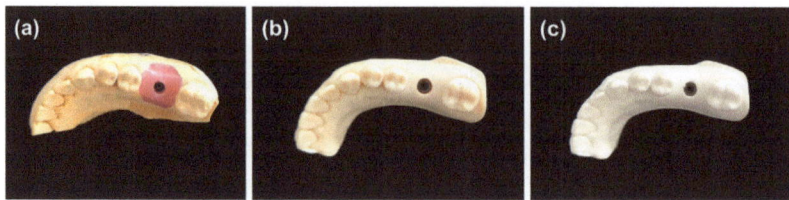

Figure 1. Different types of constructed models. (**a**) A silicone impression was made on the mother model, the lab analog was attached to the impression coping, and plaster was injected to make a plaster model. (**b**) Impressions were taken on the base model using Trios3®, and resin models were fabricated using cara Print 4.0 pro based on the obtained STL data. (**c**) Impressions were taken on the base model using Trios3®, and PLA models were fabricated using Moment M350 based on the obtained STL data. STL: stereolithography.

2.1. STL Data Acquisition for Plaster Implant Models

Precision impressions were made on base models with impression copings using silicone (Aquasil Ultra®; Dentsply Sirona, York, PA, USA). The lab analog was then mounted on an impression coping, and plaster (New Fujirock®; GC, Tokyo, Japan) was poured to fabricate the implant model. A scan body (S-WAVE, Shofu, Tokyo, Japan) was attached, scanned with a 3D scanner, and converted to STL data.

2.2. STL Date Acquisition for Resin Implant Models

Digital impressions were made by the IOS (Trios® 3; 3shape, Copenhagen, Denmark) on the base model with the scan body attached, and then DLP (cara® Print 4.0 pro; Kulzer Japan Co., Ltd., Tokyo, Japan) and light-curing resin (dima® Print Stone; Kulzer Japan Co., Ltd., Tokyo, Japan) were used to fabricate the resin models. The layer thickness was 50 µm. The resin model was fitted with a scan body and converted to STL data using a 3D scanner.

2.3. STL Data Acquisition for PLA Implant Models

Digital impressions of the base model were taken with the scan body attached; FFF (Moment® M350; Moment Co., Ltd., Seoul, Republic of Korea) and a 1.75 mm PLA filament from Moment® (Moment Co., Ltd., Seoul, Republic of Korea) were used to fabricate the PLA models. The fabrication conditions were as follows: modeling temperature of the material = 230 °C and layer thickness = 100 µm. The PLA model was fitted with a scan body and converted to STL data using a 3D scanner. No surface polishing or chemical treatment was performed after printing. The specifications of the 3D printers are shown in Table 1.

Table 1. Specifications of the 3D printers used in this study.

3D Printing Technique	3D Printer Used	Specifications
DLP [†]	cara Print 4.0 pro (Kulzer Japan Co., Ltd., Tokyo, Japan)	Pixel size: XY 65.0 µm Laminating pitch: 30–150 µm Modeling size: 127 mm × 70 mm × 130 mm
FFF [‡]	Moment M350 (Moment Co., Ltd., Seoul, Republic of Korea)	XYZ accuracy: XY 12 µm, Z 0.625 µm Laminating pitch: 0.05–0.3 mm Modeling size: 350 mm × 190 mm × 196 mm Nozzle: 0.4 mm

Resin models were constructed using cara Print 4.0 pro, and PLA models were constructed using Moment M350. [†] Digital light processing, [‡] fused filament fabrication.

2.4. Measurement of Accuracy

After obtaining the STL data for each model, the accuracy of the scanned body of plaster, resin, and PLA models was measured using Geomagic® Control (3D Systems, Washington, DC, USA) based on the STL data of the base model. The superimposing of STL data was performed after trimming the excess data, followed by manual alignment based on three landmarks, and best-fit registration was used for greater accuracy. The average of the results was obtained by randomly selecting three points from the superimposed scan body data (Figure 2). The scan bodies were all in the same orientation. Five models were designed for each. Accuracy was measured in two directions, viz. horizontal and vertical.

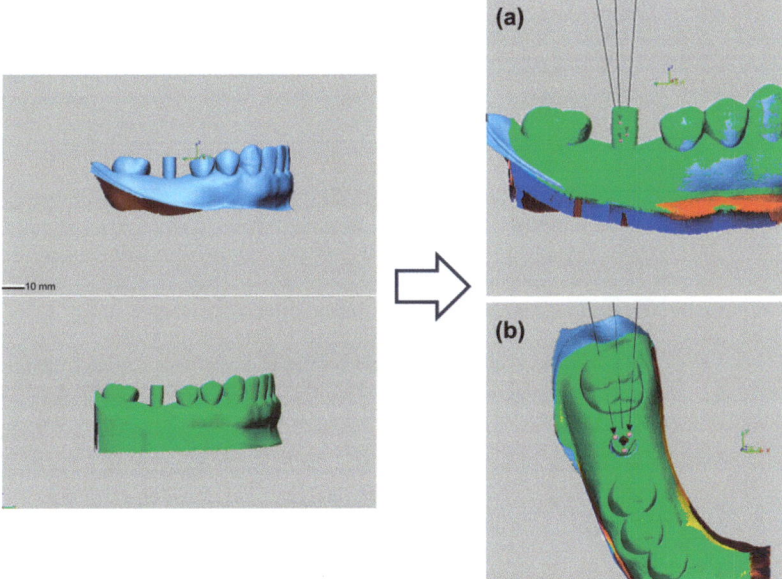

Figure 2. Stereolithography (STL) of the base model superimposed on each of the models to measure accuracy. For horizontal and vertical accuracies, three points were randomly selected, and their average was used as the result. (**a**) Horizontal and (**b**) vertical accuracy.

2.5. Statistical Analysis

The accuracy of the model was verified through the Tukey–Kramer method using a bell curve in Excel (Social Survey Research Information Co., Ltd., Tokyo, Japan). Continuous data are expressed as mean ± standard deviation. Differences with a p value < 0.05 were considered statistically significant.

3. Results and Discussion

In this study, horizontal accuracies of 53.4 ± 9.4, 54.3 ± 23.4, and 97.2 ± 48.4 µm were obtained for plaster, resin, and PLA, respectively ($p < 0.05$), while the corresponding vertical accuracies were 61.8 ± 10.1, 60 ± 13.8, and 115.5 ± 15.1 µm ($p < 0.001$). In both cases, PLA had the lowest accuracy. Significant differences in horizontal accuracies were found between PLA and plaster and PLA and resin. Vertical accuracies were similarly significantly different between PLA and resin (Figure 3).

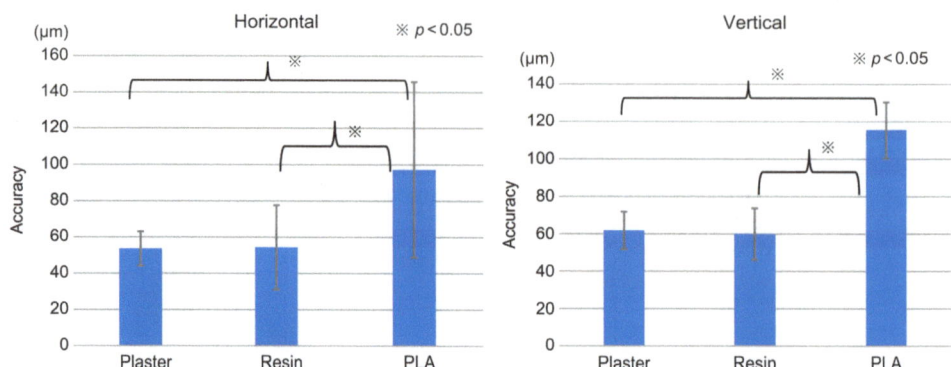

Figure 3. Comparison of the horizontal and vertical accuracies of the three models. We can observe significant differences in both horizontal and vertical accuracies between plaster and polylactic acid (PLA) and resin and PLA.

The findings of this study demonstrate that the accuracy of PLA models was inferior to that of the resin and plaster models both vertically and horizontally. However, with the improved accuracy of 3D printers, PLA could be used as a new material in dentistry. Furthermore, due to the advantages of its characteristics, PLA can be reused to reduce industrial waste and carbon dioxide emissions [50].

Reports on model-less prosthetic fittings are scarce; a systematic review by Joda et al. found only two reports on model-less crown fits and one on implant superstructure fit [51]. Joda et al. also compared the accuracy of 10 superstructures fabricated without models and 10 superstructures with models and reported that the model-less superstructures required less adjustment and time to fit [52]. However, Mühlemann et al. reported that the fabrication of fittings with digital models should be considered as these were more accurate than those made with conventional plaster models [53].

When fabricating a superstructure, a model is necessary for creating the bond between the zirconia and the titanium base. Particularly in the case of single-tooth implants, the titanium base has an anti-rotation mechanism, and if a model is not used, minor misalignments may prevent the implant from fitting in the mouth. Therefore, the accuracy of the model is important. Geomagic® Control, which was used to measure the accuracy in this study, is widely used in dentistry to verify the crown fit and IOS accuracy by comparing STL data [54–56].

Hanon et al. fabricated cylindrical specimens using FFF and reported that the modeling accuracy was as high as 98.56–99.64% [57]. The results of this study show that the accuracy of the PLA model was lower than that of the other models. We hypothesize that the accuracy loss of the PLA model was due to the difference in layer thickness between the two 3D printers. However, Kamio et al. [58] reported that the layer thickness of the FFF did not cause a significant decrease in accuracy. Additionally, FFF is limited in its ability to model detailed areas [59]. George et al. [60] reported that models fabricated with FFF are susceptible to shrinkage and warping deformation during the cooling process of the thermoplastic resin, and that geometric inaccuracies occur when models of vertebral bodies and other spinous processes are fabricated. When an implant model is fabricated using a 3D printer, a lab analog corresponding to the implant is inserted from the basal surface after the modeling. In contrast to the smooth insertion of the resin and plaster models, the PLA models could not be inserted without grinding with a laboratory bur, which could be the reason for the lower accuracy of the PLA models. It is necessary to verify whether the accuracy of dental models can be improved by using more accurate FFF or changing the modeling direction [61,62].

With respect to the fit of screw-retained implant frames, Katsoulis et al. used scanning electron microscopy to evaluate the micro-gap between the screw-retained zirconia frame and the implant using the one-screw test [63]. They reported that the micro-gap of the cast cobalt chrome frame was 236 μm, while that of the zirconia frame was 18 μm, and an acceptable distortion of <50–120 μm was noted. Al-Meraikhi et al. [64] measured the fit of the implant to the zirconia frame using an industrial computed tomography (CT) scanner and volume graphics analysis software and found that the fit was 93.8 ± 30 μm. The passive fit was reported to be acceptable at 135 μm. Yilmaz et al. [65] also reported that the marginal discrepancy of screw-fixed titanium and zirconia frameworks and abutments were 102 μm and 94 μm, respectively, measured using an industrial CT scanner and 3D volume software; they also reported clinically acceptable misfit values ranging from 10 μm to 150 μm. Many other researchers have reported misfit limits of < 150 μm for the precision of fit of screw-retained implants [66–68].

With respect to the accuracy of scan bodies using Geomagic® control, Mühlemann et al. [53] measured the accuracy of impressions using IOSs in five patients with a single missing tooth and teeth on both sides of the edentulous space. Three consecutive impressions were taken with each IOS to measure for accuracy. They reported that the scan body misfit was 57.2 ± 32.6 and 88.6 ± 46 μm for the iTero and Trios systems, respectively. Gedrimiene et al. [69] used conventional silicone-based impressions and IOS-based digital impressions and reported that the scan body misfit was 70.8 ± 59 μm. The horizontal and vertical accuracies of PLA models in our study were 97.2 ± 48.4 μm and 115.5 ± 15.1 μm, respectively. The accuracy of PLA models was found to be lower than that of the resin and plaster models. However, resin and plaster models cannot be reused and eventually become industrial waste. Since the misfit of the screw-fixed implant frame was <150 μm, PLA models can be used as implant models. Reusing PLA models may lead to a reduction in industrial waste and carbon dioxide emissions. The accuracy can be further improved by using a verification jig [70]. Although its accuracy needs to be verified in clinical practice, we believe that in the future, the use of PLA can contribute to reducing dental waste.

Three-dimensional printers are gaining popularity in medicine, but there are some concerns. SLA and DLP produce toxic substances and odors during the production process [71]. PLA is known to release volatile organic compounds (VOCs) during printing as well. Chan et al. [72] measured the concentration of VOCs in one printer and in a printing room when three printers were operating simultaneously. Total VOC concentrations were reported, with isopropyl alcohol being the primary VOC and both being below occupational exposure limits. Wojtyła et al. [73] reported that during PLA molding, methyl methacrylate was detected as a compound, accounting for 44% of total VOC emissions. Thus, ventilation and protection of the printing room are important because the emission of hazardous substances has been confirmed, even if within acceptable limits, during FFF modeling [74]. There is also much debate regarding the sterilization methods for PLA. Currently, the three most common industrially used sterilization methods for medical devices are ethylene oxide, gamma irradiation, and steam sterilization, which can significantly alter the properties of PLA. PLA cannot withstand steam sterilization due to its low heat resistance. Gamma irradiation and ethylene oxide have lower sterilization temperatures and can be applied to heat-sensitive materials such as PLA. However, gamma irradiation degrades polymers, and ethylene oxide is toxic, carcinogenic, and allergenic, among other drawbacks [75–77]. There are reports that FFF is self-sterilizing due to the high-temperature, high-pressure extrusion process [78]. Davila et al. [79] report that there is no specific technology that can be applied to all materials used in biomedical devices and that new processes are needed to avoid these problems. They also report that hydrogen peroxide gas plasma and supercritical carbon dioxide are effective sterilization methods.

A limitation of this study is that only one type of FFF was used. We believe that further detailed and extensive studies can help in better comparing the accuracy of multiple FDMs in the future. It is also important to measure how much industrial waste can be reduced by using PLA for dental treatment, compared to other materials.

4. Conclusions

We hypothesized that the characteristics of PLA could be exploited to reuse it and reduce industrial waste in dentistry. This study compared the accuracy of implant models made of PLA with that of models made of plaster and resin. The PLA models were less accurate than the other two models but considering that the misfit of the screw-fixed superstructure was <150 μm, it could be used as a new material.

However, no clear method has been established regarding the reuse of PLA. Additionally, due to the mechanical properties of PLA, an exact sterilization method has not been determined. Solving these problems will make PLA reuse a reality.

Author Contributions: Conceptualization, K.N. and H.K.; Data curation, T.N. and M.A.; Formal analysis, H.T.; Writing—original draft, K.W. and K.N. All authors have read and agreed to the published version of the manuscript.

Funding: This research received no external funding.

Institutional Review Board Statement: Not applicable.

Informed Consent Statement: Not applicable.

Data Availability Statement: The datasets used and/or analyzed during the current study are available from the corresponding author upon reasonable request.

Conflicts of Interest: The authors declare no conflict of interest.

References

1. Abraham, C.M. A Brief Historical Perspective on Dental Implants, Their Surface Coatings and Treatments. *Open Dent. J.* **2014**, *16*, 50–55. [CrossRef]
2. Glauser, R.; Ree, A.; Lundgren, A.; Gottlow, J.; Hammerle, C.H.; Scharer, P. Immediate Occlusal Loading of Brånemark Implants Applied in Various Jawbone Regions: A Prospective, 1-Year Clinical Study. *Clin. Implant. Dent. Relat. Res.* **2001**, *3*, 204–213. [CrossRef] [PubMed]
3. Bornstein, M.M.; Schmid, B.; Belser, U.C.; Lussi, A.; Buser, D. Early loading of non-submerged titanium implants with a sandblasted and acid-etched surface. 5-year results of a prospective study in partially edentulous patients. *Clin. Oral Implant. Res.* **2005**, *16*, 631–638. [CrossRef]
4. Bergkvist, G.; Koh, K.-J.; Sahlholm, S.; Klintström, E.; Lindh, C. Bone density at implant sites and its relationship to assessment of bone quality and treatment outcome. *Int. J. Oral Maxillofac. Implant.* **2010**, *25*, 321–328.
5. Oates, T.W.; Valderrama, P.; Bischof, M.; Nedir, R.; Jones, A.; Simpson, J.; Toutenburg, H.; Cochran, D.L. Enhanced implant stability with a chemically modified SLA surface: A randomized pilot study. *Int. J. Oral Maxillofac. Implant.* **2007**, *22*, 755–760.
6. Cheng, Y.-C.; Ewers, R.; Morgan, K.; Hirayama, M.; Murcko, L.; Morgan, J.; Bergamo, E.T.P.; Bonfante, E.A. Antiresorptive therapy and dental implant survival: An up to 20-year retrospective cohort study in women. *Clin. Oral Investig.* **2022**, *26*, 6569–6582. [CrossRef]
7. Andrade, C.A.S.; Paz, J.L.C.; de Melo, G.S.; Mahrouseh, N.; Januário, A.L.; Capeletti, L.R. Survival rate and peri-implant evaluation of immediately loaded dental implants in individuals with type 2 diabetes mellitus: A systematic review and meta-analysis. *Clin. Oral Investig.* **2022**, *26*, 1797–1810. [CrossRef] [PubMed]
8. Chackartchi, T.; Romanos, G.E.; Parkanyi, L.; Schwarz, F.; Sculean, A. Reducing errors in guided implant surgery to optimize treatment outcomes. *Periodontology 2000* **2022**, *88*, 64–72. [CrossRef] [PubMed]
9. Derksen, W.; Wismeijer, D.; Flügge, T.; Hassan, B.; Tahmaseb, A. The accuracy of computer-guided implant surgery with tooth-supported, digitally designed drill guides based on CBCT and intraoral scanning. A prospective cohort study. *Clin. Oral Implant. Res.* **2019**, *30*, 1005–1015. [CrossRef]
10. Wang, X.; Shaheen, E.; Shujaat, S.; Meeus, J.; Legrand, P.; Lahoud, P.; Gerhardt, M.D.N.; Politis, C.; Jacobs, R. Influence of experience on dental implant placement: An in vitro comparison of freehand, static guided and dynamic navigation approaches. *Int. J. Implant. Dent.* **2022**, *8*, 42. [CrossRef]
11. Russo, L.L.; Caradonna, G.; Biancardino, M.; De Lillo, A.; Troiano, G.; Guida, L. Digital versus conventional workflow for the fabrication of multiunit fixed prostheses: A systematic review and meta-analysis of vertical marginal fit in controlled in vitro studies. *J. Prosthet. Dent.* **2019**, *122*, 435–440. [CrossRef] [PubMed]
12. Aktas, G.; Özcan, N.; Aydin, D.H.; Şahin, E.; Akça, K. Effect of digitizing techniques on the fit of implant-retained crowns with different antirotational abutment features. *J. Prosthet. Dent.* **2014**, *111*, 367–372. [CrossRef]
13. Nagata, K.; Fuchigami, K.; Okuhama, Y.; Wakamori, K.; Tsuruoka, H.; Nakashizu, T.; Hoshi, N.; Atsumi, M.; Kimoto, K.; Kawana, H. Comparison of digital and silicone impressions for single-tooth implants and two- and three-unit implants for a free-end edentulous saddle. *BMC Oral Health* **2021**, *21*, 464. [CrossRef] [PubMed]

14. Valenzuela-Levi, N. Poor performance in municipal recycling: The case of Chile. *Waste Manag.* **2021**, *133*, 49–58. [CrossRef] [PubMed]
15. Antoniadou, M.; Varzakas, T.; Tzoutzas, I. Circular Economy in Conjunction with Treatment Methodologies in the Biomedical and Dental Waste Sectors. *Circ. Econ. Sustain.* **2021**, *1*, 563–592. [CrossRef]
16. Mandalidis, A.; Topalidis, A.; Voudrias, E.A.; Iosifidis, N. Composition, production rate and characterization of Greek dental solid waste. *Waste Manag.* **2018**, *75*, 124–130. [CrossRef]
17. Koolivand, A.; Gholami-Borujeni, F.; Nourmoradi, H. Investigation on the characteristics and management of dental waste in Urmia, Iran. *J. Mater. Cycles Waste Manag.* **2015**, *17*, 553–559. [CrossRef]
18. Sabbahi, D.A.; El-Naggar, H.M.; Zahran, M.H. Management of dental waste in dental offices and clinics in Jeddah, Saudi Arabia. *J. Air Waste Manag. Assoc.* **2020**, *70*, 1022–1029. [CrossRef]
19. Papi, P.; Di Murro, B.; Penna, D.; Pompa, G. Digital prosthetic workflow during COVID-19 pandemic to limit infection risk in dental practice. *Oral Dis.* **2020**, *27*, 723–726. [CrossRef]
20. Frahdian, T.; Hasratiningsih, Z.; Karlina, E.; Herdiyantoro, D.; Takarini, V. Dental alginate impression waste as additional fertiliser for plant yields and soil quality. *Padjadjaran J. Dent.* **2018**, *30*, 12. [CrossRef]
21. Alharbi, N.; Osman, R.; Wismeijer, D. Effects of build direction on the mechanical properties of 3D-printed complete coverage interim dental restorations. *J. Prosthet. Dent.* **2016**, *115*, 760–767. [CrossRef] [PubMed]
22. Srinivasan, M.; Kalberer, N.; Kamnoedboon, P.; Mekki, M.; Durual, S.; Özcan, M.; Müller, F. CAD-CAM complete denture resins: An evaluation of biocompatibility, mechanical properties, and surface characteristics. *J. Dent.* **2021**, *114*, 103785. [CrossRef]
23. Ishida, Y.; Miura, D.; Miyasaka, T.; Shinya, A. Dimensional Accuracy of Dental Casting Patterns Fabricated Using Consumer 3D Printers. *Polymers* **2020**, *12*, 2244. [CrossRef] [PubMed]
24. Kim, S.-Y.; Shin, Y.-S.; Jung, H.-D.; Hwang, C.-J.; Baik, H.-S.; Cha, J.-Y. Precision and trueness of dental models manufactured with different 3-dimensional printing techniques. *Am. J. Orthod. Dentofac. Orthop.* **2018**, *153*, 144–153. [CrossRef]
25. Borrello, J.; Nasser, P.; Iatridis, J.C.; Costa, K.D. 3D printing a mechanically-tunable acrylate resin on a commercial DLP-SLA printer. *Addit. Manuf.* **2018**, *23*, 374–380. [CrossRef]
26. Maspero, C.; Tartaglia, G.M. 3D Printing of Clear Orthodontic Aligners: Where We Are and Where We Are Going. *Materials* **2020**, *13*, 5204. [CrossRef]
27. Wegmüller, L.; Halbeisen, F.; Sharma, N.; Kühl, S.; Thieringer, F.M. Consumer vs. High-End 3D Printers for Guided Implant Surgery—An In Vitro Accuracy Assessment Study of Different 3D Printing Technologies. *J. Clin. Med.* **2021**, *10*, 4894. [CrossRef] [PubMed]
28. Hopewell, J.; Dvorak, R.; Kosior, E. Plastics recycling: Challenges and opportunities. *Philos. Trans. R. Soc. Lond. B Biol. Sci.* **2009**, *364*, 2115–2126. [CrossRef]
29. Kristiawan, R.B.; Imaduddin, F.; Ariawan, D.; Arifin, Z. A review on the fused deposition modeling (FDM) 3D printing: Filament processing, materials, and printing parameters. *Open Eng.* **2021**, *11*, 639–649. [CrossRef]
30. Micó-Vicent, B.; Perales, E.; Huraibat, K.; Martínez-Verdú, F.M.; Viqueira, V. Maximization of FDM-3D-Objects Gonio-Appearance Effects Using PLA and ABS Filaments and Combining Several Printing Parameters: "A Case Study". *Materials* **2019**, *12*, 1423. [CrossRef]
31. D'anna, A.; Arrigo, R.; Frache, A. PLA/PHB Blends: Biocompatibilizer Effects. *Polymers* **2019**, *11*, 1416. [CrossRef]
32. Farah, S.; Anderson, D.G.; Langer, R. Physical and mechanical properties of PLA, and their functions in widespread applications—A comprehensive review. *Adv. Drug Deliv. Rev.* **2016**, *107*, 367–392. [CrossRef]
33. Gai, M.; Li, W.; Frueh, J.; Sukhorukov, G.B. Polylactic acid sealed polyelectrolyte complex microcontainers for controlled encapsulation and NIR-Laser based release of cargo. *Colloids Surf. B Biointerfaces* **2018**, *173*, 521–528. [CrossRef] [PubMed]
34. Li, Z.; Wu, T.; Chen, Y.; Gao, X.; Ye, J.; Jin, Y.; Chen, B. Oriented homo-epitaxial crystallization of polylactic acid displaying a biomimetic structure and improved blood compatibility. *J. Biomed. Mater. Res. A* **2021**, *110*, 684–695. [CrossRef] [PubMed]
35. Ahuja, R.; Kumari, N.; Srivastava, A.; Bhati, P.; Vashisth, P.; Yadav, P.; Jacob, T.; Narang, R.; Bhatnagar, N. Biocompatibility analysis of PLA based candidate materials for cardiovascular stents in a rat subcutaneous implant model. *Acta Histochem.* **2020**, *122*, 151615. [CrossRef] [PubMed]
36. Benli, M.; Eker-Gümüş, B.; Kahraman, Y.; Huck, O.; Özcan, M. Can polylactic acid be a CAD/CAM material for provisional crown restorations in terms of fit and fracture strength? *Dent. Mater. J.* **2021**, *40*, 772–780. [CrossRef]
37. Molinero-Mourelle, P.; Canals, S.; Gómez-Polo, M.; Solá-Ruiz, M.; Highsmith, J.D.R.; Viñuela, A. Polylactic Acid as a Material for Three-Dimensional Printing of Provisional Restorations. *Int. J. Prosthodont.* **2018**, *31*, 349–350. [CrossRef] [PubMed]
38. Crenn, M.-J.; Rohman, G.; Fromentin, O.; Benoit, A. Polylactic acid as a biocompatible polymer for three-dimensional printing of interim prosthesis: Mechanical characterization. *Dent. Mater. J.* **2022**, *41*, 110–116. [CrossRef] [PubMed]
39. Park, S.-M.; Park, J.-M.; Kim, S.-K.; Heo, S.-J.; Koak, J.-Y. Flexural Strength of 3D-Printing Resin Materials for Provisional Fixed Dental Prostheses. *Materials* **2020**, *13*, 3970. [CrossRef]
40. Koske, D.; Ehrmann, A. Advanced Infill Designs for 3D Printed Shape-Memory Components. *Micromachines* **2021**, *12*, 1225. [CrossRef]
41. Yang, Y.; Xiong, Z.; Zhang, L.; Tang, Z.; Zhang, R.; Zhu, J. Isosorbide dioctoate as a "green" plasticizer for poly(lactic acid). *Mater. Des.* **2016**, *91*, 262–268. [CrossRef]

42. Muta, S.; Ikeda, M.; Nikaido, T.; Sayed, M.; Sadr, A.; Suzuki, T.; Tagami, J. Chairside fabrication of provisional crowns on FDM 3D-printed PVA model. *J. Prosthodont. Res.* **2020**, *64*, 401–407. [CrossRef] [PubMed]
43. Wang, X.; Su, J. Evaluation of Precision of Custom Edentulous Trays Fabricated with 3D Printing Technologies. *Int. J. Prosthodont.* **2021**, *34*, 109–117. [CrossRef]
44. Lagazzo, A.; Moliner, C.; Bosio, B.; Botter, R.; Arato, E. Evaluation of the Mechanical and Thermal Properties Decay of PHBV/Sisal and PLA/Sisal Biocomposites at Different Recycle Steps. *Polymers* **2019**, *11*, 1477. [CrossRef] [PubMed]
45. Vidakis, N.; Petousis, M.; Tzounis, L.; Maniadi, A.; Velidakis, E.; Mountakis, N.; Kechagias, J.D. Sustainable Additive Manufacturing: Mechanical Response of Polyamide 12 over Multiple Recycling Processes. *Materials* **2021**, *14*, 466. [CrossRef]
46. Anderson, I. Mechanical Properties of Specimens 3D Printed with Virgin and Recycled Polylactic Acid. *3D Print. Addit. Manuf.* **2017**, *4*, 110–115. [CrossRef]
47. Majgaonkar, P.; Hanich, R.; Malz, F.; Brüll, R. Chemical Recycling of Post-Consumer PLA Waste for Sustainable Production of Ethyl Lactate. *Chem. Eng. J.* **2021**, *423*, 129952. [CrossRef]
48. Hegedus, T.; Kreuter, P.; Kismarczi-Antalffy, A.A.; Demeter, T.; Banyai, D.; Vegh, A.; Geczi, Z.; Hermann, P.; Payer, M.; Zsembery, A.; et al. User Experience and Sustainability of 3D Printing in Dentistry. *Int. J. Environ. Res. Public Health* **2022**, *19*, 1921. [CrossRef]
49. Nagata, K.; Muromachi, K.; Kouzai, Y.; Inaba, K.; Inoue, E.; Fuchigami, K.; Nihei, T.; Atsumi, M.; Kimoto, K.; Kawana, H. Fit accuracy of resin crown on a dental model fabricated using fused deposition modeling 3D printing and a polylactic acid filament. *J. Prosthodont. Res.* **2023**, *67*, 144–149. [CrossRef] [PubMed]
50. Tagliaferri, V.; Trovalusci, F.; Guarino, S.; Venettacci, S. Environmental and Economic Analysis of FDM, SLS and MJF Additive Manufacturing Technologies. *Materials* **2019**, *12*, 4161. [CrossRef] [PubMed]
51. Joda, T.; Zarone, F.; Ferrari, M. The complete digital workflow in fixed prosthodontics: A systematic review. *BMC Oral Health* **2017**, *17*, 124. [CrossRef] [PubMed]
52. Joda, T.; Brägger, U. Time-efficiency analysis of the treatment with monolithic implant crowns in a digital workflow: A randomized controlled trial. *Clin. Oral Implant. Res.* **2016**, *27*, 1401–1406. [CrossRef]
53. Mühlemann, S.; Greter, E.A.; Park, J.-M.; Hämmerle, C.H.F.; Thoma, D.S. Precision of digital implant models compared to conventional implant models for posterior single implant crowns: A within-subject comparison. *Clin. Oral Implant. Res.* **2018**, *29*, 931–936. [CrossRef] [PubMed]
54. Chiu, A.; Chen, Y.-W.; Hayashi, J.; Sadr, A. Accuracy of CAD/CAM Digital Impressions with Different Intraoral Scanner Parameters. *Sensors* **2020**, *20*, 1157. [CrossRef]
55. Ren, S.; Jiang, X.; Lin, Y.; Di, P. Crown Accuracy and Time Efficiency of Cement-Retained Implant-Supported Restorations in a Complete Digital Workflow: A Randomized Control Trial. *J. Prosthodont.* **2021**, *31*, 405–411. [CrossRef] [PubMed]
56. Al Hamad, K.Q.; Al-Rashdan, R.B.; Al-Rashdan, B.A.; Baba, N.Z. Effect of Milling Protocols on Trueness and Precision of Ceramic Crowns. *J. Prosthodont.* **2021**, *30*, 171–176. [CrossRef]
57. Hanon, M.M.; Zsidai, L.; Ma, Q. Accuracy investigation of 3D printed PLA with various process parameters and different colors. *Mater. Today* **2021**, *42*, 3089–3096. [CrossRef]
58. Kamio, T.; Hayashi, K.; Onda, T.; Takaki, T.; Shibahara, T.; Yakushiji, T.; Shibui, T.; Kato, H. Utilizing a low-cost desktop 3D printer to develop a "one-stop 3D printing lab" for oral and maxillofacial surgery and dentistry fields. *3D Print. Med.* **2018**, *4*, 6. [CrossRef]
59. Chen, L.; He, Y.; Yang, Y.; Niu, S.; Ren, H. The research status and development trend of additive manufacturing technology. *Int. J. Adv. Manuf. Technol.* **2016**, *89*, 3651–3660. [CrossRef]
60. George, E.; Liacouras, P.; Rybicki, F.J.; Mitsouras, D. Measuring and Establishing the Accuracy and Reproducibility of 3D Printed Medical Models. *Radiographics* **2017**, *37*, 1424–1450. [CrossRef]
61. Rybachuk, M.; Mauger, C.A.; Fiedler, T.; Öchsner, A. Anisotropic mechanical properties of fused deposition modeled parts fabricated by using acrylonitrile butadiene styrene polymer. *J. Polym. Eng.* **2017**, *37*, 699–706. [CrossRef]
62. Mohamed, O.A.; Masood, S.H.; Bhowmik, J.L. Modeling, analysis, and optimization of dimensional accuracy of FDM-fabricated parts using definitive screening design and deep learning feedforward artificial neural network. *Adv. Manuf.* **2021**, *9*, 115–129. [CrossRef]
63. Katsoulis, J.; Mericske-Stern, R.; Rotkina, L.; Zbären, C.; Enkling, N.; Blatz, M.B. Precision of fit of implant-supported screw-retained 10-unit computer-aided-designed and computer-aided-manufactured frameworks made from zirconium dioxide and titanium: An in vitro study. *Clin. Oral Implant. Res.* **2014**, *25*, 165–174. [CrossRef] [PubMed]
64. Al-Meraikhi, H.; Yilmaz, B.; McGlumphy, E.; Brantley, W.; Johnston, W.M. In vitro fit of CAD-CAM complete arch screw-retained titanium and zirconia implant prostheses fabricated on 4 implants. *J. Prosthet. Dent.* **2017**, *119*, 409–416. [CrossRef]
65. Yilmaz, B.; Kale, E.; Johnston, W.M. Marginal discrepancy of CAD-CAM complete-arch fixed implant-supported frameworks. *J. Prosthet. Dent.* **2018**, *120*, 65–70. [CrossRef] [PubMed]
66. Presotto, A.G.C.; Bhering, C.L.B.; Mesquita, M.F.; Barão, V.A.R. Marginal fit and photoelastic stress analysis of CAD-CAM and overcast 3-unit implant-supported frameworks. *J. Prosthet. Dent.* **2017**, *117*, 373–379. [CrossRef]
67. Yilmaz, B.; Alshahrani, F.A.; Kale, E.; Johnston, W.M. Effect of feldspathic porcelain layering on the marginal fit of zirconia and titanium complete-arch fixed implant-supported frameworks. *J. Prosthet. Dent.* **2018**, *120*, 71–78. [CrossRef]

68. Molinero-Mourelle, P.; Cascos-Sanchez, R.; Yilmaz, B.; Lam, W.Y.H.; Pow, E.H.N.; Highsmith, J.D.R.; Gómez-Polo, M. Effect of Fabrication Technique on the Microgap of CAD/CAM Cobalt–Chrome and Zirconia Abutments on a Conical Connection Implant: An In Vitro Study. *Materials* **2021**, *14*, 2348. [CrossRef]
69. Gedrimiene, A.; Adaskevicius, R.; Rutkunas, V. Accuracy of digital and conventional dental implant impressions for fixed partial dentures: A comparative clinical study. *J. Adv. Prosthodont.* **2019**, *11*, 271–279. [CrossRef]
70. De La Cruz, J.E.; Funkenbusch, P.; Ercoli, C.; Moss, M.E.; Graser, G.N.; Tallents, R.H. Verification jig for implant-supported prostheses: A comparison of standard impressions with verification jigs made of different materials. *J. Prosthet. Dent.* **2002**, *88*, 329–336. [CrossRef]
71. Krechmer, J.E.; Phillips, B.; Chaloux, N.; Shomberg, R.; Daube, C.; Manchanda, G.; Murray, S.; McCarthy, A.; Fonseca, R.; Thakkar, J.; et al. Chemical Emissions from Cured and Uncured 3D-Printed Ventilator Patient Circuit Medical Parts. *ACS Omega* **2021**, *6*, 30726–30733. [CrossRef] [PubMed]
72. Chan, F.L.; Hon, C.-Y.; Tarlo, S.M.; Rajaram, N.; House, R. Emissions and health risks from the use of 3D printers in an occupational setting. *J. Toxicol. Environ. Health A* **2020**, *83*, 279–287. [CrossRef] [PubMed]
73. Wojtyła, S.; Klama, P.; Baran, T. Is 3D printing safe? Analysis of the thermal treatment of thermoplastics: ABS, PLA, PET, and nylon. *J. Occup. Environ. Hyg.* **2017**, *14*, D80–D85. [CrossRef]
74. Dobrzyńska, E.; Kondej, D.; Kowalska, J.; Szewczyńska, M. State of the art in additive manufacturing and its possible chemical and particle hazards—Review. *Indoor Air* **2021**, *31*, 1733–1758. [CrossRef]
75. Qiu, Q.Q.; Sun, W.Q.; Connor, J. *Sterilization of Biomaterials of Synthetic and Biological Origin*; Elsevier Ltd.: Amsterdam, The Netherlands, 2017.
76. Tipnis, N.P.; Burgess, D.J. Sterilization of implantable polymer-based medical devices: A review. *Int. J. Pharm.* **2018**, *544*, 455–460. [CrossRef]
77. Ribeiro, N.; Soares, G.C.; Santos-Rosales, V.; Concheiro, A.; Alvarez-Lorenzo, C.; García-González, C.A.; Oliveira, A.L. A new era for sterilization based on supercritical CO_2 technology. *J. Biomed. Mater. Res. Part B Appl. Biomater.* **2019**, *108*, 399–428. [CrossRef] [PubMed]
78. Dai, Z.; Ronholm, J.; Tian, Y.; Sethi, B.; Cao, X. Sterilization techniques for biodegradable scaffolds in tissue engineering applications. *J. Tissue Eng.* **2016**, *7*, 2041731416648810. [CrossRef] [PubMed]
79. Davila, S.P.; Rodríguez, L.G.; Chiussi, S.; Serra, J.; González, P. How to Sterilize Polylactic Acid Based Medical Devices? *Polymers* **2021**, *13*, 2115. [CrossRef] [PubMed]

Disclaimer/Publisher's Note: The statements, opinions and data contained in all publications are solely those of the individual author(s) and contributor(s) and not of MDPI and/or the editor(s). MDPI and/or the editor(s) disclaim responsibility for any injury to people or property resulting from any ideas, methods, instructions or products referred to in the content.

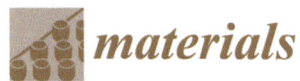 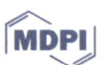

Article

Restorative Dental Resin Functionalized with Calcium Methacrylate with a Hydroxyapatite Remineralization Capacity

Xin Zhang [1], Yuxuan Zhang [2], Ying Li [1], Xiaoming Wang [3] and Xueqin Zhang [1,*]

[1] College of Chemistry and Materials Engineering, Beijing Technology and Business University, Beijing 100048, China
[2] FuYang Sineva Materials Technology Co., Ltd., Beijing 100176, China; zhangyuxuan@sineva.com.cn
[3] Shuozhou Comprehensive Inspection and Testing Center, Shuozhou 036000, China
* Correspondence: zhangxueqin@btbu.edu.cn

Abstract: The ability of dental materials to induce the mineralization of enamel like hydroxyapatite (HA) is of great importance. In this article, a novel kind of dental restorative material characterized by a mineralization ability was fabricated by photopolymerization. Calcium methacrylate (CMA) was introduced into the classical bisphenol A-glycidyl methacrylate (Bis-GMA) and triethylene glycol dimethacrylate (TEGDMA) dental resin formulation. This functional dental resin (BTCM) was calcium-rich and can be prepared simply by one-step photopolymerization. The influence of CMA on the photopolymerization kinetics, the dental resin's mechanical properties, and its capacity to induce dynamic in situ HA mineralization were examined. Real-time FTIR, compression modulus, scanning electron microscopy, X-ray spectroscopy, MTT assay, and cell attachment test were carried out. The obtained data were analyzed for statistical significance using analysis of variance (ANOVA). Double bond conversion could be completed in less than 300 s, while the compression modulus of BTCM decreased with the increase in CMA content (30 wt%, 40 wt%, and 50 wt%). After being soaked in $Ca(NO_3)_2$ and Na_2HPO_4 solutions alternatively, dense HA crystals were found on the surface of the dental resin which contained CMA. The amount of HA increased with the increase in CMA content. The MTT results indicated that BTCM possesses good biocompatibility, while the cell adhesion and proliferation investigation demonstrated that L929 cells can adhere and proliferate well on the surface of BTM. Thus, our approach provides a straightforward, cost-effective, and environmentally friendly solution that has the potential for immediate clinical use.

Keywords: dentistry; dental materials; dental resin; photopolymerization; hydroxyapatite; calcium methacrylate; remineralization

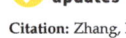

Citation: Zhang, X.; Zhang, Y.; Li, Y.; Wang, X.; Zhang, X. Restorative Dental Resin Functionalized with Calcium Methacrylate with a Hydroxyapatite Remineralization Capacity. *Materials* 2023, *16*, 6497. https://doi.org/10.3390/ma16196497

Academic Editors: Josip Kranjčić and Tina Poklepovic Pericic

Received: 29 August 2023
Revised: 24 September 2023
Accepted: 27 September 2023
Published: 29 September 2023

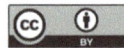

Copyright: © 2023 by the authors. Licensee MDPI, Basel, Switzerland. This article is an open access article distributed under the terms and conditions of the Creative Commons Attribution (CC BY) license (https://creativecommons.org/licenses/by/4.0/).

1. Introduction

Enamel serves as the outermost protective layer of teeth, primarily comprising inorganic minerals, with hydroxyapatite (HA) being the predominant component, making up approximately 96% to 98% of its composition [1,2]. Enamel mineralization is a complex extracellular process regulated by matrix proteins, especially enamel proteins, which control the nucleation, growth, and self-assembly of crystals [3]. However, enamel is vulnerable to demineralization due to acid erosion or mechanical wear, leading to enamel loss and the formation of cavities [4]. Mature enamel is non-vital tissue, which means that it lacks the ability for rapid self-repair once cavities have formed [5]. Given the importance of enamel in tooth protection and oral health, the repair of enamel defects is of significant importance. Enamel can be effectively restored using biomimetic repair strategies, which focus on chemical consistency and structural restoration. The traditional dental restoration strategy, which employs materials such as metal [6,7], ceramic [8], and composite resin [9], primarily follows a dislocated repair approach. In contrast, biomimetic mineralization repair represents an in situ repair strategy, allowing the regeneration of calcium phosphate crystals in the mineral-deficient area [10–12]. Incorporating the component with the ability to bind with Ca^{2+} or PO_4^{3-} into the dental restorative materials can enhance the remineralization capacity of enamel lesions caused by dental caries. Moreover, releasing Ca^{2+} and PO_4^{3-} around the carious region to increase the oversaturation of HA can lead to more Ca^{2+} and PO_4^{3-} from saliva being deposited onto the carious lesion [13,14]. Historically, fluoride was the first and has long been used as a highly effective agent for inhibiting the formation of dental caries and promoting enamel remineralization [15,16]. Fluoride can directly react with HA crystals in the solution to form fluoroapatite (FHAP) or fluorapatite (FAP) [17]. Recently, various biomimetic systems containing ACP (amorphous calcium phosphate) nanoparticles which significantly enhance enamel remineralization have been developed [18]. There has been significant research focused on commercialized casein phosphopeptide-ACP (CPP-ACP) [19–21]. CPP-ACP can promote enamel remineralization, and its synergistic effect with fluoride further enhances the remineralization process [22]. In addition, biomimetic HA is a highly effective enamel repair material due to its similar chemical composition to enamel [23,24]. Clinical trials demonstrated that biomimetic HA paste can effectively reduce dental sensitivity and improve enamel integrity [25]. In addition, dental resin composites incorporated with one or a variety of reinforcing fillers such as bioactive glass [26,27], zeolites [28–30], HA [31,32], ACC [33,34], silica [35], calcium fluoride [36], CPP-ACP [14,37] and so on, have found widespread use in repairing decayed teeth due to their enhanced HA regeneration ability, substantial mechanical strength, excellent aesthetic results, minimal health concerns, and ease of handling properties [38–40]. A typical composition for dental resin composites includes a resin matrix composed of monomers such as bisphenol A-glycidyl methacrylate (Bis-GMA) and triethylene glycol dimethacrylate (TEGDMA) [41]. Liu et al. [42] developed a poly (Bis-GMA)-grafted HA-whisker-reinforced Bis-GMA/TEGDMA dental resin with a reduced volume shrinkage and enhanced flexural strength. Sandomierski et al. [43] fabricated Bis-GMA/TEGDMA filled with a calcium montmorillonite filler coated with HA, demonstrating its capacity to promote HA mineralization. Qin et al. [31] prepared a salinized HA nanofiber filler loaded with erythromycin (s-HAFs@EM) to reinforce Bis-GMA/TEGDMA resin. The addition of s-HAFs@EM imparted the dental composite with an excellent antibacterial activity and HA remineralization capacity. Jardim et al. [44] incorporated HA nanoparticles (HANPs) into Bis-GMA/TEGDMA dental resin matrix. This composite was capable of releasing Ca^{2+} and PO_4^{3-} ions, thereby enhancing the remineralization ability.

Nonetheless, the complex oral environment and the impact from chewing can result in irrevocable or enduring loss of fillers in the restorative composite, further reducing their ability to induce HA regeneration. Calcium methacrylate (CMA, Figure 1), a bifunctional monomer and the calcium salt of methacrylic acid, can also be employed as a monomer for photopolymerization [45]. The photopolymerization product of CMA can not only serve as a binding site for PO_4^{3-} in the oral environment but also release Ca^{2+}, facilitating the deposition of HA on its surface. When CMA is copolymerized within the Bis-GMA/TEGDMA resin system, the resulting polymer gains the capability to induce HA remineralization. Even if the surface is abraded, it retains the ability to promote HA remineralization because CMA is copolymerized within the resin network.

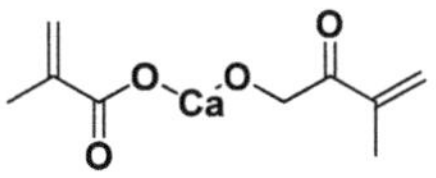

Figure 1. Chemical structure of CMA.

Thus, in this work, a novel dental restorative material characterized by a mineralization ability was fabricated by photopolymerization. CMA was introduced into the classical Bis-GMA/TEGDMA dental resin formulation. This functional dental resin Bis-

GMA/TEGDMA/CMA (BTCM) was calcium-rich and could be prepared simply by one-step photopolymerization. Through copolymerization with CMA, the resulting BTCM could induce the mineralization of a dense HA layer and could continue to stimulate the in situ generation of HA even if the surface layer was damaged. The primary purpose of this work is to endow dental restorative resin with the ability to regenerate HA and achieve self-repair in an oral environment by constructing a calcium-rich 3D polymer network structure. Another objective is to establish a simple and controllable method for the production of dental resin, facilitating scalable applications.

2. Materials and Methods

2.1. Materials

Bisphenol A-glycidyl methacrylate (Bis-GMA) and triethylene glycol dimethacrylate (TEGDMA) were kindly supplied by Sartomer Company (Warrington, PA, USA). Calcium methacrylate (CMA) and methacrylic acid (MAA) were purchased from Sigma-Aldrich (St. Louis, MO, USA). Camphorquinon (CQ) was obtained from Runtec Co., Ltd. (Jintan, Jiangsu, China). Ethyl 4-dimethylaminobenzoate (EDAB), calcium nitrate anhydrous ($Ca(NO_3)_2 \bullet 4H_2O$, analytical reagent), sodium dihydrogen phosphate ($Na_2HPO_4 \bullet 12H_2O$, analytical reagent), hydrochloric acid (HCl, 37.5%), and sodium hydroxide (NaOH, analytical reagent) were purchased from Sinopharm Chemical Reagent Co., Ltd. (Shanghai, China). 3-(4,5-dimethylthiazol-2-yl)-2,5-diphenyltetrazolium bromide tetrazole (MTT), Dulbecco's modified eagle medium (DMEM), fetal calf serum (FBS), and phosphate-buffered saline (PBS) were purchased from Sigma-Aldrich (St. Louis, MO, USA). Dimethyl sulfoxide (DMSO) and toluene were purchased from InnoChem Science & Technology Co., Ltd. (Beijing, China).

2.2. Methods

2.2.1. The Fabrication of Calcium Poly(methyl methacrylate) (BTCM)-Based Dental Material

Bis-GMA, TEGDMA, CMA, MAA, and the photoinitiation system (CQ and EDAB) were mixed in specific ratios as indicated in Table 1. Notably, the weight ratios of Bis-GMA to TEGDMA and CQ to EDAB were maintained at 7:3 and 1:1, respectively. The mixture was intensely stirred for 20 min and then subjected to 15 min of sonication to eliminate any air inside the container. The resulting mixture was subsequently added into a polytetrafluoroethylene (PTFE) cylindrical mold. Photocrosslinking was carried out for 10 min by using an LED light with an emission wavelength at 460 nm, and the light intensity was set to 50 mW cm^{-2} [46]. The sample BTCM-1, without adding any CMA, was used as the control group. The preparation steps are illustrated in Figure 2.

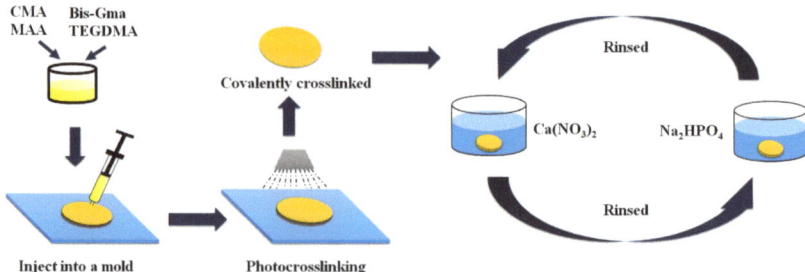

Figure 2. Diagram illustrating the process of mineralization of BTCM.

Table 1. The formulation of the BTCM samples.

Sample	Bis-GMA (g)	TEGDMA (g)	CMA (g)	MAA (g)	CQ (g)	EDAB (g)
BTCM-1	7	3	0	0	0.1	0.1
BTCM-2	3.85	1.65	3	1.5	0.1	0.1
BTCM-3	2.8	1.2	4	2	0.1	0.1
BTCM-4	1.75	0.75	5	2.5	0.1	0.1

2.2.2. The Mineralization of BTCM

The remineralization of HA induced by BTCM was achieved via alternative soaking process (ASP) [47]. A Ca(NO$_3$)$_2$ solution of 0.5 mol L^{-1} and a Na$_2$HPO$_4$ solution of 0.3 mol L^{-1} were prepared by dissolving the calculated amount of Ca(NO$_3$)$_2$ and Na$_2$HPO$_4$ in deionized water, respectively. By using 1 mol L^{-1} NaOH, the pH of the Ca(NO$_3$)$_2$ and Na$_2$HPO$_4$ solutions was adjusted to 10. The photopolymerized BTCMs were preconditioned in deionized water for 60 s and then soaked in the Ca(NO$_3$)$_2$ solution for 4 h. Afterward, the samples were taken out and rinsed with deionized water for 60 s before being soaked in the Na$_2$HPO$_4$ solution for 4 h. This entire process constituted one cycle of ASP (Figure 2). Three cycles of ASP were performed for the mineralization of each BTCM sample. Following these three cycles of ASP, BTCM samples were washed with deionized water and placed in a vacuum dryer at 50 °C for 24 h.

2.2.3. Remineralization of HA on the Abraded BTCM Matrixes

To simulate the abrasion of the HA layer, the surface of each BTCM matrix, which was already mineralized with HA, were polished using sandpaper. After polishing, the mineralized HA was removed, and the inner polymer was exposed. All polished BTCM samples were then set to three cycles of ASP [47] to induce the remineralization of HA (Figure 2). Each cycle lasted for 8 h. The BTCM samples obtained from three cycles of ASP were washed with deionized water and placed in a vacuum dryer at 50 °C for 24 h.

2.3. Characterization

2.3.1. Photopolymerization Kinetics

The kinetics analysis of photopolymerization reactions was investigated using Realtime-FTIR (Nicolet 5700, Nicolet Instrument Corp., Madison, WI, USA), equipped with an MCT/A KBr detector [48,49]. The BTCM mixtures with varying compositions were applied between two layers of KBr salt plates using a capillary and placed on a real-time infrared horizontal sample stage. An LED light with an emission wavelength of 460 nm was utilized as the light source for photopolymerization. The infrared absorption peak of the C=C double bonds in CMA was observed around 1640 cm^{-1}, while the absorption peak of the C=C double bonds in Bis-GMA/TEGDMA was observed around 1680 cm^{-1}. Information about the progress of the reaction was obtained by monitoring changes in its peak area. The final conversion rate of the polymerization reaction was calculated using Equation (1), with data processing carried out using the OMNIC 7.5 infrared software (Thermo Fisher Scientific, Wilmington, MA, USA) and the ORIGIN 8.0 (OriginLab Corporation, Norwood, MA, USA) data processing software.

$$DC(\%) = \frac{A_0 - A_t}{A_0} 100\% \tag{1}$$

where DC is the conversion of C=C double bonds at t time, A_0 represents the peak area of C=C double bonds before photopolymerization, and A_t represents the peak area of C=C double bonds after photopolymerization at time t.

2.3.2. Thermogravimetric Analysis

The thermal stability of the BTCM dental resin with different CMA concentrations was investigated using a TA Q500 thermogravimetric analyzer (TA Instruments, New Castle,

DE, USA) [50]. The BTCM samples were ground into a powder, and 5 mg was weighed and placed in a platinum sample pan for testing. Under a nitrogen atmosphere, the sample was heated from room temperature to 800 °C at a ramp rate of 10 °C/min. The nitrogen flow rate was set to 40 mL/min.

2.3.3. X-ray Diffraction Analysis (XRD)

The crystallinity of the crystals obtained from BTCM after three cycles of ASP was examined by an X-ray diffraction analysis. An X-ray diffractometer with Cu Kα radiation (λ = 0.154 nm), a 40 kV voltage, and a 40 mA current (Rigaku D/Max2500VB^{2+}/Pc diffract meter, Rigaku Company, Tokyo, Japan), was used [50]. The scanning range was from 10° to 70°, with a scanning speed of 5°/min.

2.3.4. Mechanical Compression Test

The mechanical properties of the BTCM samples were investigated using an Instron 4505 universal materials testing machine (Instron, High Wycombe, UK) with a 10 kN load cell [51]. The samples were cylindrical columns with a diameter of 8 mm and a depth of 12 mm. The Instron testing machine's probe was programmed to descend at a rate of 5 mm/min, and the load was applied until the specimen's height was reduced by 30%. Testing was conducted using three samples for each composition.

2.3.5. Scanning Electron Microscopy (SEM)

The morphology of the BTCM samples, before and after three cycles of ASP, was observed by utilizing a Hitachi S-4700 (Hitachi, Tokyo, Japan) scanning electron microscope [51]. The BTCM samples were cut into the required shapes and placed on the sample stage, followed by gold coating before observation.

2.3.6. In Vitro Cell Cytotoxicity

The biocompatibility of the BTCM dental material was assessed through MTT cytotoxicity assays [46]. Prior to cell incubation, the BTCM slices were immersed in ultrapure water and ethanol for 18 h, respectively, to remove monomers and residual small molecules. The samples, which had undergone ultrapure water and ethanol soaking, were then subjected to high-pressure steam sterilization for sterilization and disinfection.

L929 mouse fibroblast cells were seeded in a sterile 96-well plate, and the density was 1×10^4 cells per well. After 24 h of culturing at 37 °C in an incubator with a humid atmosphere, 5% carbon dioxide, and a temperature of 37 °C, 100 μL of DMEM cell suspension was added to each well of the 96-well plate. The prepared BTCM samples were subsequently put into the confluent layer of L929 cells and further incubated under the same conditions. A PBS solution of 5 mg/mL MTT was prepared, and 20 μL of this solution was added to the 96-well plate after 24 h, 48 h, and 72 h of incubation, followed by another 4 h of incubation. Then, DMSO was added to the 96-well plate, and the formed MTT was dissolved by DMSO. Once the MTT had dissolved, the optical density (OD) at 595 nm was examined by using an enzyme-linked immunosorbent assay (ELISA) reader (Multiskan FC instrument, Thermo Fisher Scientific, Waltham, MA, USA), for each time point (24 h, 48 h, and 72 h). The biocompatibility of BTCM was determined by comparing the OD values of the sample group with those of the negative and positive control groups. In this context, toluene served as the positive control, while DMEM with 0.1% DMSO served as the negative control. Testing was conducted using three samples for each composition.

2.3.7. Cell Adhesion and Proliferation Investigation

The adhesion and proliferation of L929 cells on the BTCM surfaces were investigated using SEM [51]. Firstly, the BTCM samples were sterilized by autoclaving, and then these samples were affixed onto glass slides and placed in sterilized 24-well plates. Sterilized PBS buffer was added to the 24-well plate, followed by the addition of 1 mL of L929 cell suspension at a density of 1.5×10^4 cells mL^{-1}. After incubation in a humidified atmosphere with 5% carbon dioxide at 37 °C for 24 h, the cell-populated samples were removed and washed with PBS solution. The cells on the BTCM surfaces were fixed using a 2.5% glutaraldehyde solution and underwent a gradual dehydration process. After drying, the BTCM samples were gold-coated and then examined using SEM.

2.3.8. Statistical Analysis

IBM SPSS 25 (IBM Corp., Armonk, NY, USA) was used to analyze variance (ANOVA) for statistical analysis. All quantitative data are denoted in the form of "mean ± standard deviation". The compression test and MTT test were repeated three times independently, and a p-value <0.05 was considered statistically significant.

3. Results and Discussion

3.1. Photopolymerization Kinetics

The plots showing the double bond conversion (DC) versus irradiation time of Bis-GMA and TEGDMA incorporating different concentrations of CMA, irradiated by 460 nm wavelength light with an intensity of 50 mW cm^{-2}, are displayed in Figure 3. As shown in Figure 3, the DC of BTCM-1, BTCM-2, BTCM-3, and BTCM-4 all reached approximately 100% within 300 s (Table 2). This indicates that the double bonds in all samples were completely polymerized, forming C-C covalent bonds, ensuring the absence of small monomer molecule residues in the system. This is essential for BTCM's use as a dental material. With the increase in CMA concentration, the photopolymerization speed decreased, and the induction time of the photopolymerization system increased. This can be attributed to the positive charge of Ca^{2+} in CMA, which reduces the electron density in the double bond of CMA, thereby reducing the reactivity of the C=C double bond and leading to a decrease in the photopolymerization rate and an increase in the induction time. It is worth noting that the photopolymerization rate increased when 30% CMA (BTCM-2) was added to the resin system, while it decreased when 40% and 50% CMA (BTCM-3 and BTCM-4) were added to the resin system. This variation in the photopolymerization rate can be assigned to the joint effect of CMA and MAA on the viscosity of the resin mixture. By adding CMA and MAA into the formulation, the viscosity of the photopolymerization system decreased, leading to a higher molecule mobility and an increased reaction rate. However, excessive CMA in the formulation led to a reduction in the reaction rate, primarily due to the decreased electron density of the C=C bond.

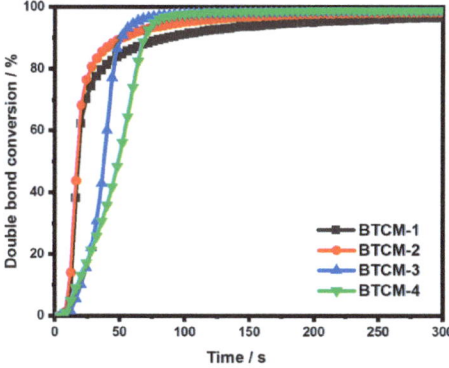

Figure 3. Photopolymerization kinetics of BTCM with different compositions.

Table 2. Double bond conversion of BTCM.

Sample Code	DC/%		
	60 s	150 s	300 s
BTCM-1	87.12	93.72	96.79
BTCM-2	92.18	96.76	98.41
BTCM-3	95.58	98.21	98.59
BTCM-4	82.56	98.58	99.02

3.2. Thermogravimetric Analysis (TGA)

The thermal degradation properties of the BTCM samples were explored through TGA. Figure 4 shows the TG curves for BTCM samples with different compositions. BTCM-1 exhibited a residual mass of 4.6%, primarily attributable to the remaining carbon content, while BTCM-2, BTCM-3, and BTCM-4 exhibited a residual mass of 7.7%, 10.1%, and 12.3% at 800 °C, respectively (Table 3). The remaining weight represented both the calcium and residual carbon content. The residual mass increased with the increase in CMA concentration. During the heating process, the copolymer breaks down and converts into small molecules, such as carbon dioxide, alkanes, and alkenes, which exit the reaction furnace at high temperatures. Simultaneously, the calcium present in the system undergoes transformation into $CaCO_3$ and ultimately decomposes into CaO, which remains in the heating furnace. A higher calcium content in the system leads to a higher final residual mass after heating.

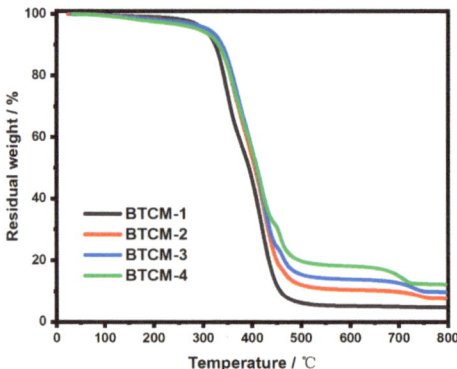

Figure 4. TGA curves of BTCM-1, BTCM-2, BTCM-3, and BTCM-4, respectively.

Table 3. The thermogravimetric analysis of the BTCM samples.

Sample Code	Residual Mass (%)
BTCM-1	4.67
BTCM-2	7.7
BTCM-3	10.1
BTCM-4	12.3

3.3. Compression Modulus Analysis

The mechanical characteristics of dental materials are crucial in the long-term durability of biomaterials. The compression moduli of the BTCM samples are depicted in Figure 5 and Table 4. As can be seen, the compression moduli of BTCM-1, BTCM-2, BTCM-3, and BTCM-4 were found to be 905.36 ± 10.68, 701.58 ± 20.13, 625.71 ± 25.69, and 537.43 ± 23.45 MPa (Table 4), respectively. The samples contained CMA showed statistically significant differences from BTCM-1 ($p = 0.000 < 0.005$). This indicates that the presence of CMA in the system has a substantial impact on the mechanical properties of BTCM. As the concentration of CMA increased, the compression modulus decreased. Since both CMA and MAA are present in the photopolymerization system, the mechanical properties of their polymerization product were significantly lower than those of BTCM-1, resulting in a decrease in the compression modulus.

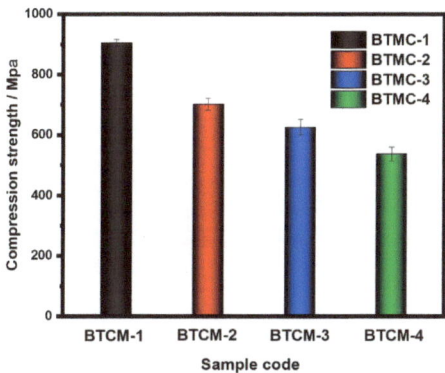

Figure 5. Compression moduli of BTCM samples with different compositions. The error bars represent the standard deviation of three replicates.

Table 4. The compression moduli of BTCM-1, BTCM-2, BTCM-3, and BTCM-4 after photopolymerization.

Sample Code	Compression Modulus
	Mean ± Standard Deviation (MPa)
BTCM-1	905.36 ± 10.68
BTCM-2	701.58 ± 20.13 ***
BTCM-3	625.71 ± 25.69 ***
BTCM-4	537.43 ± 23.45 ***

*** BTCM-2, BTCM-3, and BTCM-4 showed a statistically significant difference from BTCM-1, $p = 0.000 < 0.005$.
*** $p < 0.001$.

3.4. X-ray Diffraction (XRD) Analysis

Figure 6 displays the XRD patterns of the BTCM dental materials after three cycles of ASP. BTCM-1 exhibited a broad diffraction peak between 10° and 25°, indicating that BTCM-1 was amorphous and lacked bioactivity to induce the mineralization of HA. In contrast, BTCM-2, BTCM-3, and BTCM-4 all exhibited characteristic peaks of HA after three cycles of ASP, appearing at 2θ = 25.7°, 31.56°, 39.48°, 46.42°, and 53.38°, corresponding to the (002), (211), (310), (203), and (004) diffraction planes of HA (JCPDS #9-432), respectively [52,53]. Furthermore, BTCM-3 and BTCM-4 demonstrated better bioactivity, as mineralization of HA could be achieved within 24 h. Furthermore, BTCM-3 and BTCM-4 displayed diffraction peaks with higher intensities than BTCM-2, which indicated that the HA content was higher on BTCM-3 and BTCM-4. This is attributed to the higher calcium content in the polymerized materials. The greater the calcium content, the more HA can be generated.

To investigate the ability of BTCM to induce a dynamic HA regeneration, the surface of BTCM, which was covered with a layer of HA, was polished to expose the polymer once again, in order to simulate the damage or erosion of enamel. Subsequently, another three cycles of ASP were conducted, and the XRD patterns of BTCM after the ASP experiments are shown in Figure 7. The polished BTCM samples subjected to three new cycles of ASP exhibited similar crystallinity to the BTCM samples after the first three cycles of ASP. BTCM-1, once again, displayed a broad peak at 2θ = 10–25°, indicating its amorphous nature and low bioactivity. BTCM-2, BTCM-3, and BTCM-4 all exhibited diffraction peaks identical to those observed in the first round of ASP, specifically at 2θ = 25.7°, 31.56°, 39.48°,

46.42°, and 53.38°, corresponding to the (002), (211), (310), (203), and (004) diffraction planes of HA (JCPDS #9-432). The results indicate that the prepared BTCM dental materials possess a robust ability to stimulate HA regeneration, suggesting their potential in clinical utility as dental materials.

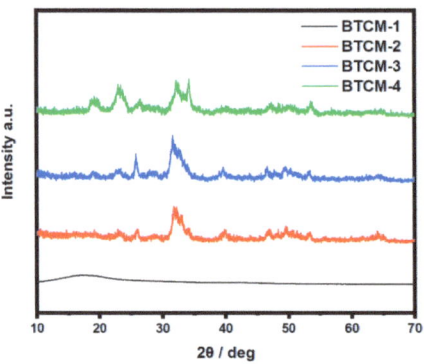

Figure 6. XRD patterns of the BTCM samples after three cycles of ASP.

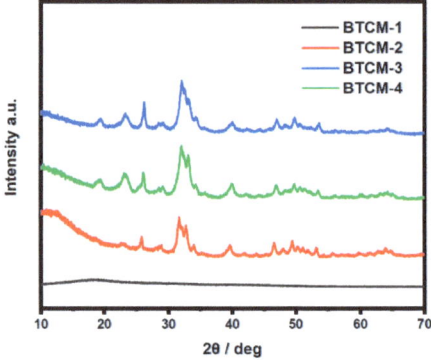

Figure 7. XRD patterns of the polished BTCM samples after 3 cycles of ASP.

3.5. Morphology Analysis by Scanning Electron Microscopy (SEM)

The morphology of the BTCM samples after three cycles of ASP was investigated by SEM, and the corresponding images are shown in Figure 8. As can be seen, with the increase in CMA concentration, a crystal growth evolution from spheroidal sediment to flocculent crystal sediment on the surface of BTCM can be observed. After three cycles of ASP, the surface of BTCM-1 appeared flat and smooth, which is consistent with the XRD patterns. This observation suggests that BTCM cannot induce the mineralization of HA due to the absence of binding sites for Ca^{2+} or PO_4^{3-}, which is required for mineralization. BTCM-2, BTCM-3, and BTCM-4 all exhibited strong bioactivity. After one cycle of mineralization, BTCM-2 exhibited spheroidal sediment on its surface. Meanwhile, BTCM-3 and BTCM-4 exhibited flocculent sediment composed of spheroidal crystals on their surfaces. After three cycles of mineralization, densely packed clusters of spheroids were found on the surfaces of BTCM-2, BTCM-3, and BTCM-4, indicating the excellent bioactivity of BTCM.

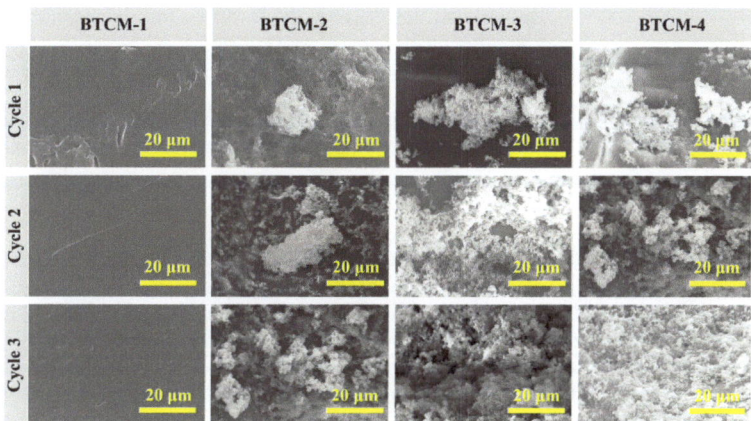

Figure 8. SEM images showing the evolution of the HA layer on BTCM samples with different compositions after 3 cycles of mineralization (scale bar: 20 μm).

To further investigate the ability of BTCM in inducing dynamic HA regeneration, the mineralized BTCM samples were polished and set to three new cycles of ASP and the mineralization results are shown in Figure 9. BTCM-1 showed no capacity to induce the mineralization of HA, while BTCM-2, BTCM-3, and BTCM-4 exhibited a similar trend to that observed during the first three cycles of mineralization. After the first cycle, spheroids of crystals appeared on the surfaces of BTCM-2, BTCM-3, and BTCM-4. As time progressed, thick layers of clustered spheroidal crystals developed on the surfaces of BTCM-2, BTCM-3, and BTCM-4, once again indicating the ability of the BTCM materials to induce a dynamic mineralization of HA on their surfaces. These results indicate that the calcium-rich BTCM dental restorative resin can effectively induce a dynamic and in situ remineralization of HA.

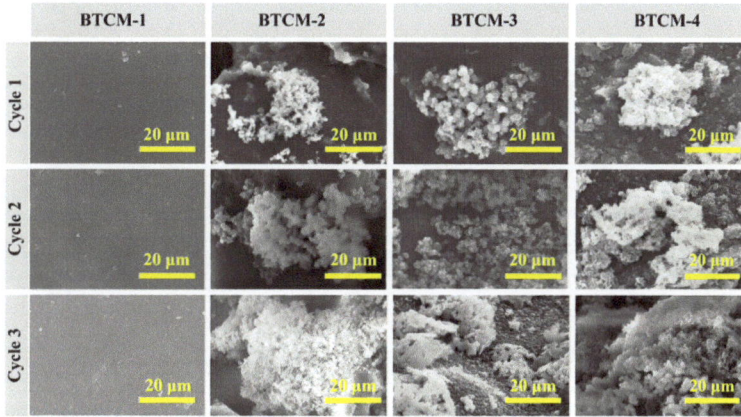

Figure 9. SEM images showing the evolution of the HA layer on BTCM samples with different compositions after 3 cycles of remineralization (scale bar: 20 μm).

Based on the XRD patterns and SEM images of the mineralized BTCM samples, an underlying HA growth mechanism could be inferred. Within the BTCM matrix, there are large quantities of calcium ions and carboxyl groups that serve as nucleation sites and binding sites for Ca^{2+} and PO_4^{3-} during the mineralization of HA. In the early stages, when BTCM was immersed in a solution containing PO_4^{3-}, the PO_4^{3-} ions rapidly accumulate around the positively charged Ca^{2+} ions, forming a locally supersaturated calcium phosphate solution (Figure 10a). When the system's Gibbs free energy decreased to a critical value, nucleation of crystals occurred. Subsequently, when PO_4^{3-}-bounded BTCM was immersed in $Ca(NO_3)_2$ solution, the substrate bound with the Ca^{2+} in the solution to generate amorphous calcium phosphate precursors. After three cycles of mineralization, more minerals, which were identified as HA (Figures 6 and 7), were generated. Moreover, when the HA-rich matrix was abraded and the former mineralized HA was removed, the Ca^{2+}- and carboxyl group-rich matrix could once again induce HA mineralization. Consequently, the matrix is covered by HA after immersion in the appropriate environment (Figures 9 and 10b). Enamel demineralization refers to the dissolution of the HA mineral, hydroxyapatite mineral, in the teeth under acidic conditions in the oral cavity, while enamel remineralization refers to the reprecipitation of calcium, phosphate, and other mineral ions on the surface of the teeth in situations of normal or localized demineralization. Enamel in a healthy oral environment with the presence of saliva is relatively stable, and demineralization and remineralization are continuous and alternating processes that occur [54]. Thus, BTCM can simulate the dynamic mineralization and demineralization processes that occur in the oral cavity, making it a potential dental material capable of inducing the dynamic mineralization of HA in the oral environment.

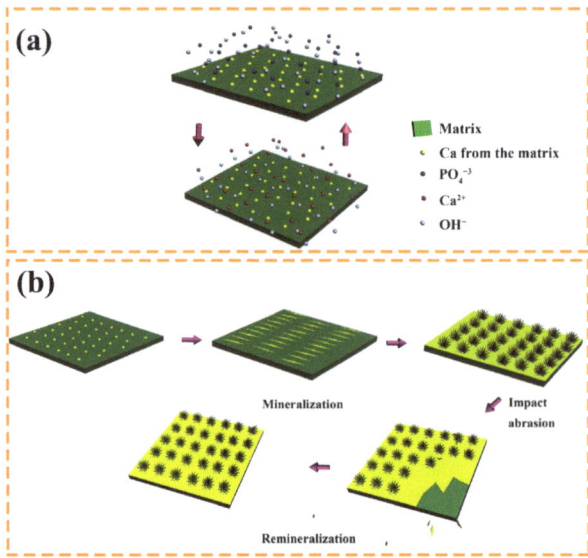

Figure 10. The mechanism of the dynamic mineralization of HA on BTCM samples. (**a**) PO_4^{3-} and Ca^{2+} accumulate around the BTCM matrix and lead to the mineralization of HA during the ASP process; (**b**) Abraded HA-rich matrix could again induce HA mineralization.

3.6. MTT Toxicity Assay

An ideal dental material should not release toxic substances or induce harmful reactions within the human oral cavity. An MTT cytotoxicity assay was employed to investigate the toxicity of the BTCM dental materials. In this test, the viability of L929 cells was assessed after 24 h, 48 h, and 72 h of in vitro culture to evaluate the material for potential toxicity, and the results are shown in Figure 11 and Table 5. After 24 h of cultivation, the viability of all L929 cells was high, and there was no significant difference ($p > 0.05$) between BTCM-1, BTCM-2, BTCM-3, BTCM-4, and the negative control group, while there were statistically differences between the BTCM samples and the negative control group ($p = 0.000 < 0.005$). After 48 h, the OD values for all four groups had increased, suggesting cell proliferation during this period. The absorbance values of the four BTCM samples were not significantly different from the negative control group. After 72 h of cultivation, the L929 cell viability on the surfaces of BTCM-1, BTCM-2, BTCM-3, and BTCM-4 slightly increased, suggesting that BTCM was non-toxic to L929 cells and was unlikely to pose toxicity concerns for oral tissues upon implantation. Therefore, BTCM dental materials demonstrate good biocompatibility and hold promise for clinical applications.

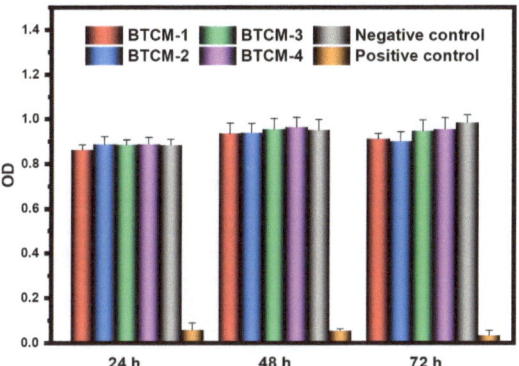

Figure 11. Cell viability study of different BTCM dental resins. The error bars represent the standard deviation of three samples.

Table 5. The OD values measured for L929 cells cultivated on BTCM samples at 24 h, 48 h, and 72 h, respectively.

Sample Code	OD Values (Mean ± Standard Deviation)		
	24 h	48 h	72 h
BTCM-1	0.863 ± 0.021	0.936 ± 0.046	0.911 ± 0.024
BTCM-2	0.888 ± 0.033	0.959 ± 0.042	0.902 ± 0.041
BTCM-3	0.886 ± 0.023	0.965 ± 0.049	0.948 ± 0.048
BTCM-4	0.888 ± 0.030	0.954 ± 0.044	0.955 ± 0.052
Positive control	0.883 ± 0.027	0.942 ± 0.045	0.985 ± 0.034
Negative control	0.057 ± 0.03 ***	0.054 ± 0.009 ***	0.034 ± 0.0218 ***

BTCM-1, BTCM-2, BTCM-3, BTCM-4, and positive control showed a statistically significance difference from the negative control, $p = 0.000 < 0.005$. *** $p < 0.001$.

3.7. Cell Adhesion and Proliferation Analysis

The SEM photos in Figure 12 depict L929 cells adhering to BTCM samples prepared with varying concentrations of CMA following 72 h of cultivation. As can be seen, the L929 cells were evenly distributed on the surfaces of the BTCM samples, and the cell population was higher on the BTCM samples with higher CMA content. Notably, on the surfaces of BTCM-3 and BTCM-4, L929 cells spread completely across the material surfaces. Moreover, cells at various growth stages were observed. These results indicated that as the CMA content increased, the biocompatibility of BTCM improved. In conclusion, BTCM exhibited excellent cell adhesion properties. Cross-linked CMA showed no toxicity to cells, and with the increase in calcium content in the system, the biocompatibility also increased. Therefore, the BTCM dental material is non-toxic and demonstrates exceptional biocompatibility.

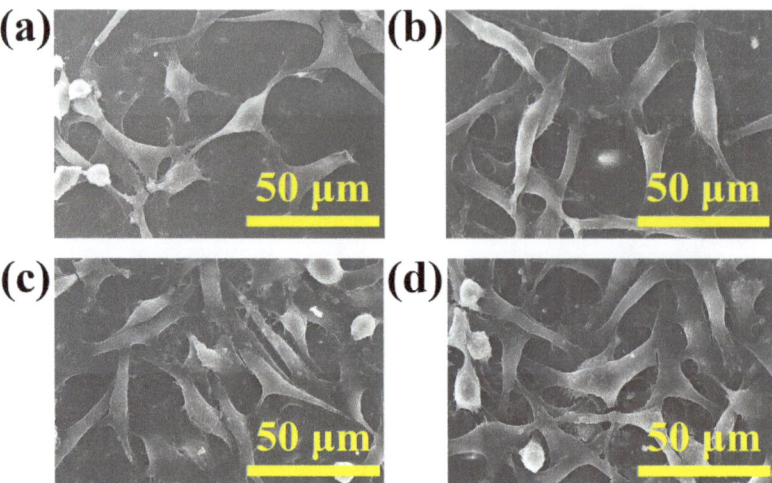

Figure 12. The morphology of L929 cells attached on BTCM: (**a**) BTCM-1; (**b**) BTCM-2; (**c**) BTCM-3; and (**d**) BTCM-4 (scale bar: 50 μm).

4. Discussion

The self-repair ability of tooth enamel is quite limited when the enamel is damaged by acid erosion or cavities. As enamel plays a vital role in the protection of oral health, the significance of enamel restoration is substantial. Integrating components with photoactivity and remineralization properties into the classical dental resin Bis-GMA/TEGDMA formulation is an effective strategy for improving the remineralization property of dental restorative resin. Former studies usually realized the mineralization of Bis-GMA/TEGDMA dental resin by incorporating fillers or coatings with a remineralization ability to the resin formulation [9,55,56]. In this study, a bifunctional monomer called CMA, which is the calcium salt of methacrylic acid, was incorporated into the Bis-GMA/TEGDMA dental resin formulation to develop a bioactive dental restorative resin. The photopolymerization product BTCM was calcium-rich and demonstrated an excellent HA regeneration ability.

Photopolymerization efficiency and double-bond conversion are two important factors for dental resin. Although the addition of CMA led to a decrease in photopolymerization speed to some extent due to the lower reactivity of CMA, the photopolymerization can still be completed in less than 300 s, demonstrating the high photoactivity of the BTCM dental resin. However, the double-bond conversion of BTCM slightly increased with the increase in CMA. This is caused by the decreased viscosity of the formulation, which can lead to a higher mobility of the molecules, allowing more double bonds to polymerize. Tian et al. [57] incorporated nano fibrillar silicate (FS) in Bis-GMA/TEGDMA dental resin which also exhibited a high double-bond conversion and a high photopolymerization speed.

Although the compression modulus decreased with an increase in CMA content, BTCM still exhibited sufficient mechanical properties for dental restoration applications [58,59]. To obtain a transparent mixture of Bis-GMA/TEGDMA/CMA when prepare the BTCM formulation, MAA has to be added into the formulation so that CMA can be dissolved completely. The photopolymerization product of MAA is often used as a hydrogel [60], drug carrier [61], polyelectrolyte [62] and so on. Thus, the incorporation of MAA can lead to the decrease in the compression modulus of BTCM. In a study conducted by Liu et al. [42], Bis-GMA and TEGDMA were grafted onto the surface of HA whiskers. These whiskers were subsequently utilized as fillers in Bis-GMA/TEGDMA dental restorative resin composites, resulting in an enhanced compression modulus.

Combined with the XRD results, the mineralization findings showed that the BTCM restorative dental resin exhibited good bioactivity. When immersed alternately in $Ca(NO_3)_2$

and Na_2HPO_4 solutions, the surface of the BTCM samples became covered with HA crystals, and the layer became denser with increasing immersion time. This is because the surface of BTCM contains large amounts of calcium and carboxyl groups which can bind with PO_4^{3-} and Ca^{2+} to generate HA crystals. The CMA content has a significant influence on the bioactivity of BTCM. With an increase in CMA concentration, the mineralized HA layer on the surface of BTCM is thicker due to the increased binding sites for Ca^{2+} and PO_4^{3-}. Enamel primarily consists of HA crystals with complex hierarchical structure [63,64]. Within enamel, HA crystals run parallel to each other along the long axis, forming enamel rods that interlock internally. This unique arrangement is vital for enhancing enamel's mechanical strength and resistance to fissures. As a result, it is also important to control the structure of the mineralized HA crystals. However, the HA crystals in our work were not well arranged. Shao [65] designed a material composed of calcium phosphate ion clusters (CPICs) that can result in a precursor layer with a continuous mineralization interface, inducing epitaxial crystal growth of enamel HA, which mimics the biomineralization crystal-precursor frontier of enamel development. Furthermore, in combination with the cell adhesion results, all BTCM samples demonstrated excellent bioactivity, as evidenced by the high viability of L929 cells cultivated on their surfaces. There were no statistically significant differences between the BTCM samples and the positive control group.

5. Conclusions

CMA-functionalized bis-GMA/TEGDMA dental resin with the ability to induce the remineralization of HA was fabricated in this work. The calcium-rich restorative dental material with good bioactivity could be obtained by photopolymerization. The photopolymerization kinetics were investigated by real-time FTIR. The photopolymerization rate increased first with the increase in CMA concentration, but then decreased with higher CMA concentrations. The compression test results indicated a negative impact of CMA on the compression modulus of BTCM. The bioactivity which showed the HA mineralization ability of BTCM was confirmed through SEM and XRD patterns. Calcium within the BTCM matrix played a significant role in this bioactivity. With three cycles of ASP, BTCM-2, BTCM-3, and BTCM-4 all exhibited densely clustered spheroids of HA on their surfaces. The mineralization speed and amount of HA on the BTCM surfaces are closely related to the calcium content in the BTCM matrix. Additionally, MTT assays showed that the BTCM samples are non-toxic to L929 cells, indicating that the BTCM samples have good biocompatibility. Cell adhesion experiments revealed that BTCM with higher CMA content can promote the attachment and proliferation of L929 cells. Thus, BTCM can simulate the dynamic mineralization and demineralization processes that occur in the oral cavity, making it a potential dental material capable of inducing the dynamic mineralization of HA in the oral environment. The novel CMA-based dental restorative resin showed remarkable bioactivity and biocompatibility, which makes it a promising dental restorative resin for use in dental restorative procedures and the field of biomedicine.

Author Contributions: Conceptualization, X.Z. (Xueqin Zhang) and Y.Z.; methodology, X.Z. (Xin Zhang), Y.Z. and Y.L.; formal analysis, X.Z. (Xin Zhang) and Y.Z.; investigation, X.Z. (Xin Zhang) and X.W.; resources, X.Z. (Xin Zhang), Y.Z. and Y.L.; data curation, X.Z. (Xin Zhang), Y.Z., and Y.L.; writing—original draft preparation, X.Z. (Xin Zhang); writing—review and editing, X.Z. (Xueqin Zhang), Y.Z. and X.W.; supervision, X.Z. (Xueqin Zhang). All authors have read and agreed to the published version of the manuscript.

Funding: This research received no external funding.

Data Availability Statement: Not applicable.

Conflicts of Interest: The authors declare no conflict of interest.

References

1. Mohring, S.; Cieplik, F.; Hiller, K.A.; Ebensberger, H.; Ferstl, G.; Hermens, J.; Zaparty, M.; Witzgall, R.; Mansfeld, U.; Buchalla, W.; et al. Elemental Compositions of Enamel or Dentin in Human and Bovine Teeth Differ from Murine Teeth. *Materials* **2023**, *16*, 1514. [CrossRef] [PubMed]
2. Besnard, C.; Marie, A.; Sasidharan, S.; Bucek, P.; Walker, J.M.; Parker, J.E.; Spink, M.C.; Harper, R.A.; Marathe, S.; Wanelik, K.; et al. Multi-resolution Correlative Ultrastructural and Chemical Analysis of Carious Enamel by Scanning Microscopy and Tomographic Imaging. *ACS Appl. Mater. Interfaces* **2023**, *15*, 37259–37273. [CrossRef] [PubMed]
3. Seredin, P.; Goloshchapov, D.; Emelyanova, A.; Buylov, N.; Kashkarov, V.; Lukin, A.; Ippolitov, Y.; Khmelevskaia, T.; Mahdy, I.A.; Mahdy, M.A. Engineering of biomimetic mineralized layer formed on the surface of natural dental enamel. *Results Eng.* **2022**, *15*, 100583. [CrossRef]
4. Aldhaian, B.A.; Balhaddad, A.A.; Alfaifi, A.A.; Levon, J.A.; Eckert, G.J.; Hara, A.T.; Lippert, F. In vitro demineralization prevention by fluoride and silver nanoparticles when applied to sound enamel and enamel caries-like lesions of varying severities. *J. Dent.* **2021**, *104*, 103536. [CrossRef]
5. Grohe, B.; Mittler, S. Advanced non-fluoride approaches to dental enamel remineralization: The next level in enamel repair management. *Biomater. Biosyst.* **2021**, *4*, 100029. [CrossRef]
6. Yip, H.K.; Li, D.K.; Yau, D.C. Dental amalgam and human health. *Int. Dent. J.* **2003**, *53*, 464–468. [CrossRef]
7. Roach, M. Base metal alloys used for dental restorations and implants. *Dent. Clin. N. Am.* **2007**, *51*, 603–627. [CrossRef]
8. Giordano Ii, R. Ceramics overview. *Br. Dent. J.* **2022**, *232*, 658–663. [CrossRef]
9. Pratap, B.; Gupta, R.K.; Bhardwaj, B.; Nag, M. Resin based restorative dental materials: Characteristics and future perspectives. *Jpn. Dent. Sci. Rev.* **2019**, *55*, 126–138. [CrossRef]
10. Singer, L.; Fouda, A.; Bourauel, C. Biomimetic approaches and materials in restorative and regenerative dentistry: Review article. *BMC Oral Health* **2023**, *23*, 105. [CrossRef]
11. Pandya, M.; Diekwisch, T.G.H. Enamel biomimetics-fiction or future of dentistry. *Int. J. Oral Sci.* **2019**, *11*, 8. [CrossRef] [PubMed]
12. Clift, F. Artificial methods for the remineralization of hydroxyapatite in enamel. *Mater. Today Chem.* **2021**, *21*, 100498.
13. Shahid, S.; Hassan, U.; Billington, R.W.; Hill, R.G.; Anderson, P. Glass ionomer cements: Effect of strontium substitution on esthetics, radiopacity and fluoride release. *Dent. Mater.* **2014**, *30*, 308–313.
14. Goncalves, F.M.C.; Delbem, A.C.B.; Gomes, L.F.; Emerenciano, N.G.; Pessan, J.P.; Romero, G.D.A.; Cannon, M.L.; Danelon, M. Effect of fluoride, casein phosphopeptide-amorphous calcium phosphate and sodium trimetaphosphate combination treatment on the remineralization of caries lesions: An in vitro study. *Arch. Oral Biol.* **2021**, *122*, 105001. [CrossRef] [PubMed]
15. Zampetti, P.; Scribante, A. Historical and bibliometric notes on the use of fluoride in caries prevention. *Eur. J. Paediatr. Dent.* **2020**, *21*, 148–152. [PubMed]
16. Amaechi, B.T.; AbdulAzees, P.A.; Alshareif, D.O.; Shehata, M.A.; Lima, P.; Abdollahi, A.; Kalkhorani, P.S.; Evans, V. Comparative efficacy of a hydroxyapatite and a fluoride toothpaste for prevention and remineralization of dental caries in children. *BDJ Open* **2019**, *5*, 18. [CrossRef] [PubMed]
17. Wang, M.; Zhang, H.-Y.; Xiang, Y.-Y.; Qian, Y.-P.; Ren, J.-N.; Jia, R. How does fluoride enhance hydroxyapatite? A theoretical understanding. *Appl. Surf. Sci.* **2022**, *586*, 152753. [CrossRef]
18. Ionescu, A.C.; Degli Esposti, L.; Iafisco, M.; Brambilla, E. Dental tissue remineralization by bioactive calcium phosphate nanoparticles formulations. *Sci. Rep.* **2022**, *12*, 5994. [CrossRef]
19. Fallahzadeh, F.; Heidari, S.; Najafi, F.; Hajihasani, M.; Noshiri, N.; Nazari, N.F. Efficacy of a Novel Bioactive Glass-Polymer Composite for Enamel Remineralization following Erosive Challenge. *Int. J. Dent.* **2022**, *2022*, 6539671. [CrossRef]
20. Hani, T.B.; O'Connell, A.C.; Duane, B. Casein phosphopeptide-amorphous calcium phosphate products in caries prevention. *Evid. Based Dent.* **2016**, *17*, 46–47. [CrossRef]
21. Alkarad, L.; Alkhouli, M.; Dashash, M. Remineralization of teeth with casein phosphopeptide-amorphous calcium phosphate: Analysis of salivary pH and the rate of salivary flow. *BDJ Open* **2023**, *9*, 16. [CrossRef]
22. Srinivasan, N.; Kavitha, M.; Loganathan, S.C. Comparison of the remineralization potential of CPP-ACP and CPP-ACP with 900 ppm fluoride on eroded human enamel: An in situ study. *Arch. Oral Biol.* **2010**, *55*, 541–544. [CrossRef] [PubMed]
23. Li, L.; Pan, H.; Tao, J.; Xu, X.; Mao, C.; Gu, X.; Tang, R. Repair of enamel by using hydroxyapatite nanoparticles as the building blocks. *J. Mater. Chem.* **2008**, *18*, 4079–4084. [CrossRef]
24. Anil, A.; Ibraheem, W.I.; Meshni, A.A.; Preethanath, R.S.; Anil, S. Nano-Hydroxyapatite (nHAp) in the Remineralization of Early Dental Caries: A Scoping Review. *Int. J. Environ. Res. Public Health* **2022**, *19*, 5629. [CrossRef]
25. Butera, A.; Pascadopoli, M.; Pellegrini, M.; Trapani, B.; Gallo, S.; Radu, M.; Scribante, A. Biomimetic hydroxyapatite paste for molar-incisor hypomineralization: A randomized clinical trial. *Oral. Dis.* **2022**. [CrossRef] [PubMed]
26. Tian, J.; Wu, Z.; Wang, Y.; Han, C.; Zhou, Z.; Guo, D.; Lin, Y.; Ye, Z.; Fu, J. Multifunctional dental resin composite with antibacterial and remineralization properties containing nMgO-BAG. *J. Mech. Behav. Biomed. Mater.* **2023**, *141*, 105783. [CrossRef] [PubMed]
27. Par, M.; Gubler, A.; Attin, T.; Tarle, Z.; Tarle, A.; Taubock, T.T. Ion release and hydroxyapatite precipitation of resin composites functionalized with two types of bioactive glass. *J. Dent.* **2022**, *118*, 103950. [CrossRef] [PubMed]
28. Sandomierski, M.; Buchwald, Z.; Koczorowski, W.; Voelkel, A. Calcium forms of zeolites A and X as fillers in dental restorative materials with remineralizing potential. *Microporous Mesoporous Mater.* **2020**, *294*, 109899. [CrossRef]

29. Han, X.; Erkan, A.; Xu, Z.; Chen, Y.; Boccaccini, A.R.; Zheng, K. Organic solvent-free synthesis of dendritic mesoporous bioactive glass nanoparticles with remineralization capability. *Mater. Lett.* **2022**, *320*, 132366. [CrossRef]
30. Choi, A.; Yoo, K.H.; Yoon, S.Y.; Park, S.B.; Choi, Y.K.; Kim, Y.I. Enhanced antimicrobial and remineralizing properties of self-adhesive orthodontic resin containing mesoporous bioactive glass and zwitterionic material. *J. Dent. Sci.* **2022**, *17*, 848–855. [CrossRef]
31. Qin, L.; Yao, S.; Meng, W.; Zhang, J.; Shi, R.; Zhou, C.; Wu, J. Novel antibacterial dental resin containing silanized hydroxyapatite nanofibers with remineralization capability. *Dent. Mater.* **2022**, *38*, 1989–2002. [CrossRef] [PubMed]
32. Reis, D.P.; Filho, J.D.N.; Rossi, A.L.; de Almeida Neves, A.; Portela, M.B.; da Silva, E.M. Remineralizing potential of dental composites containing silanized silica-hydroxyapatite (Si-HAp) nanoporous particles charged with sodium fluoride (NaF). *J. Dent.* **2019**, *90*, 103211. [CrossRef]
33. Skrtic, D.; Antonucci, J.M.; Eanes, E.D.; Eidelman, N. Dental composites based on hybrid and surface-modified amorphous calcium phosphates. *Biomaterials* **2004**, *25*, 1141–1150. [CrossRef]
34. Tao, S.; Su, Z.; Xiang, Z.; Xu, H.H.K.; Weir, M.D.; Fan, M.; Yu, Z.; Zhou, X.; Liang, K.; Li, J. Nano-calcium phosphate and dimethylaminohexadecyl methacrylate adhesive for dentin remineralization in a biofilm-challenged environment. *Dent. Mater.* **2020**, *36*, e316–e328. [CrossRef]
35. Chen, W.C.; Wu, H.Y.; Chen, H.S. Evaluation of reinforced strength and remineralized potential of resins with nanocrystallites and silica modified filler surfaces. *Mater. Sci. Eng. C Mater. Biol. Appl.* **2013**, *33*, 1143–1151. [CrossRef] [PubMed]
36. Mitwalli, H.; AlSahafi, R.; Albeshir, E.G.; Dai, Q.; Sun, J.; Oates, T.W.; Melo, M.A.S.; Xu, H.H.K.; Weir, M.D. Novel Nano Calcium Fluoride Remineralizing and Antibacterial Dental Composites. *J. Dent.* **2021**, *113*, 103789. [CrossRef] [PubMed]
37. Veeramani, R.; Shanbhog, R.; Priyanka, T.; Bhojraj, N. Remineralizing effect of calcium-sucrose-phosphate with and without fluoride on primary and permanent enamel: Microhardness and quantitative-light-induced-fluorescence™ based in vitro study. *Pediatr. Dent. J.* **2021**, *31*, 51–59. [CrossRef]
38. Mai, S.; Zhang, Q.; Liao, M.; Ma, X.; Zhong, Y. Recent Advances in Direct Adhesive Restoration Resin-Based Dental Materials with Remineralizing Agents. *Front. Dent. Med.* **2022**, *3*, 868651. [CrossRef]
39. Cheng, L.; Zhang, K.; Zhang, N.; Melo, M.A.S.; Weir, M.D.; Zhou, X.D.; Bai, Y.X.; Reynolds, M.A.; Xu, H.H.K. Developing a New Generation of Antimicrobial and Bioactive Dental Resins. *J. Dent. Res.* **2017**, *96*, 855–863. [CrossRef]
40. Toledano, M.; Aguilera, F.S.; Osorio, E.; Toledano-Osorio, M.; Escames, G.; Medina-Castillo, A.L.; Toledano, R.; Lynch, C.D.; Osorio, R. Melatonin-doped polymeric nanoparticles reinforce and remineralize radicular dentin: Morpho-histological, chemical and biomechanical studies. *Dent. Mater.* **2021**, *37*, 1107–1120. [CrossRef]
41. Charton, C.; Falk, V.; Marchal, P.; Pla, F.; Colon, P. Influence of Tg, viscosity and chemical structure of monomers on shrinkage stress in light-cured dimethacrylate-based dental resins. *Dent. Mater.* **2007**, *23*, 1447–1459. [CrossRef] [PubMed]
42. Liu, F.; Wang, R.; Cheng, Y.; Jiang, X.; Zhang, Q.; Zhu, M. Polymer grafted hydroxyapatite whisker as a filler for dental composite resin with enhanced physical and mechanical properties. *Mater. Sci. Eng. C Mater. Biol. Appl.* **2013**, *33*, 4994–5000. [CrossRef] [PubMed]
43. Sandomierski, M.; Buchwald, Z.; Voelkel, A. Calcium montmorillonite and montmorillonite with hydroxyapatite layer as fillers in dental composites with remineralizing potential. *Appl. Clay Sci.* **2020**, *198*, 105822. [CrossRef]
44. Jardim, R.N.; Rocha, A.A.; Rossi, A.M.; de Almeida Neves, A.; Portela, M.B.; Lopes, R.T.; Pires Dos Santos, T.M.; Xing, Y.; Moreira da Silva, E. Fabrication and characterization of remineralizing dental composites containing hydroxyapatite nanoparticles. *J. Mech. Behav. Biomed. Mater.* **2020**, *109*, 103817. [CrossRef] [PubMed]
45. Noble, B.B.; Coote, M.L. Isotactic Regulation in the Radical Polymerization of Calcium Methacrylate: Is Multiple Chelation the Key to Stereocontrol? *J. Polym. Sci.* **2019**, *58*, 52–61. [CrossRef]
46. Zhang, X.; Ma, G.; Nie, J.; Wang, Z.; Wu, G.; Yang, D. Restorative dental resin functionalized with methacryloxy propyl trimethoxy silane to induce reversible in situ generation of enamel-like hydroxyapatite. *J. Mater. Sci.* **2018**, *53*, 16183–16197. [CrossRef]
47. Wang, C.; Xie, Y.; Li, A.; Shen, H.; Wu, D.; Qiu, D. Bioactive nanoparticle through postmodification of colloidal silica. *ACS Appl. Mater. Interfaces* **2014**, *6*, 4935–4939. [CrossRef]
48. Zhang, M.; Jiang, S.; Gao, Y.; Nie, J.; Sun, F. UV-Nanoimprinting Lithography Photoresists with No Photoinitiator and Low Polymerization Shrinkage. *Ind. Eng. Chem. Res.* **2020**, *59*, 7564–7574. [CrossRef]
49. Zhang, Y.; He, Y.; Yang, J.; Zhang, X.; Bongiovanni, R.; Nie, J. A fluorinated compound used as migrated photoinitiator in the presence of air. *Polymer* **2015**, *71*, 93–101. [CrossRef]
50. Kang, Z.; Zhang, X.; Chen, Y.; Akram, M.Y.; Nie, J.; Zhu, X. Preparation of polymer/calcium phosphate porous composite as bone tissue scaffolds. *Mater. Sci. Eng. C Mater. Biol. Appl.* **2017**, *70 Pt 2*, 1125–1131. [CrossRef]
51. Zhang, X.; Zhang, Y.; Ma, G.; Yang, D.; Nie, J. The effect of the prefrozen process on properties of a chitosan/hydroxyapatite/poly(methyl methacrylate) composite prepared by freeze drying method used for bone tissue engineering. *RSC Adv.* **2015**, *5*, 79679–79686. [CrossRef]
52. Petropoulou, K.; Platania, V.; Chatzinikolaidou, M.; Mitraki, A. A Doubly Fmoc-Protected Aspartic Acid Self-Assembles into Hydrogels Suitable for Bone Tissue Engineering. *Materials* **2022**, *15*, 8928. [CrossRef] [PubMed]
53. El Boujaady, H.; Mourabet, M.; Abdelhadi, E.R.; Bennani-Ziatni, M.; El Hamri, R.; Abderrahim, T. Adsorption of a textile dye on synthesized calcium deficient hydroxyapatite (CDHAp): Kinetic and thermodynamic studies. *J. Mater. Environ. Sci.* **2016**, *7*, 4049–4063.
54. Aoba, T. Solubility properties of human tooth mineral and pathogenesis of dental caries. *Oral Dis.* **2004**, *10*, 249–257. [CrossRef]

55. da Silva Meirelles Doria Maia, J.N.; Portela, M.B.; Sanchez Candela, D.R.; Neves, A.A.; Noronha-Filho, J.D.; Mendes, A.O.; Barros, M.A.; Moreira da Silva, E. Fabrication and characterization of remineralizing dental composites containing calcium type pre-reacted glass-ionomer (PRG-Ca) fillers. *Dent. Mater.* **2021**, *37*, 1325–1336. [CrossRef]
56. Liu, F.; Jiang, X.; Zhang, Q.; Zhu, M. Strong and bioactive dental resin composite containing poly(Bis-GMA) grafted hydroxyapatite whiskers and silica nanoparticles. *Compos. Sci. Technol.* **2014**, *101*, 86–93. [CrossRef]
57. Tian, M.; Gao, Y.; Liu, Y.; Liao, Y.; Hedin, N.E.; Fong, H. Fabrication and evaluation of Bis-GMA/TEGDMA dental resins/composites containing nano fibrillar silicate. *Dent. Mater.* **2008**, *24*, 235–243. [CrossRef]
58. Sadananda, V.; Shetty, C.M.; Hegde, M.N.; Bhat, G.S. Alkasite restorative material: Flexural and compressive strength evaluation. *Res. J. Pharm. Biol. Chem. Sci.* **2018**, *9*, 2179.
59. Naz, F.; Samad Khan, A.; Kader, M.A.; Al Gelban, L.O.S.; Mousa, N.M.A.; Asiri, R.S.H.; Hakeem, A.S. Comparative evaluation of mechanical and physical properties of a new bulk-fill alkasite with conventional restorative materials. *Saudi Dent. J.* **2021**, *33*, 666–673. [CrossRef]
60. Kaith, B.S.; Sharma, K.; Kumar, V.; Kalia, S.; Swart, H.C. Fabrication and characterization of gum ghatti-polymethacrylic acid based electrically conductive hydrogels. *Synth. Met.* **2014**, *187*, 61–67. [CrossRef]
61. Sajeesh, S.; Sharma, C.P. Cyclodextrin-insulin complex encapsulated polymethacrylic acid based nanoparticles for oral insulin delivery. *Int. J. Pharm.* **2006**, *325*, 147–154. [CrossRef] [PubMed]
62. Sulatha, M.S.; Natarajan, U. Molecular Dynamics Simulations of PAA–PMA Polyelectrolyte Copolymers in Dilute Aqueous Solution: Chain Conformations and Hydration Properties. *Ind. Eng. Chem. Res.* **2012**, *51*, 10833–10839.
63. Cui, F.Z.; Ge, J. New observations of the hierarchical structure of human enamel, from nanoscale to microscale. *J. Tissue Eng. Regen. Med.* **2007**, *1*, 185–191. [CrossRef]
64. Beniash, E.; Stifler, C.A.; Sun, C.Y.; Jung, G.S.; Qin, Z.; Buehler, M.J.; Gilbert, P. The hidden structure of human enamel. *Nat. Commun.* **2019**, *10*, 4383. [CrossRef]
65. Shao, C.; Jin, B.; Mu, Z.; Lu, H.; Zhao, Y.; Wu, Z.; Yan, L.; Zhang, Z.; Zhou, Y.; Pan, H.; et al. Repair of tooth enamel by a biomimetic mineralization frontier ensuring epitaxial growth. *Sci. Adv.* **2019**, *5*, eaaw9569. [CrossRef] [PubMed]

Disclaimer/Publisher's Note: The statements, opinions and data contained in all publications are solely those of the individual author(s) and contributor(s) and not of MDPI and/or the editor(s). MDPI and/or the editor(s) disclaim responsibility for any injury to people or property resulting from any ideas, methods, instructions or products referred to in the content.

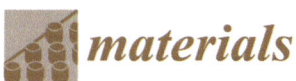

Article

Polyvinylpyrrolidone—Alginate—Carbonate Hydroxyapatite Porous Composites for Dental Applications

Anna A. Forysenkova [1], Inna V. Fadeeva [1], Dina V. Deyneko [2,3], Alevtina N. Gosteva [4], Georgy V. Mamin [5], Darya V. Shurtakova [5], Galina A. Davydova [6], Viktoriya G. Yankova [7], Iulian V. Antoniac [8,9] and Julietta V. Rau [7,10,*]

1. A.A. Baikov Institute of Metallurgy and Material Science RAS, Leninsky, 49, 119334 Moscow, Russia; aforysenkova@gmail.com (A.A.F.); fadeeva_inna@mail.ru (I.V.F.)
2. Chemistry Department, Lomonosov Moscow State University, Leninskie Gory 1, 119991 Moscow, Russia; deynekomsu@gmail.com
3. Laboratory of Arctic Mineralogy and Material Sciences, Kola Science Centre RAS, 14 Fersman Str., 184209 Apatity, Russia
4. Tananaev Institute of Chemistry, Kola Science Centre RAS, Akademgorodok 26A, 184209 Apatity, Russia; angosteva@list.ru
5. Institute of Physics, Kazan Federal University, Kremlevskaya 18, 420008 Kazan, Russia; georgemamin@gmail.com (G.V.M.); darja-shurtakva@mail.ru (D.V.S.)
6. Institute of Theoretical and Experimental Biophysics of RAS, Institutskaya 3, Puschino, 142290 Moscow, Russia; davidova_g@mail.ru
7. Department of Analytical, Physical and Colloid Chemistry, Institute of Pharmacy, I.M. Sechenov First Moscow State Medical University, Trubetskaya 8, Build. 2, 119991 Moscow, Russia; yankova_v_g@staff.sechenov.ru
8. Faculty of Materials Science and Engineering, University Politehnica of Bucharest, 313 Splaiul Independentei Street, District 6, 060042 Bucharest, Romania; antoniac.iulian@gmail.com
9. Academy of Romanian Scientists, 54 Splaiul Independentei Street, District 5, 050094 Bucharest, Romania
10. Istituto di Struttura della Materia, Consiglio Nazionale delle Ricerche (ISM-CNR), Via del Fosso del Cavaliere, 100, 00133 Rome, Italy
* Correspondence: giulietta.rau@ism.cnr.it

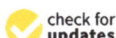

Citation: Forysenkova, A.A.; Fadeeva, I.V.; Deyneko, D.V.; Gosteva, A.N.; Mamin, G.V.; Shurtakova, D.V.; Davydova, G.A.; Yankova, V.G.; Antoniac, I.V.; Rau, J.V. Polyvinylpyrrolidone—Alginate—Carbonate Hydroxyapatite Porous Composites for Dental Applications. *Materials* **2023**, *16*, 4478. https:// doi.org/10.3390/ma16124478

Academic Editor: George Eliades

Received: 29 May 2023
Revised: 13 June 2023
Accepted: 18 June 2023
Published: 20 June 2023

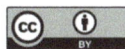

Copyright: © 2023 by the authors. Licensee MDPI, Basel, Switzerland. This article is an open access article distributed under the terms and conditions of the Creative Commons Attribution (CC BY) license (https:// creativecommons.org/licenses/by/ 4.0/).

Abstract: An alternative approach for the currently used replacement therapy in dentistry is to apply materials that restore tooth tissue. Among them, composites, based on biopolymers with calcium phosphates, and cells can be applied. In the present work, a composite based on polyvinylpyrrolidone (PVP) and alginate (Alg) with carbonate hydroxyapatite (CHA) was prepared and characterized. The composite was investigated by X-ray diffraction, infrared spectroscopy, electron paramagnetic resonance (EPR) and scanning electron microscopy methods, and the microstructure, porosity, and swelling properties of the material were described. In vitro studies included the MTT test using mouse fibroblasts, and adhesion and survivability tests with human dental pulp stem cells (DPSC). The mineral component of the composite corresponded to CHA with an admixture of amorphous calcium phosphate. The presence of a bond between the polymer matrix and CHA particles was shown by EPR. The structure of the material was represented by micro- (30–190 μm) and nano-pores (average 8.71 ± 4.15 nm). The swelling measurements attested that CHA addition increased the polymer matrix hydrophilicity by 200%. *In vitro* studies demonstrated the biocompatibility of PVP-Alg-CHA (95 ± 5% cell viability), and DPSC located inside the pores. It was concluded that the PVP-Alg-CHA porous composite is promising for dentistry applications.

Keywords: composite; hydroxyapatite; carbonate hydroxyapatite; alginate; polyvinylpyrrolidone

1. Introduction

One of most common oral diseases is dental caries, which affects more than 90% of the population in Western countries [1,2]. Starting as enamel damage, caries eventually affects the soft tissues of the tooth (pulp), which leads to inflammation and necrosis [3]. In the most cases, the treatment of caries consists of the removal of necrotic tissues and their replacement with various restorative materials [3]. For these purposes, cements and ceramic materials based on calcium phosphates (CaP) are widely used [4]; in particular, hydroxyapatite (HA, $Ca_{10}(PO_4)_6(OH)_2$)) is used due to its similarity with the mineral component of the hard tissues of teeth [5,6].

Recently, the development of new methods of treatment that take into account the tissue structure of teeth, namely the combination of mineralized and non-mineralized components, dentin and pulp, has become relevant [1]. This approach implies the restoration of tooth function and the extension to the period during which teeth appear healthy [7]. In perspective, these issues can be solved by porous composites based on biopolymers with CaP [6,8].

To prepare composites, a variety of polymers, both synthetic and natural, can be used, including polylactic acid derivatives, polyacrylate, polyvinyl alcohol, collagen, chitosan, alginate (Alg), etc. [9]. These polymers have their own advantages and disadvantages. In particular, synthetic polymers are bioinert and non-immunogenic, but do not undergo bioresorption [10]. Natural polymers are capable of bioresorption, but, as a rule, have lower strength characteristics [11]. The optimal solution is to combine various polymers to obtain materials with unique properties.

CaP is available in the form of cements [12], granules [13] or powders [14]. CaP may contain substituting ions [15–17] to impart osteoinductive (Sr) [18] or antibacterial (Cu, Zn, Ag, Mn, Gd) [19–23] properties. For dental applications, carbonate hydroxyapatite (CHA, $Ca_{10}(PO_4)_6(CO_3)_{0.5}(OH)$ is a good choice, because of its similar composition to the mineral component of dentin [24].

Porous structures are required for better bio-integration and angiogenesis [25,26]. They can be obtained by freeze-drying of gels [27]. In this way, such composite materials as collagen-HA [28], chitosan-HA [29], and gelatine-HA have been generated [30]. Therefore, gel-forming natural or synthetic hydrophilic polymers need to be employed [31], such as alginate and polyvinylpyrrolidone (polyvidone, povidone) (PVP), described in [11]. Alginate is a natural polysaccharide that forms viscous gels [32]. PVP is a synthetic polymer that is highly soluble in water [33]. Separately, these polymers as well as composites based on them have been studied [34,35]. However, literature data on their mixtures possessing unique properties, as well as composite materials based on them, are scarce. Previously, we reported film materials based on PVP-Alg-HA [14], with HA prepared *in situ*.

In the present work, a composite based on the mixture of PVP and Alg with CHA obtained by gel freeze-drying was developed. CHA was synthesized *ex situ*. The composition, structure and physico-chemical properties of the material were studied by X-ray diffraction (XRD), Fourier transform infrared spectroscopy (FT-IR), electron paramagnetic resonance (EPR), and scanning electron microscopy (SEM) methods. The porosity and swelling properties of the material were investigated. Its biocompatibility was assessed by the MTT test, applying the NCTC clone L-929 fibroblast of mouse subcutaneous connective tissue. The adhesion and viability of dental pulp stem cells (DPSC) on the composite surface were investigated, and perspectives for its applications in dentistry were described.

2. Materials and Methods

2.1. PVP-Alg-CHA Preparation

CHA and HA (prepared for EPR studies described in Section 2.4) were synthesized *ex situ* by precipitation in accordance with Equation (1):

$$10Ca(NO_3)_2 + 6(NH_4)_2HPO_4 + 0.5(NH_4)_2CO_3 + 7NH_4OH \rightarrow$$
$$\rightarrow Ca_{10}(PO_4)_6(CO_3)_{0.5}(OH)\downarrow + 20NH_4NO_3 + 6H_2O \quad (1)$$

The resulting suspension was filtered on a Buchner funnel using a vacuum pump and dried at 110 °C to a constant mass.

To obtain composite materials, CHA powder was milled to ≤50 μm and mixed with powders of PVP (360 kDa, Sigma-Aldrich, St. Louis, MO, USA) and Alg (pure, Reakhim, Moscow, Russia) polymers at a concentration of 5 wt.%. The powder mixture was dissolved in water to obtain a gel with a PVP-Alg-CHA content of 2.5 wt.%. The resulting gel was mixed until a homogeneous mixture was obtained using a top-drive agitator at a speed of 700 rpm. To obtain porous materials, the resulting gel was whipped at a speed of 7000 rpm. The foam obtained was squeezed out through a syringe into a pre-prepared solution of 0.1 mol/L $CaCl_2$ (Khimed, Moscow, Russia) for cross-linking of Alg [36]. After 5 min, materials were pulled out from the solution, frozen at a temperature of −10 °C and then dried in an LS-1000 freeze dryer (Prointech, St. Petersburg, Russia). The sample obtained was named PVP-Alg-CHA. The preparation scheme is presented in Figure 1.

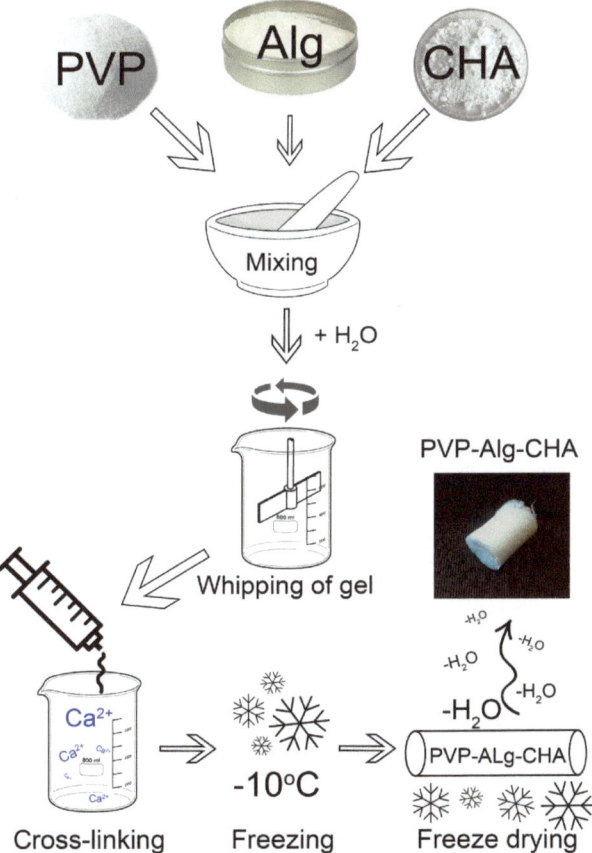

Figure 1. The scheme of PVP-Alg-CHA composite preparation.

2.2. XRD Analysis

Powder X-ray diffraction (PXRD) patterns were collected on a Rigaku SmartLab SE diffractometer (Rigaku, Wilmington, MA, USA) with a 3 kW sealed X-ray tube, D/teX Ultra 250 silicon strip detector, vertical type θ-θ geometry, and HyPix-400 (2D HPAD) detector. PXRD data were collected at room temperature in the 2θ range of 3° to 110° with a step interval of 0.02°. PXRD patterns were plotted using the Crystallographica Search-Match (Version 2, 0, 3, 1.) and the PFD#2 database.

2.3. FT-IR Spectroscopy

Absorption spectra of the samples were recorded on an FT-803 Fourier spectrometer (Simeks Research and Production Company 2022 Novosibirsk, Russia) in the wavenumber region of 4000–400 cm^{-1}, with 1 cm^{-1} spectral resolution. The standard KBr disc method was applied to obtained the spectra.

2.4. EPR Spectroscopy

Electron paramagnetic resonance studies were carried out with non-carbonated HA, since the CO_3^{2-} groups displace the NO_3^- groups (coming from residual impurity) from the HA structure, as discussed in an earlier ref. [37]. The EPR studies were carried out by means of a Bruker Elexsys E580 spectrometer (Bruker, Germany) (X-range, ν = 9.61 GHz) and E680 (W—range, ν = 94 GHz) at 200 and 297 K. In pulse mode, the Khan sequence was used: $\pi/2$-τ-π-τ – (electronic spin echo (ESE)); where time $\pi/2$ = 64 ns, τ = 248 ns. The EPR spectra were obtained by measuring the integral intensity of the ESE with a continuous extension of the magnetic field B_0. The samples were subjected to X-ray irradiation for 1 h on the URS-55 device with an absorption dose of 15 kGy at room temperature to create stable radiation centers.

2.5. SEM

The microstructure of PVP-Alg-CHA composite was studied by scanning electron microscopy using the TescanVegaII microscope (Tescan, Brno, Czech Republic).

2.6. Porosity Measurements

The porosity of the PVP-Alg-CHA composite was determined using a TriStar 3000 porosimeter (Micromeritics, Norcross, GA, USA) by low-temperature nitrogen adsorption [38].

2.7. Swelling Measurements

Swelling behavior of the porous PVP-Alg-CHA composite was determined by the change in mass after its immersion in deionized water.

2.8. In Vitro Cell Tests

The MTT test was used for evaluation of the cytotoxicity of extracts from the investigated materials. It was carried out using cells of the NCTC clone L-929 fibroblast of mouse subcutaneous connective tissue. The 3 day extracts were prepared in accordance with the requirements of GOST R ISO 10993.12-15 [39].

The adhesion and proliferation of the DPSC was investigated by direct contact, as described earlier in the ref. [14]. The cells were spread on the surface of the test samples and placed in the wells of a 24-well plate with a layer density of 40,000 cm^{-2}. The viability of DPSC cells on the surface of the composite was assessed by differentiated fluorescent staining of living and dead cells using of an Axiovert 200 inverted microscope (Zeiss, Jena, Germany). The fluorescent dye SYTO9 turns green after the interaction with DNA and RNA of living and dead cells (λ_{ex} = 450–490 nm, λ_{emiss} = 515–565 nm), and propidium iodide (PI) turns red after the interaction with DNA and RNA of dead cells (λ_{ex} = 546 nm, λ_{emiss} = 575–640 nm).

The statistical analysis of the experimental data on DPSC adhesion was carried out. A set of 24 composite samples was placed in a 24-well plate. The extracts from each well were analyzed, and the mean values and corresponding standard deviations were presented. For the adhesion test, the nuclei of dead cells were stained using the intercalating reagent PI (λ_{ex} = 546 nm, λ_{emiss} = 575–640 nm).

3. Results and Discussion

3.1. Powder X-ray Diffraction (PXRD) Study

The PXRD patterns of the CHA sample obtained by precipitation and of the composite material are shown in Figure 2. The profiles of the patterns correspond to poor crystallized HA phase due to the broadening of the reflections. The broad lines on the PXRD patterns at $2\theta° = 15$–35 were attributed to amorphous calcium phosphate formed according to Equation (2):

$$x\text{Ca}^{2+} + y\text{HPO}_4^{2-} + y\text{OH}^- + (n - y)\text{H}_2\text{O} \rightarrow \text{Ca}_x(\text{PO}_4)_y \cdot n\text{H}_2\text{O}\downarrow \quad (2)$$

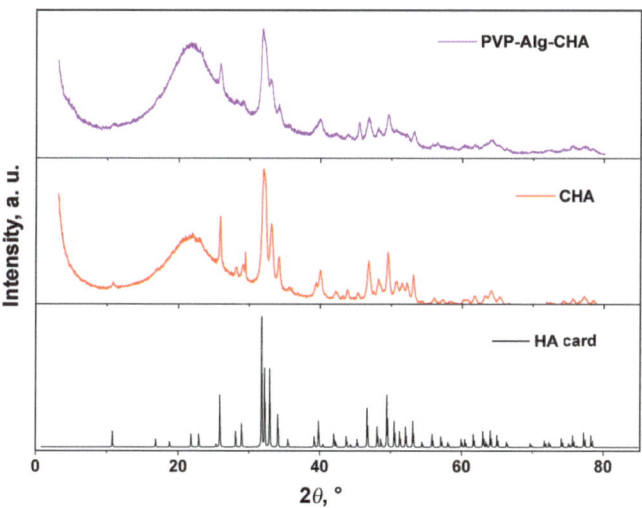

Figure 2. PXRD patterns of CHA obtained by precipitation and of composite PVP-Alg-CHA material, along with HA (card PDF#4 No 00-009-0432).

In ref. [40], it was shown that amorphous calcium phosphate transforms into HA upon aging [41].

The broad rage at $2\theta° = 3$–40 can be attributed to the polymer matrix of the composite (Figure 2, PVP-Alg-CHA pattern). PVP and Alg have some crystallinity and demonstrate broad lines at 10.9 and 21.1 $2\theta°$ (PVP) [42,43], and at 13.73 and 21.71 $2\theta°$ (Alg) [44].

3.2. FT-IR Spectroscopy Investigation

The chemical composition of the synthesized CHA and PVP-Alg-CHA composites were confirmed by FT-IR spectroscopy (Figure 3). The characteristic oscillation frequencies are given in Table 1.

Table 1. Vibration modes of CHA and PVP-Alg-CHA composite in the FT-IR spectra.

Assignment	Frequencies, cm^{-1}	
	CHA	PVP-Alg-CHA
$\nu_{as}[\text{OH}^-] + \nu_s[\text{OH}^-]$	3562	3544
bending vibration [OH$^-$]	3399	3378
$\nu_2[\text{CO}_3^{2-}]$	2922	2916
$\nu_{as}[\text{CH}_2]$		2916, 2942
$\nu_s[\text{CH}_2]$		2847
amide I (C=O ν-s with molecular bond δ)		1738
$\delta[\text{CH}_2]$		1425, 1466
$\omega[\text{CH}_2]$		1323, 1367
$\tau[\text{CH}_2]$		1250, 1289

Table 1. *Cont.*

Assignment	Frequencies, cm^{-1}	
	CHA	PVP-Alg-CHA
bending vibration ν_4(O–P–O) in [PO$_4^{3-}$]	565, 603	563, *606*
ν_{3as}[P–O]	1034	*1038*
ν[C–C]		1038
ν_2[PO$_4^{3-}$]	433, 470	417, 438, 469
ν_2 [NO$_3^-$]	822	826
ν_s[P–O–P] in P$_2$O$_7^{4-}$		718, 1211
ν_3[NO$_3^-$]	1350	1367
bending vibration O–C–O bands in [CO$_3^{2-}$]	873	872
bending vibration [H–O–H] in H$_2$O	1636	*1663*
carbonyl band of PVP		1663
ν_{3as}[C–O] in [CO$_3^{2-}$] of B-type	1418, 1458	*1425, 1466, 1495*
δ[C–N]		*1425, 1466, 1495*
ν[C–N]		1289
ν [C–N] partial double bond of PVP		1425, 1466, 1495
ν_{3as} [PO$_4^{3-}$]	1103	1092
ν_{1s} and ν_{3s} of [P–O] in PO$_4^{3-}$	963	*959*
δ[OH$^-$]	603	606
ρ[C–H$_2$]		*872*
ν[C–C] + ρ[CH$_2$]		959
ν_{as}[O–C=O] in COO$^-$ of Alg		1590
ν_s[O–C=O] in COO$^-$ of Alg		1411
ν [O–C–O] ring		1078

The intervals of characteristic bands for the [PO$_4^{3-}$] and [C–C], [CO$_3^{2-}$] and [CH$_2$], [C–N] and [CH$_2$], [PO$_4^{3-}$] and [OH$^-$] groups partially overlap with each other [45–54]. Therefore, it is difficult to make an unambiguous attribution. The authors consider that it is acceptable to have a double identification of characteristic values. Repeated frequencies are italicized.

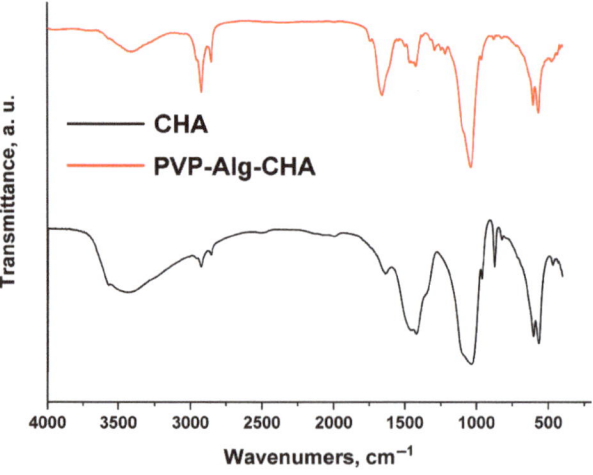

Figure 3. FT-IR spectra of CHA and PVP-Alg-CHA composite.

The OH⁻ ions were present in both the samples. In addition, the banding vibration of water is fixed in CHA and PVP-Alg-CHA. The presence of C−O bond oscillation bands (1420, 1460 cm^{-1}) indicated the substitution of PO_4^{3-}–tetrahedra by carbonate ions. This is called the substitution of B-type HA with a low V cell. The absence of the 1550 cm^{-1} band indicated that the OH⁻ groups were not replaced by carbonate ions in the channels of the HA structure. This showed the absence of HA of A-type with a large V cell [45,49]. The presence of amide group in PVP was confirmed by the absorption band at 1738 cm^{-1} [47]. The peak at 1425 cm^{-1} was ascribed to the stretching mode of the C=N partial double bond of PVP [50]. The carbonyl band of PVP appeared at 1663 cm^{-1} [55]. The frequencies of functional groups of Alg (carboxyl group – 1590 cm^{-1}, 1411 cm^{-1}, ring oxygen 1078 cm^{-1}) correspond to calcium alginate [54], which was formed as a result of cross-linking by $CaCl_2$.

However, a small amount of NO_3^- ions was detected in CHA. This can be explained by the peculiarity of synthesis by precipitation, often characterized by the presence of a small amount of impurities of initial reagents. A small amount of pyrophosphate was also found in the developed composition of PVP-Alg-CHA [22].

3.3. EPR Spectroscopy Investigation

The interaction between the polymer matrix with HA was detected by EPR spectroscopy. The interaction between the phases in the composite is a significant characteristic, described in the ref. [8].

As mentioned in Section 2.4, the use of carbonate HA in the EPR method is not appropriate and, therefore, non-carbonated HA was synthesized *ex situ*, and a composite of PVP-Alg-HA was obtained and investigated by EPR.

The EPR signal was not observed due to the absence of paramagnetic centers (PCs) in the structure of HA and composite samples. After X-ray irradiation, in the HA sample in the X- and W-ranges, three lines of the EPR spectrum characteristic of powders appeared (Figure 4, black lines). The parameters of this spectrum (shown in Table 2) allowed us to confirm the presence of NO_3^{2-} radicals in the HA structure [56]. PVP-Alg samples after X-ray irradiation were also investigated (Figure 4, red lines). In the W-range, the spectrum of the free radical was observed. In this spectrum, there were three EPR lines, which showed the localization of the unpaired electron on the nitrogen atom of PVP with the constant $A_{||} = 106 \pm 10$ MHz (Table 2). This constant is characteristic of nitrogen radicals in undissolved spin labels. In the X-band, this splitting was hidden in the line-width.

As can be seen from Figure 4 (blue lines), the EPR spectrum of PVP-Alg-HA accounts for the presence of NO_3^{2-} radicals in HA, and the polymeric mixture components were not observed. This means that the radiation-induced centers in PVP-Alg have a competitive electron trap channel, which is possible only if there is a chemical bond between the components of the composite. In addition, mixing HA with PVP-Alg somewhat changed the hyperfine interaction constants $A_\perp$ and $A_{||}$ upwards, and also increased the distribution of the constants $\Delta A_\perp$ and $\Delta A_{||}$ (Table 2). Analysis of changes in $A_\perp$ and $A_{||}$ showed that the isotropic part of the hyperfine interaction increased by 3.7 MHz, which corresponds to an increase in the electron density at the nitrogen nucleus in the HA NO_3^{2-} complex by 2%. It can be assumed that, when HA is added *ex situ*, PVP-Alg molecules form a positively charged layer around the HA particles with the formation of a chemical bond, which increases the electron density in its near-surface layer. Due to electrical neutrality, the charge on the outer surface of the PVP-Alg shell will be negative.

It should be noted that in our previous work [14], the interaction between PVP and HA phases (HA was synthesized *in situ*) was also detected by EPR spectroscopy. In the present work, despite the fact that HA was synthesized *ex situ*, the interaction between the polymer matrix and HA was also confirmed by EPR.

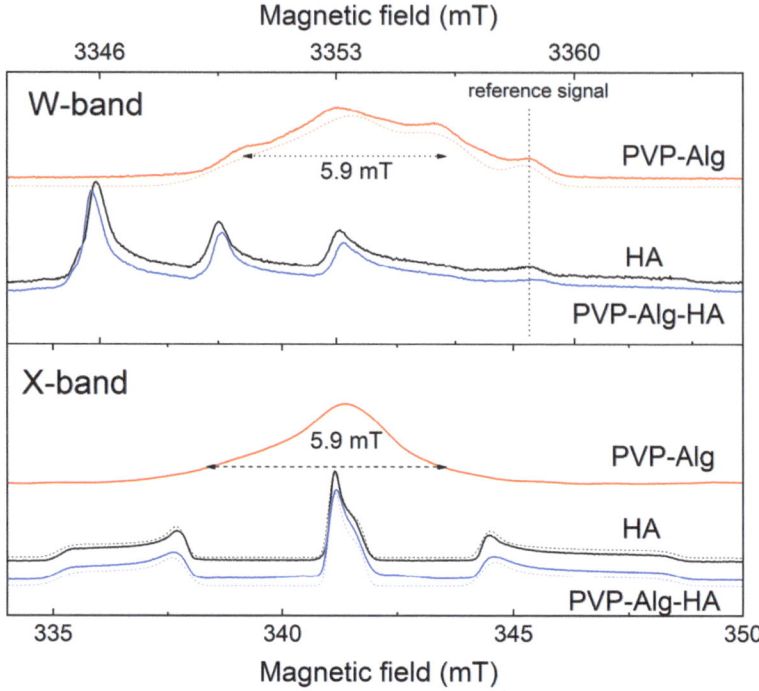

Figure 4. EPR spectra obtained by ESE detection of HA, PVP-Ag, and PVP-Alg-HA samples subjected to X-ray irradiation. W-range at the top; X-range at the bottom. The red lines show the spectra of PVP-Alg, the black lines are referred to HA, and the blue lines to PVP-Alg-HA. The dotted lines show the approximation of the EPR spectra. The approximation parameters are given in Table 2.

Table 2. EPR spectroscopic parameters of the HA and composite.

Sample	$g_\perp$	$g_{||}$	$A_\perp$ MHz	$A_{||}$ MHz	$\Delta A_\perp$ MHz	$\Delta A_{||}$ MHz
PVP-Alg	2.0022 (2)	2.0026(2)	38 ± 8	106 ± 10	-	-
HA	2.0011(1)	2.0052(1)	92.4 ± 0.5	186 ± 1	7 ± 1	12 ± 1
PVP-Alg-HA	2.0011(1)	2.0052(1)	93.6 ± 0.5	191 ± 1	13 ± 1	18 ± 1

3.4. Microstructure

SEM images of PVP-Alg and PVP-Alg-CHA samples are presented in Figure 5. The microstructure of PVP-Alg is represented by the large pores with an average size from about 10 to 50 μm, whereas the PVP-Alg-CHA sample has larger pores with an average size from about 30 to 190 μm. This observation is interesting because in the case of film samples of similar composition described in our previous work [14], the introduction of HA led to the reduction of pores. Instead, in this work, the addition of CHA resulted in a significant increase in the pore size. This is likely related to the methods of material preparation. To obtain films, the gels were dried in the air by the evaporation of moisture and spontaneous removal of air bubbles. In contrast, during the preparation of porous composite, the gel whipped into foam was first fixed by partial cross-linking in a calcium solution, and then frozen and dried by freeze-drying. As a result, the porous structure of the gel was saved.

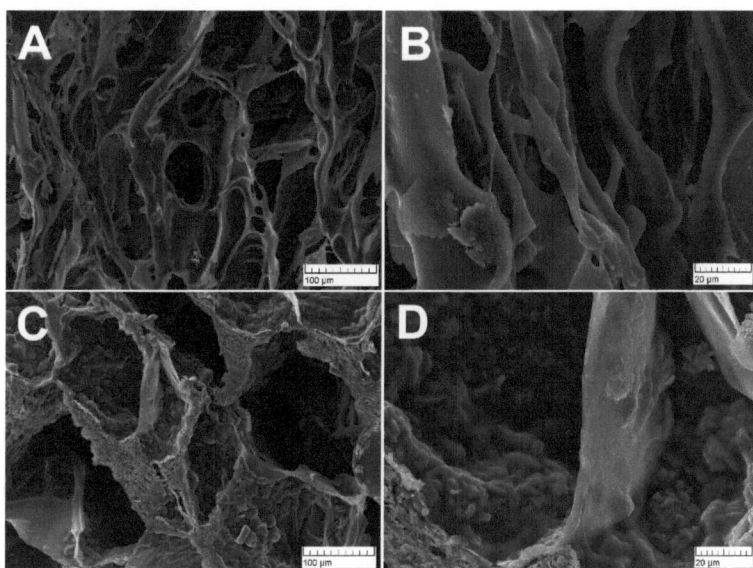

Figure 5. SEM images of PVP-Alg sample (**A**,**B**) and PVP-Alg-CHA sample (**C**,**D**).

The PVP-polyvinylalcohol(PVA) scaffold characterized by round pores with smooth walls was described in the ref. [57], such morphology being similar to the one obtained in this work for PVP-Alg (see Figure 5A). A similar porous composite structure, such as the one presented in Figure 5C, was observed for the Alg-HA scaffold frozen at −10 °C, as described in ref. [58]. There is a different effect of HA on the size and distribution of the pores. In ref. [57], the increase in HA content synthesized *in situ* (1.5–4.5 wt.%) led to a decrease in the pore size, which was explained by agglomeration of HA particles and their heterogeneous distribution in the gel. In ref. [59], a scaffold made of pure alginate obtained by freeze-drying was characterized by large pores in the order of 500 μm. The addition of HA (6–10 wt.%) also led to a reduction in the pore size to 200–300 μm, whereas in ref. [58], the addition of HA (25 and 50 wt.%) to an alginate-based scaffold did not lead to changes in pore characteristics. It is worth emphasizing here that in the present work, the CHA addition to PVP-Alg led to an increase in pore size. Thus, it is likely that the pore size parameter is influenced by many different factors, including synthesis conditions, etc.

3.5. Porosity

The porosity data obtained by the BET method are presented in Figure 6 and Table 3. The presence of a hysteresis loop with a characteristic S-shape (Figure 6) indicates the presence of slit-like micropores in the material, which is confirmed by the SEM data (Figure 6). The BET method allowed us to determine the nanoporosity of the developed composite material in terms of total pore volume, average diameter, and specific surface area (Table 3). It should be mentioned that the presence of nanopores can be useful for drug loading [60].

Table 3. BET data of PVP-Alg-CHA.

Total Pore Volume, cm^3/g	Average Pore Diameter, nm	Specific Surface Area, m^2/g
0.0094	8.71 ± 4.15	4.31

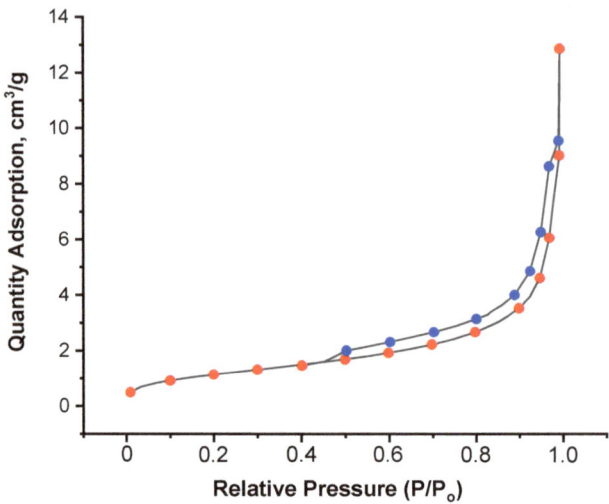

Figure 6. Isotherms of N_2 adsorption (red dotes) and desorption (blue dotes) on PVP-Alg-CHA.

The formation of nano-pores was influenced by the composition of the gel, namely by the polymers forming it. The nanoporosity of an alginate scaffold is affected by the method of alginate cross-linking, as shown in ref. [61]. The nanopores of freeze-dried alginate gel were preserved when the gel was cross-linked with calcium in the solution before freezing, in contrast to the cross-linking of the already dried scaffold (in this latter case, the pores were not preserved) [61]. Thus, the method we have chosen for obtaining the composite—gel cross-linking before freezing allowed us to preserve the nanoporous structure.

3.6. Swelling Behavior

In our previous study [14], it was shown that the introduction of HA led to the reduction of porosity and, consequently, this also reduced the swelling properties of PVP-Alg-HA films. In the case of the porous composite samples developed in this work, a different result was obtained. The swelling curves of PVP-Alg and PVP-Alg-CHA are shown in Figure 7. As can be seen, the degree of swelling was lower for the sample without CHA. This experimental result can be explained by the fact that CHA contains hydrophilic OH^- groups in its structure, which are able to bind water through hydrogen bonds. Thus, the introduction of CHA leads to an increase in the degree of swelling of the composite with porous structure. In ref. [57], the swelling of PVP-PVA-HA scaffolds in water, saline, and dextran solution was investigated. It was shown that the increase in the HA content led to an increase in the swelling rate in water, contrary to saline and dextran solutions [57]. This may confirm our assumption that HA also binds water due to the presence of the OH^- groups. Although in ref. [59], a sharp decrease in the swelling degree of the Alg-HA hydrogel was demonstrated upon the addition of HA at a concentration of 2 wt.% or more.

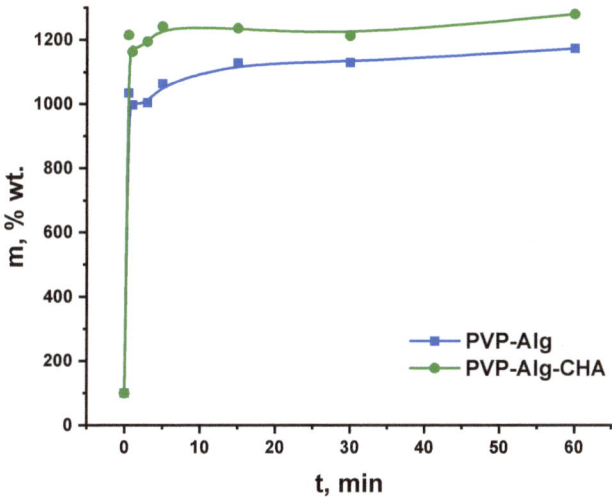

Figure 7. Swelling curves of PVP-Alg and PVP-Alg-CHA in water.

3.7. In Vitro Cell Tests

The MTT test, revealing the biocompatibility of PVP-Alg and PVP-Alg-CHA materials, was carried out using the NCTC clone L-929 of mouse fibroblast cells. As can be seen from the data shown in Figure 8, the cells' survivability was similar to the control in both samples, and there were no statistically significant differences between PVP-Alg and PVP-Alg-CHA.

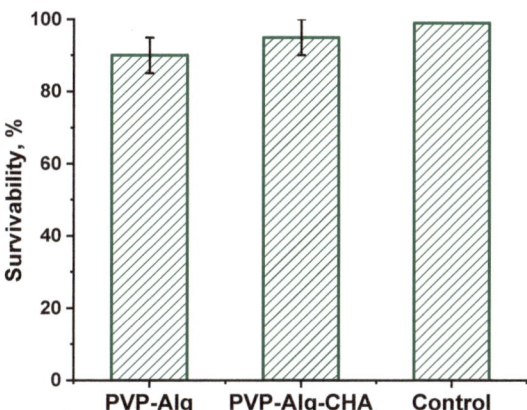

Figure 8. Survivability of NCTC mouse fibroblast cells on PLP-Alg and PVP-Alg-CHA samples.

The images of DPSC on the surface of PVP-Alg and PVP-Alg-CHA samples are presented in Figure 9. It is clearly visible that the cells have a spherical shape, and many of them are out of the focus of the microscope. This is due to the fact that the composite samples are porous, and the cells were located in the pores (white circles on Figure 9(A1,B1)). The spherical shape of the cells indicated a low adhesion of the cells to the surface of the materials [62]. This property of alginate and PVP, like of many other polymers, is useful for creation of anti-adhesive devices that prevent scarring of wounds and promote normal healing [63]. In the context of this work, this property can also be useful. Low adhesion of the material can prevent fibrosis and improper tissue fusion, and CHA can serve as a material for the functioning of osteoclasts and the growth of new bone tissue. Cell location in the pores of the samples can be also useful from the point of view of the bio-integration of the material.

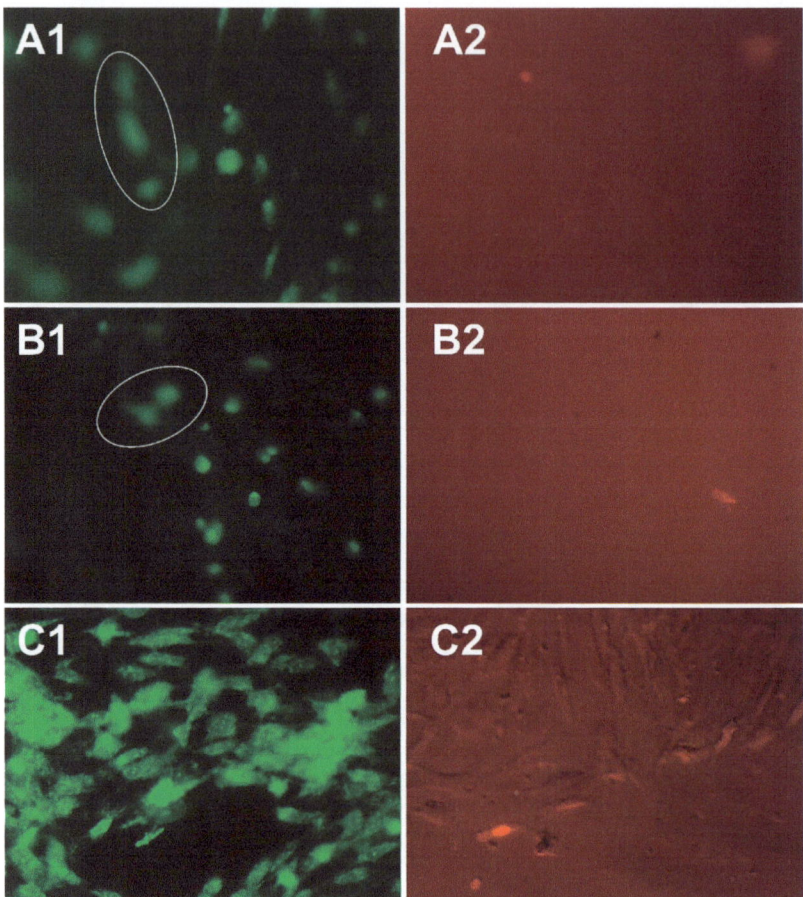

Figure 9. Images of DPSC after 24 h of seeding: green—all cells, red—dead cells. (**A1,A2**)—PVP-Alg, (**B1,B2**)—PVP-Alg-CHA, (**C1,C2**)—control.

Cell spheroids shown in Figure 10 were also observed on the surface of porous Alg-HA composite reported in ref. [58]. It can be seen that the cells are located inside the pores (Figure 10). The growth of the cell population was associated with an increase in HA content [58]. This effect was also confirmed in our previous research on the biocompatibility of PVP-Alg and PVP-Alg-HA film materials [14].

The developed PVP-Alg-CHA composite has all the necessary characteristics for a possible application in dentistry to eliminate the effects of caries. Since PVP-Alg-CHA is a bulk scaffold, it is supposed to be used in the treatment of deep caries of the posterior teeth [64], but can also be used for anteriors [65]. Since the composite is white, aesthetic problems should not arise.

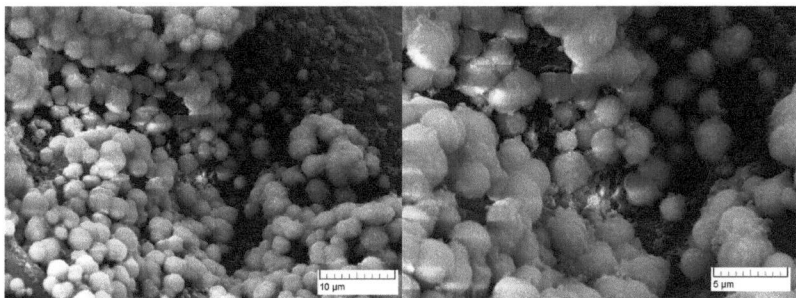

Figure 10. SEM images of DPSC spheroids on the PVP-Alg-CHA surface.

CHA present in the composite is not only very close to the mineral composition of dentin, but also has a higher resorbability with respect to HA [66]. Alginate, cross-linked with calcium ions, could be an additional source of calcium ions for bone tissue cells and, therefore, also promotes mineralization [67]. In addition, the cross-linked alginate allows the scaffold microstructure to be preserved when in contact with liquids. This, in turn, is necessary for the biointegration of the material namely, for the colonization of cells [68]. A porous microstructure is essential for teeth vascularization [69]. The PVP in the scaffold reduces its mechanical stiffness and, being non-crosslinked, will be removed faster than the alginate mesh, creating more space for tissue growth. The hydrophilic nature of polymers prevents cell adhesion [68,70]; their attachment will proceed gradually as the matrix dissolves and mineralizes. Due to the high swelling capacity of the composite, the scaffold can be used as a local hemostatic agent [71]. In this case, the material will be loaded with blood proteins necessary for cell proliferation and tissue repair. Finally, the nanoporosity of the scaffold can be used for drug delivery.

4. Conclusions

Porous composite material based on the mixture of PVP and Alg polymers with CHA, prepared by freeze-drying of the gel, was obtained and characterized. The mineral component of the developed composite was mainly represented by the B-type carbonate hydroxyapatite, according to XRD and IR spectroscopy data. The microstructure of PVP-Alg-CHA was characterized by large pores of about 30–190 μm, and the swelling was 1200 wt.%. The BET method showed that along with micropores, the composite has nanopores, the total volume of which is 0.0094 cm^3/g, and average size is 8.71 ± 4.15 nm. MTT test studies showed that the developed composite material is biocompatible. The DPSC seeded on the surface of the composite penetrated into its pores, while maintaining a spherical shape.

It can be concluded that the combination of material properties (phase composition, porous microstructure, swelling, nanoporosity, and cell integration) allows us to consider it as a promising material for caries treatment and regenerative therapy in dentistry.

Author Contributions: Conceptualization, A.A.F. and I.V.F.; methodology, I.V.F., D.V.D., A.N.G., G.V.M., G.A.D., V.G.Y., I.V.A. and J.V.R.; validation, V.G.Y., I.V.A. and J.V.R.; formal analysis, I.V.F., D.V.D. and G.V.M.; investigation, D.V.D., A.N.G., G.V.M., D.V.S. and G.A.D.; resources, I.V.F., D.V.D., A.N.G., G.V.M. and G.A.D.; data curation, A.A.F.; writing—original draft preparation, A.A.F., D.V.D., G.V.M. and J.V.R.; writing—review and editing, A.A.F. and J.V.R.; visualization, A.A.F., D.V.D., D.V.S. and G.A.D.; supervision, I.V.F. and J.V.R.; project administration, I.V.F.; funding acquisition, I.V.F., D.V.D. and J.V.R. All authors have read and agreed to the published version of the manuscript.

Funding: This research was funded by Russian Scientific Fund, grant number 22-23-00278. The X-ray study was carried out in accordance with the state of the Russian Federation, state registration number 122011300125-2.

Institutional Review Board Statement: The experiments with dental pulp stem cells were carried out in accordance with good clinical practice and ethical principles of the current version of the Declaration of Helsinki and approved by the Ethics Committee of the Institute of Theoretical and Experimental Biophysics of the Russian Academy of Sciences (Pushchino, Moscow Region, Russian Federation), Protocol No. 35 from 5 March 2022. Postnatal human DPSCs were extracted from the third molar of a human donor (18-year-old donor). The tooth was removed in accordance with the dental indications of the Central Research Institute of Dentistry and Maxillofacial Surgery of the Ministry of Health (Moscow, Russia), in accordance with the Ethics Committee, after the consent was signed by the patient's parents.

Informed Consent Statement: Informed consent was obtained from all subjects involved in the study.

Data Availability Statement: The experimental data on the results reported in this manuscript are available upon a reasonable request to corresponding author.

Acknowledgments: Authors are grateful to the Anatoly A. Konovalov for carrying out the porosity measurements and Olga S. Antonova for carrying out the SEM measurements.

Conflicts of Interest: The authors declare no conflict of interest.

References

1. Franca, C.M.; Balbinot, G.d.S.; Cunha, D.; Saboia, V.d.P.A.; Ferracane, J.; Bertassoni, L.E. In-Vitro Models of Biocompatibility Testing for Restorative Dental Materials: From 2D Cultures to Organs on-a-Chip. *Acta Biomater.* **2022**, *150*, 58–66. [CrossRef] [PubMed]
2. Ramburrun, P.; Pringle, N.A.; Dube, A.; Adam, R.Z.; D'souza, S.; Aucamp, M. Recent Advances in the Development of Antimicrobial and Antifouling Biocompatible Materials for Dental Applications. *Materials* **2021**, *14*, 3167. [CrossRef] [PubMed]
3. Cavalcanti, B.N.; Zeitlin, B.D.; Nör, J.E. A Hydrogel Scaffold That Maintains Viability and Supports Differentiation of Dental Pulp Stem Cells. *Dent. Mater.* **2013**, *29*, 97–102. [CrossRef]
4. Vadalà, G.; Russo, F.; Ambrosio, L.; Denaro, V. *Handbook of Bioceramics and Biocomposites*; Antoniac, I.V., Ed.; Springer: Berlin/Heidelberg, Germany, 2016; ISBN 9783319124605.
5. Ridi, F.; Meazzini, I.; Castroflorio, B.; Bonini, M.; Berti, D.; Baglioni, P. Functional Calcium Phosphate Composites in Nanomedicine. *Adv. Colloid Interface Sci.* **2017**, *244*, 281–295. [CrossRef]
6. Chen, I.H.; Lee, T.M.; Huang, C.L. Biopolymers Hybrid Particles Used in Dentistry. *Gels* **2021**, *7*, 31. [CrossRef] [PubMed]
7. Bertassoni, L.E. Progress and Challenges in Microengineering the Dental Pulp Vascular Microenvironment. *J. Endod.* **2020**, *46*, S90–S100. [CrossRef]
8. Furko, M.; Balázsi, K.; Balázsi, C. Calcium Phosphate Loaded Biopolymer Composites—A Comprehensive Review on the Most Recent Progress and Promising Trends. *Coatings* **2023**, *13*, 360. [CrossRef]
9. Xu, X.; He, L.; Zhu, B.; Li, J.; Li, J. Advances in Polymeric Materials for Dental Applications. *Polym. Chem.* **2017**, *8*, 807–823. [CrossRef]
10. Anisha, A.D.; Shegokar, R. Expert Opinion on Drug Delivery Polyethylene Glycol (PEG): A Versatile Polymer for Pharmaceutical Applications. *Expert Opin. Drug Deliv.* **2016**, *13*, 1257–1275. [CrossRef]
11. Kheilnezhad, B.; Hadjizadeh, A. Biomaterials Science from a Biomaterial Perspective. *Biomater. Sci.* **2021**, *9*, 2850–2873. [CrossRef]
12. Fadeeva, I.V.; Deyneko, D.V.; Knotko, A.V.; Olkhov, A.A.; Slukin, P.V.; Davydova, G.A.; Trubitsyna, T.A.; Preobrazhenskiy, I.I.; Gosteva, A.N.; Antoniac, I.V.; et al. Antibacterial Composite Material Based on Polyhydroxybutyrate and Zn-Doped Brushite Cement. *Polymers* **2023**, *15*, 2106. [CrossRef] [PubMed]
13. Pietrzykowska, E.; Romelczyk-Baishya, B.; Wojnarowicz, J.; Sokolova, M.; Szlazak, K.; Swieszkowski, W.; Locs, J.; Lojkowski, W. Preparation of a Ceramic Matrix Composite Made of Hydroxyapatite Nanoparticles and Polylactic Acid by Consolidation of Composite Granules. *Nanomaterials* **2020**, *10*, 1060. [CrossRef] [PubMed]
14. Fadeeva, I.V.; Trofimchuk, E.S.; Forysenkova, A.A.; Ahmed, A.I.; Gnezdilov, O.I.; Davydova, G.A.; Kozlova, S.G.; Antoniac, A.; Rau, J.V. Composite Polyvinylpyrrolidone—Sodium Alginate—Hydroxyapatite Hydrogel Films for Bone Repair and Wound Dressings Applications. *Polymers* **2021**, *13*, 3989. [CrossRef]
15. Albulescu, R.; Popa, A.C.; Enciu, A.M.; Albulescu, L.; Dudau, M.; Popescu, I.D.; Mihai, S.; Codrici, E.; Pop, S.; Lupu, A.R.; et al. Comprehensive in Vitro Testing of Calcium Phosphate-Based Bioceramics with Orthopedic and Dentistry Applications. *Materials* **2019**, *12*, 3704. [CrossRef]
16. Rau, J.V.; Fadeeva, I.V.; Forysenkova, A.A.; Davydova, G.A.; Fosca, M.; Filippov, Y.Y.; Antoniac, I.V.; Antoniac, A.; D'Arco, A.; Di Fabrizio, M.; et al. Strontium Substituted Tricalcium Phosphate Bone Cement: Short and Long-Term Time-Resolved Studies and In Vitro Properties. *Adv. Mater. Interfaces* **2022**, *9*, 2200803. [CrossRef]
17. Tite, T.; Popa, A.C.; Balescu, L.M.; Bogdan, I.M.; Pasuk, I.; Ferreira, J.M.F.; Stan, G.E. Cationic Substitutions in Hydroxyapatite: Current Status of the Derived Biofunctional Effects and Their in Vitro Interrogation Methods. *Materials* **2018**, *11*, 2081. [CrossRef]
18. Neves, N.; Linhares, D.; Costa, G.; Ribeiro, C.C.; Barbosa, M.A. In Vivo and Clinical Application of Strontium-Enriched Biomaterials for Bone Regeneration. *Bone Jt. Res.* **2017**, *6*, 366–375. [CrossRef] [PubMed]

19. Graziani, G.; Barbaro, K.; Fadeeva, I.V.; Ghezzi, D.; Fosca, M.; Sassoni, E.; Vadalà, G.; Cappelletti, M.; Valle, F.; Baldini, N.; et al. Ionized Jet Deposition of Antimicrobial and Stem Cell Friendly Silver-Substituted Tricalcium Phosphate Nanocoatings on Titanium Alloy. *Bioact. Mater.* **2021**, *6*, 2629–2642. [CrossRef]
20. Fadeeva, I.V.; Goldberg, M.A.; Preobrazhensky, I.I.; Mamin, G.V.; Davidova, G.A.; Agafonova, N.V.; Fosca, M.; Russo, F.; Barinov, S.M.; Cavalu, S.; et al. Improved Cytocompatibility and Antibacterial Properties of Zinc-Substituted Brushite Bone Cement Based on β-Tricalcium Phosphate. *J. Mater. Sci. Mater. Med.* **2021**, *32*, 99. [CrossRef]
21. Rau, J.V.; Fadeeva, I.V.; Fomin, A.S.; Barbaro, K.; Galvano, E.; Ryzhov, A.P.; Murzakhanov, F.; Gafurov, M.R.; Orlinskii, S.B.; Antoniac, I.V. Sic Parvis Magna: Manganese-Substituted Tricalcium Phosphate and Its Biophysical Properties. *ACS Biomater. Sci. Eng.* **2019**, *5*, 6632–6644. [CrossRef]
22. Fadeeva, I.V.; Deyneko, D.V.; Barbaro, K.; Davydova, G.A.; Sadovnikova, M.A.; Murzakhanov, F.F.; Fomin, A.S.; Yankova, V.G.; Antoniac, I.V.; Barinov, S.M.; et al. Influence of Synthesis Conditions on Gadolinium-Substituted Tricalcium Phosphate Ceramics and Its Physicochemical, Biological, and Antibacterial Properties. *Nanomaterials* **2022**, *12*, 853. [CrossRef]
23. Fosca, M.; Streza, A.; Antoniac, I.V.; Vadal, G.; Rau, J.V. Ion-Doped Calcium Phosphate-Based Coatings with Antibacterial Properties. *J. Funct. Biomater.* **2023**, *14*, 250. [CrossRef]
24. Kono, T.; Sakae, T.; Nakada, H.; Kaneda, T.; Okada, H. Confusion between Carbonate Apatite and Biological Apatite (Carbonated Hydroxyapatite) in Bone and Teeth. *Minerals* **2022**, *12*, 170. [CrossRef]
25. Tavelli, L.; McGuire, M.K.; Zucchelli, G.; Rasperini, G.; Feinberg, S.E.; Wang, H.L.; Giannobile, W.V. Extracellular Matrix-Based Scaffolding Technologies for Periodontal and Peri-Implant Soft Tissue Regeneration. *J. Periodontol.* **2020**, *91*, 17–25. [CrossRef]
26. Lee, J.-H.; Parthiban, P.; Jin, G.-Z.; Knowles, J.C.; Kim, H.-W. Materials roles for promoting angiogenesis in tissue regeneration. *Prog. Mater. Sci.* **2020**, *117*, 100732. [CrossRef]
27. Qian, L.; Zhang, H. Controlled Freezing and Freeze Drying: A Versatile Route for Porous and Micro-/Nano-Structured Materials. *J. Chem. Technol. Biotechnol.* **2011**, *86*, 172–184. [CrossRef]
28. Chai, Y.; Okuda, M.; Otsuka, Y.; Ohnuma, K.; Tagaya, M. Comparison of Two Fabrication Processes for Biomimetic Collagen/Hydroxyapatite Hybrids. *Adv. Powder Technol.* **2019**, *30*, 1419–1423. [CrossRef]
29. Rogina, A.; Ressler, A.; Matić, I.; Gallego Ferrer, G.; Marijanović, I.; Ivanković, M.; Ivanković, H. Cellular Hydrogels Based on PH-Responsive Chitosan-Hydroxyapatite System. *Carbohydr. Polym.* **2017**, *166*, 173–182. [CrossRef]
30. Gelli, R.; Del Buffa, S.; Tempesti, P.; Bonini, M.; Ridi, F.; Baglioni, P. Enhanced Formation of Hydroxyapatites in Gelatin/Imogolite Macroporous Hydrogels. *J. Colloid Interface Sci.* **2018**, *511*, 145–154. [CrossRef]
31. Kyoung, J.; Hyung, K.; Kim, J.; Lee, J.C.J. Natural and Synthetic Biomaterials for Controlled Drug Delivery. *Arch. Pharm. Res.* **2014**, *37*, 60–68. [CrossRef]
32. Hernández-González, A.C.; Téllez-Jurado, L.; Rodríguez-Lorenzo, L.M. Alginate Hydrogels for Bone Tissue Engineering, from Injectables to Bioprinting: A Review. *Carbohydr. Polym.* **2020**, *229*, 115514. [CrossRef] [PubMed]
33. Bercea, M.; Morariu, S.; Teodorescu, M. Rheological Investigation of Poly(VinylAlcohol)/Poly(N-Vinyl Pyrrolidone) Mixtures in Aqueous Solution and Hydrogel State. *J. Polym. Res.* **2016**, *23*, 142. [CrossRef]
34. Yong, K.; Mooney, D.J. Progress in Polymer Science Alginate: Properties and Biomedical Applications. *Prog. Polym. Sci.* **2012**, *37*, 106–126. [CrossRef]
35. Kurakula, M.; Koteswara Rao, G.S.N. Moving Polyvinyl Pyrrolidone Electrospun Nanofibers and Bioprinted Scaffolds toward Multidisciplinary Biomedical Applications. *Eur. Polym. J.* **2020**, *136*, 109919. [CrossRef]
36. Forysenkova, A.A.; Ivanova, V.A.; Fadeeva, I.V.; Mamin, G.V.; Rau, J.V. NMR and EPR Spectroscopies Investigation of Alginate Cross-Linking by Divalent Ions. *Materials* **2023**, *16*, 2832. [CrossRef]
37. Kovaleva, E.S.; Filippov, Y.Y.; Putlyaev, V.I.; Tretyakov, Y.D.; Ivanov, V.K.; Silkin, N.I.; Galiullina, L.F.; Rodionov, A.A.; Mamin, G.V.; Orlinsky, S.B.; et al. Bioresorbable Powder Material Based on $Ca_{10-x}Na_x(PO_4)_{6-x}(CO_3)_x(OH)_2$. *Uchenyye Zap. Kazan. Gos. Univ.* **2010**, *152*, 79–98.
38. Sing, K. The Use of Nitrogen Adsorption for the Characterisation of Porous Materials. *Colloids Surf. A Physicochem. Eng. Asp.* **2001**, *187*, 3–9. [CrossRef]
39. Bicker, M.; Müller, M.; Mittermüller, M.; Haines, D.; Rothhaar, U. Comparative extractable studies for injectables and medical devices aligned with USP<1663> and ISO 10993 Guidelines. *ONdrugDelivery* **2021**, *120*, 86–95.
40. Uskoković, V.; Marković, S.; Veselinović, L.; Škapin, S.; Ignjatović, N.; Uskoković, D.P. Insights into the Kinetics of Thermally Induced Crystallization of Amorphous Calcium Phosphate. *Phys. Chem. Chem. Phys.* **2018**, *20*, 29221–29235. [CrossRef]
41. Uskokovic, V. The Role of Hydroxyl Channel in Defining Selected Physicochemical Peculiarities Exhibited by Hydroxyapatite. *RSC Adv.* **2015**, *5*, 36614–36633. [CrossRef]
42. Chaudhuri, B.; Mondal, B.; Ray, S.K.; Sarkar, S.C. A Novel Biocompatible Conducting Polyvinyl Alcohol (PVA)-Polyvinylpyrrolidone (PVP)-Hydroxyapatite (HAP) Composite Scaffolds for Probable Biological Application. *Colloids Surf. B Biointerfaces* **2016**, *143*, 71–80. [CrossRef] [PubMed]
43. Guesmi, Y.; Agougui, H.; Jabli, M.; Alsharabasy, A.M. Bioactive Composites of Hydroxyapatite/Polyvinylpyrrolidone for Bone Regeneration Applications. *Chem. Eng. Commun.* **2019**, *206*, 279–288. [CrossRef]
44. Tang, S.; Zhao, Y.; Wang, H.; Wang, Y.; Zhu, H.; Chen, Y.; Chen, S.; Jin, S.; Yang, Z.; Li, P.; et al. Preparation of the Sodium Alginate-g-(Polyacrylic Acid-Co-Allyltrimethylammonium Chloride) Polyampholytic Superabsorbent Polymer and Its Dye Adsorption Property. *Mar. Drugs* **2018**, *16*, 476. [CrossRef] [PubMed]

45. Mason, H.E.; Kozlowski, A.; Phillips, B.L. Solid-State NMR Study of the Role of H and Na in AB-Type Carbonate Hydroxylapatite. *Chem. Mater.* **2008**, *20*, 294–302. [CrossRef]
46. Jillavenkatesa, A.; Condrate, R.A. Sol-Gel Processing of Hydroxyapatite. *J. Mater. Sci.* **1998**, *33*, 4111–4119. [CrossRef]
47. Ji, Y.; Yang, X.; Ji, Z.; Zhu, L.; Ma, N.; Chen, D.; Jia, X.; Tang, J.; Cao, Y. DFT-Calculated IR Spectrum Amide I, II, and III Band Contributions of N-Methylacetamide Fine Components. *ACS Omega* **2020**, *5*, 8572–8578. [CrossRef]
48. Ansari, M.T.; Sunderland, V.B. Solid Dispersions of Dihydroartemisinin in Polyvinylpyrrolidone. *Arch. Pharm. Res.* **2008**, *31*, 390–398. [CrossRef]
49. Stathopoulou, E.T.; Psycharis, V.; Chryssikos, G.D.; Gionis, V.; Theodorou, G. Bone Diagenesis: New Data from Infrared Spectroscopy and X-Ray Diffraction. *Palaeogeogr. Palaeoclimatol. Palaeoecol.* **2008**, *266*, 168–174. [CrossRef]
50. Chen, Y.H.; Khairullin, I.I.; Suen, M.P.; Hwang, L.P. Electron Spin Resonance and Infrared Spectroscopy Study of the Polyvinylpyrrolidone-C60 Composite. *Fuller. Sci. Technol.* **1999**, *7*, 807–823. [CrossRef]
51. Malina, D.; Sobczak-Kupiec, A.; Wzorek, Z.; Kowalski, Z. Silver Nanoparticles Synthesis with Different Concentrations of Polyvinylpyrrolidone. *Dig. J. Nanomater. Biostruct.* **2012**, *7*, 1527–1534.
52. Serafim, A.; Petre, D.G.; Adriana, L.; Cioflan, H.E.; Stancu, I.C. Hybrid Hydrogels Intended as Scaffolds for Soft Tissue Repair. *Key Eng. Mater.* **2014**, *638*, 54–61. [CrossRef]
53. Wang, W.; Wang, A. Synthesis and Swelling Properties of pH-Sensitive Semi-IPN Superabsorbent Hydrogels Based on Sodium Alginate-g-Poly(Sodium Acrylate) and Polyvinylpyrrolidone. *Carbohydr. Polym.* **2010**, *80*, 1028–1036. [CrossRef]
54. Papageorgiou, S.K.; Kouvelos, E.P.; Favvas, E.P.; Sapalidis, A.A.; Romanos, G.E.; Katsaros, F.K. Metal—Carboxylate Interactions in Metal—Alginate Complexes Studied with FTIR Spectroscopy. *Carbohydr. Res.* **2010**, *345*, 469–473. [CrossRef] [PubMed]
55. Liu, M.; Yan, X.; Liu, H.; Yu, W. Investigation of the Interaction between Polyvinylpyrrolidone and Metal Cations. *React. Funct. Polym.* **2000**, *44*, 55–64. [CrossRef]
56. Gafurov, M.; Biktagirov, T.; Yavkin, B.; Mamin, G.; Filippov, Y.; Klimashina, E.; Putlayev, V.; Orlinskii, S. Nitrogen-Containing Species in the Structure of the Synthesized Nano-Hydroxyapatite. *JETP Lett.* **2014**, *99*, 196–203. [CrossRef]
57. Ma, Y.; Bai, T.; Wang, F. The Physical and Chemical Properties of the Polyvinylalcohol/Polyvinylpyrrolidone/Hydroxyapatite Composite Hydrogel. *Mater. Sci. Eng. C* **2016**, *59*, 948–957. [CrossRef]
58. Lin, H.R.; Yen, Y.J. Porous Alginate/Hydroxyapatite Composite Scaffolds for Bone Tissue Engineering: Preparation, Characterization, and in Vitro Studies. *J. Biomed. Mater. Res. Part B Appl. Biomater.* **2004**, *71*, 52–65. [CrossRef]
59. Yan, J.; Miao, Y.; Tan, H.; Zhou, T.; Ling, Z.; Chen, Y.; Xing, X.; Hu, X. Injectable Alginate/Hydroxyapatite Gel Scaffold Combined with Gelatin Microspheres for Drug Delivery and Bone Tissue Engineering. *Mater. Sci. Eng. C* **2016**, *63*, 274–284. [CrossRef]
60. Alsmadi, M.T.M.; Obaidat, R.M.; Alnaief, M.; Albiss, B.A.; Hailat, N. Development, in vitro characterization, and in vivo toxicity evaluation of chitosan-alginate nanoporous carriers loaded with cisplatin for lung cancer treatment. *AAPS PharmSciTech* **2020**, *21*, 191. [CrossRef]
61. Jin Lee, H.; Kim, G.H. Cryogenically Direct-Plotted Alginate Scaffolds Consisting of Micro/Nano-Architecture for Bone Tissue Regeneration. *RSC Adv.* **2012**, *2*, 7578–7587. [CrossRef]
62. Lee, H.P.; Gu, L.; Mooney, D.J.; Levenston, M.E.; Chaudhuri, O. Mechanical Confinement Regulates Cartilage Matrix Formation by Chondrocytes. *Nat. Mater.* **2017**, *16*, 1243–1251. [CrossRef] [PubMed]
63. Spicer, C.D. Hydrogel Scaffolds for Tissue Engineering: Polymer Chemistry Importance of Polymer Choice. *Polym. Chem.* **2020**, *11*, 184–219. [CrossRef]
64. Heintze, S.D.; Loguercio, A.D.; Hanzen, T.A.; Reis, A.; Rousson, V. Clinical efficacy of resin-based direct posterior restorations and glass-ionomer restorations—An updated meta-analysis of clinical outcome parameters. *Dent. Mater.* **2022**, *38*, e109–e135. [CrossRef] [PubMed]
65. Paolone, G.; Scolavino, S.; Gherlone, E.; Spagnuolo, G. Direct esthetic composite restorations in anterior teeth: Managing symmetry strategies. *Symmetry* **2021**, *13*, 797. [CrossRef]
66. Ressler, A.; Žužić, A.; Ivanišević, I.; Kamboj, N.; Ivanković, H. Ionic substituted hydroxyapatite for bone regeneration applications: A review. *Open Ceram.* **2021**, *6*, 100122. [CrossRef]
67. Serra-Aguado, C.I.; Llorens-Gámez, M.; Vercet-Llopis, P.; Martínez-Chicote, V.; Deb, S.; Serrano-Aroca, Á. Engineering Three-Dimensional-Printed Bioactive Polylactic Acid Alginate Composite Scaffolds with Antibacterial and In Vivo Osteoinductive Capacity. *ACS App. Mater. Interf.* **2022**, *14*, 53593–53602. [CrossRef] [PubMed]
68. Giraudo, M.V.; Di Francesco, D.; Catoira, M.C.; Cotella, D.; Fusaro, L.; Boccafoschi, F. Angiogenic Potential in Biological Hydrogels. *Biomedicines* **2020**, *8*, 436. [CrossRef] [PubMed]
69. Jazayeri, H.E.; Lee, S.M.; Kuhn, L.; Fahimipour, F.; Tahriri, M.; Tayebi, L. Polymeric scaffolds for dental pulp tissue engineering: A review. *Dent. Mater.* **2020**, *36*, e47–e58. [CrossRef]
70. Lih, E.; Oh, S.H.; Joung, Y.K.; Lee, J.H.; Han, D.K. Polymers for cell/tissue anti-adhesion. *Prog. Polym. Sci.* **2015**, *44*, 28–61. [CrossRef]
71. Guo, B.; Dong, R.; Liang, Y.; Li, M. Haemostatic materials for wound healing applications. *Nat. Rev. Chem.* **2021**, *5*, 773–791. [CrossRef]

Disclaimer/Publisher's Note: The statements, opinions and data contained in all publications are solely those of the individual author(s) and contributor(s) and not of MDPI and/or the editor(s). MDPI and/or the editor(s) disclaim responsibility for any injury to people or property resulting from any ideas, methods, instructions or products referred to in the content.

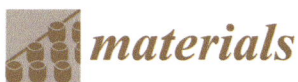

Article

Fabrication of Ciprofloxacin-Immobilized Calcium Phosphate Particles for Dental Drug Delivery

Aniruddha Pal [1], Ayako Oyane [1,*], Tomoya Inose [1], Maki Nakamura [1], Erika Nishida [2] and Hirofumi Miyaji [2]

[1] Nanomaterials Research Institute, National Institute of Advanced Industrial Science and Technology (AIST), AIST Tsukuba Central 5, 1-1-1 Higashi, Tsukuba 305-8565, Japan; aniruddhapal8@gmail.com (A.P.); t.inose@aist.go.jp (T.I.); ma-ki-nakamura@aist.go.jp (M.N.)

[2] Department of General Dentistry, Faculty of Dental Medicine, Hokkaido University, N13 W7 Kita-ku, Sapporo 060-8586, Japan; erikanishida@den.hokudai.ac.jp (E.N.); miyaji@den.hokudai.ac.jp (H.M.)

* Correspondence: a-oyane@aist.go.jp; Tel.: +81-50-3521-1018

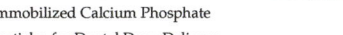

Citation: Pal, A.; Oyane, A.; Inose, T.; Nakamura, M.; Nishida, E.; Miyaji, H. Fabrication of Ciprofloxacin-Immobilized Calcium Phosphate Particles for Dental Drug Delivery. *Materials* **2024**, *17*, 2035. https://doi.org/10.3390/ma17092035

Academic Editors: Josip Kranjčić and Tina Poklepovic Pericic

Received: 8 April 2024
Revised: 19 April 2024
Accepted: 23 April 2024
Published: 26 April 2024

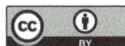

Copyright: © 2024 by the authors. Licensee MDPI, Basel, Switzerland. This article is an open access article distributed under the terms and conditions of the Creative Commons Attribution (CC BY) license (https:// creativecommons.org/licenses/by/ 4.0/).

Abstract: Calcium phosphate (CaP) particles immobilizing antibacterial agents have the potential to be used as dental disinfectants. In this study, we fabricated CaP particles with immobilized ciprofloxacin (CF), a commonly prescribed antibacterial agent, via a coprecipitation process using a supersaturated CaP solution. As the aging time in the coprecipitation process increased from 2 to 24 h, the CaP phase in the resulting particles transformed from amorphous to low-crystalline hydroxyapatite, and their Ca/P elemental ratio, yield, and CF content increased. Despite the higher CF content, the particles aged for 24 h displayed a slower release of CF in a physiological salt solution, most likely owing to their crystallized matrix (less soluble hydroxyapatite), than those aged for 2 h, whose matrix was amorphous CaP. Both particles exhibited antibacterial and antibiofilm activities along with an acid-neutralizing effect against the major oral bacteria, *Streptococcus mutans*, *Porphyromonas gingivalis*, and *Actinomyces naeslundii*, in a dose-dependent manner, although their dose–response relationship was slightly different. The aging time in the coprecipitation process was identified as a governing factor affecting the physicochemical properties of the resulting CF-immobilized CaP particles and their functionality as a dental disinfectant.

Keywords: coprecipitation; antibacterial activity; biofilm; carrier; ciprofloxacin

1. Introduction

Oral microorganisms such as bacteria, fungi, and viruses can cause oral diseases [1]. For example, certain types of oral bacteria, including *Streptococcus mutans* (*S. mutans*), *Porphyromonas gingivalis* (*P. gingivalis*), and *Actinomyces naeslundii* (*A. naeslundii*), are associated with two major oral diseases: dental caries and periodontal disease. *S. mutans* is the main component of dental plaque and the primary cause of caries [2]. The gram-negative bacterium *P. gingivalis* can cause periodontal disease, leading to tooth loss in the most severe case [3], whereas *A. naeslundii* is a major component of oral biofilms [4]. These bacteria often proliferate in narrow spaces in the mouth, such as dental fissures, pits, grooves, and periodontal pockets. Therefore, nano- and micro-carriers for local delivery of antibacterial agents are expected to be useful in controlling dental diseases caused by these bacteria [5,6].

Calcium phosphate (CaP) particles are one of the most promising carriers for dental drug delivery, because CaPs are chemically similar to the mineral fraction of human teeth [7,8], intrinsically safe, and white in color. Additionally, CaPs may promote remineralization of teeth by degrading into calcium and phosphate ions [9,10]. CaPs have long been used as biomaterials for dental care and restoration because of their good biocompatibility and osteoconductivity [11].

In the last few decades, CaP particles have been loaded with various antibacterial agents, such as silver nanoparticles [12], silver ions [13], gallium ions [14], zinc ions [15], chlorhexidine [16], and ciprofloxacin (CF) [17–19]. Among these agents, CF is particularly beneficial because it is a clinically approved fluoroquinolone antibiotic [20] that is white in color, exhibits high oral availability, and has antibacterial effects against a wide range of bacteria, including *S. mutans* [21,22], *P. gingivalis* [23,24], and *A. naeslundii* [25,26].

In previous studies, CF-immobilized CaP particles were fabricated by a coprecipitation process in a supersaturated CaP solution [18] or by an adsorption process [17,19]. The coprecipitation process can generally produce composite particles in which drugs are immobilized throughout the CaP matrix [27]. Hence, it is advantageous over the adsorption process in terms of having higher drug loading capacity [28]. CF-immobilized CaP particles prepared by the coprecipitation process showed antibacterial activity against certain types of bacteria [18]; however, their antibacterial activities against oral bacteria related to dental caries and periodontal disease have not been investigated.

In the previous coprecipitation process, the concentration of CF in the supersaturated CaP solution was varied to adjust the amount of CF immobilized in the CaP particles and to control their CF-release profile [18]. Here, we attempted a different approach based on the phase transformation of CaP to control the CF-release profile. We hypothesized that the aging time in the coprecipitation process would influence not only the amount of immobilized CF but also the CaP crystalline structure in the resulting CF-immobilized CaP particles, thereby affecting their CF-release profile. This hypothesis was based on previous results that showed that amorphous CaP particles changed into crystalline hydroxyapatite particles upon 24 h of aging during the coprecipitation process [29], and amorphous CaP particles released immobilized drugs faster than hydroxyapatite particles [30].

The first aim of the present study was to prepare CF-immobilized CaP particles with different crystalline phases and CF-release profiles by changing the aging time (2 h and 24 h) during the coprecipitation process. The second aim was to demonstrate the antibacterial and antibiofilm activities of the prepared particles against oral bacteria associated with dental caries and periodontal disease: *S. mutans*, *A. naeslundii*, and *P. gingivalis*.

2. Materials and Methods

2.1. Preparation of CF-Immobilized CaP Particles

We used four source solutions: calcium ion solution, phosphate ion solution, sodium carbonate solution, and CF solution. As calcium and phosphate ion solutions (500 mM for both), Calcium Chloride Corrective Injection 1 mEq/mL (Otsuka Pharmaceutical Co., Ltd., Tokyo, Japan) and Dibasic Potassium Phosphate Injection 20 mEq Kit (Terumo Corporation, Tokyo, Japan) were utilized, respectively. The sodium carbonate solution (500 mM) was prepared by adding sodium carbonate (FUJIFILM Wako Pure Chemical Corporation, Osaka, Japan) to ultrapure water in a glass vial, followed by sonication (VS-70RS1, AS ONE, Osaka, Japan) for a few minutes for complete dissolution. The CF solution (2 mg/mL) was prepared by dissolving CF (Fluorochem Ltd., Yokohama, Japan) in 0.0075 M HCl (FUJIFILM Wako Pure Chemical Corporation) via sonication for 5 min. Before preparing the supersaturated CaP solution, two solutions (solutions A and B) were prepared as described in a previous study [29]. Solution A was prepared by mixing the calcium ion solution (500 mM) and ultrapure water at a volume ratio of 4:21 in a 50 mL centrifuge tube. Solution B was prepared by mixing the phosphate ion solution (500 mM), sodium carbonate solution (500 mM), and ultrapure water at a volume ratio of 4:4:17 in a 50 mL centrifuge tube.

Finally, the supersaturated CaP solution was prepared by adding solution B (1 mL), followed by 2 mg/mL CF solution (1 mL), and lastly, solution A (2 mL) to a 15 mL centrifuge tube at 25 °C (Figure 1). Immediately after adding solution A, the final supersaturated CaP solution (4 mL) was vortexed for 1 min. Subsequently, the solution was aged under shaking at 150 rpm in a thermostatic shaker (M-BR-104P, TAITEC CORPORATION, Koshigaya, Japan) for 2 or 24 h at 25 °C to allow coprecipitation. The precipitate was collected by centrifugation (CN-1050, Hsiang Tai, New Taipei, Taiwan) at 6000 rpm for 5 min, followed by washing three times with ultrapure water. After washing, the product was resuspended in ultrapure water and freeze-dried for 24 h before further analysis. The resulting products were named CF-CaP2h and CF-CaP24h according to the aging times of 2 and 24 h, respectively.

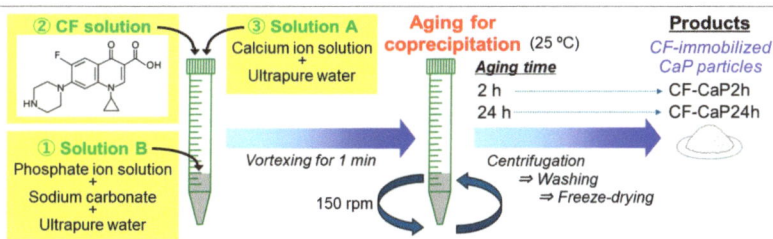

Figure 1. Schematic diagram showing the preparation of CF-immobilized CaP particles.

2.2. Characterization of the Products

The morphologies of the products were examined using field-emission scanning electron microscopy (FESEM; SU8020, Hitachi High-Tech Corporation, Tokyo, Japan). The products were sputter-coated with gold for 2 min using a sputter-coating machine (SC-701MkII, Sanyu Electron Co., Ltd., Tokyo, Japan) before FESEM analysis. The chemical compositions of the products were examined without coating using an energy-dispersive X-ray (EDX) spectrometer (AZtecOne, Oxford Instruments plc, Abingdon, UK) equipped in a tabletop SEM (TM4000Plus II, Hitachi High-Tech Corp.). Before the EDX analysis, the products were mounted on a silicon sample holder using carbon tape.

The nanostructures of the products were further investigated using a transmission electron microscope (TEM; JEM-2100, JEOL Ltd., Tokyo, Japan) operating at 200 kV. Prior to TEM analysis, the products were mounted on a formvar-supported copper grid (JEOL Ltd.) and dried under reduced pressure. The diameter of the product was determined from 100 particles in the TEM images using ImageJ software (ver. 1.54).

The crystalline structure of the products was investigated by X-ray diffractometry (XRD; Rigaku RINT-Ultima III, Tokyo, Japan) with CuKα radiation (λ = 0.154 nm) at 40 kV and 30 mA. The chemical bonds of the products were investigated using a Fourier-transform infrared (FTIR) spectrometer (FT/IR-4700, JASCO Corporation, Hachioji, Japan) equipped with an attenuated total reflection accessory and a monolithic diamond crystal.

The Ca and P contents of the products were determined by performing inductively coupled plasma optical emission spectrometry (ICP-OES; ULTIMA2, HORIBA, Ltd., Kyoto, Japan). Before the ICP-OES analysis, the products were dissolved in 0.1 mL of 6 M HCl solution (FUJIFILM Wako Pure Chemical Corporation), which was subsequently diluted with 9.9 mL of ultrapure water.

2.3. Determination of CF-Immobilization Efficiency

The immobilization efficiency of CF in the products was calculated by dividing the CF amount in the product by the total amount of CF (2.0 mg) added to the supersaturated CaP solution in the same tube, using the following equation.

$$\text{Immobilization efficiency of CF (\%)} = 100 \times \frac{\text{CF amount in the product (mg)}}{\text{CF amount in the solution (mg)}}$$

The CF amount in the product was determined as follows: After the first centrifugation following the coprecipitation process (Section 2.1), the supernatant was taken out from the tube and diluted 40 times with a physiological salt solution (pH 7.4 at 37 °C). The physiological salt solution was prepared according to a previous report [31]. The amount of CF in the diluted supernatant was determined using a UV–visible spectrophotometer (UV-2450, SHIMADZU CORPORATION, Kyoto, Japan). For measurements, 1 mL diluted supernatant was poured in a UV-transparent disposable cuvette (BrandTech® 759210, BrandTech Scientific, Essex, MA, USA), and the absorbance was measured at 270 nm, which correspond to the maximum absorption wavelength (Figure 2a). Standard solutions with various CF concentrations were prepared by diluting the 2 mg/mL CF solution described in Section 2.1 with the physiological salt solution. The absorbance of these solutions was then measured at 270 nm to obtain a calibration curve (Figure 2b). The amount of CF in the product was calculated by subtracting the amount of residual CF in the supernatant from the total amount of CF added to the supersaturated CaP solution. Six independent batches were used to obtain average and standard deviation (SD) values.

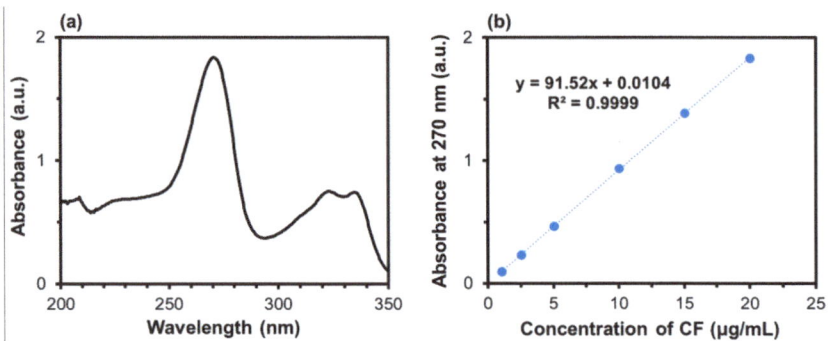

Figure 2. (a) UV absorption spectrum of the 20 µg/mL CF solution and (b) absorbance of the CF solutions with various concentrations at 270 nm.

2.4. CF-Release Assay

The release of CF from the product was studied in the physiological salt solution (pH 7.4 at 37 °C). First, the product was suspended in the appropriate amount of ultrapure water such that the concentration of CF in the suspension was 0.40 mg/mL. The suspension (0.5 mL) was poured into a dialysis tube (Bio-Tech MWCO 12000, Bio-Tech, Taoyuan, Taiwan), which was kept in 10 mL of physiological salt solution in a 25 mL tube. After incubation at 37 °C for 0, 1, 3, 5, 7, 24, 48, and 72 h, an aliquot of 1.0 mL was sampled from the physiological salt solution, and fresh physiological salt solution (1.0 mL) was added to it. The amount of CF released into the physiological salt solution was determined by measuring the absorbance at 270 nm using the UV–visible spectrophotometer as described in Section 2.3. The percentage of CF released into the physiological salt solution from the net dose of CF (0.2 mg) added to the dialysis tube was calculated using the following equation.

$$\text{Percentage of CF released } (\%) = 100 \times \frac{\text{CF amount in the physiological salt solution (mg)}}{\text{CF dose added to the dialysis tube (mg)}}$$

To investigate the diffusion of free CF through the dialysis tube, 0.40 mg/mL CF solution (0.5 mL) was poured into the dialysis tube and tested using the same procedure. Three independent batches were used to determine the average and SD values.

2.5. Antibacterial Assay

The antibacterial properties of the products were assayed against *S. mutans*, *A. naeslundii*, and *P. gingivalis*. Each bacterium was procured from the American Type Culture Collection (Manassas, VA, USA) and frozen until further analysis. First, the frozen bacterial stocks were thawed and grown on brain heart infusion (BHI) medium (Pearlcore®, Eiken Chemical, Co., Ltd., Tokyo, Japan) supplemented with 0.1% antibiotic (0.05% gramicidin D and 0.05% bacitracin, FUJIFILM Wako Pure Chemical Corporation) and 1% sucrose (FUJIFILM Wako Pure Chemical Corporation).

In a 96-well plate, *S. mutans* (1.1×10^6 CFU/200 µL/well), *A. naeslundii* (1.0×10^6 CFU/200 µL/well), and *P. gingivalis* (2.8×10^9 CFU/200 µL/well) were incubated for 24 h at 37 °C under anaerobic conditions in the BHI medium supplemented with the product at various doses: 0 (ctrl), 0.001, 0.01, and 0.1 w/v%. After incubation, the metabolic activity of the bacteria (proportional to the number of living bacteria) was assayed using a microbial viability assay kit-WST (DOJINDO Laboratories, Mashiki, Japan) according to the manufacturer's instructions, and the absorbance was measured at 450 nm using a microplate reader (Multiskan FC, Thermo Fisher Scientific, Waltham, MA, USA). The pH of each bacterial suspension was measured before and after incubation using a portable pH meter (LAQUA-PH-SE, HORIBA, Ltd., Kyoto, Japan).

2.6. Biofilm Formation Assay

The antibiofilm activity of the products was assayed against *S. mutans*. Biofilms were created on peg lids of a biofilm formation assay kit (DOJINDO Laboratories) by incubating *S. mutans* (5.5×10^6 CFU/200 µL/well) for 24 h. Subsequently, the biofilms were incubated anaerobically for 48 h in the BHI medium supplemented with the product at various doses: 0 (ctrl), 0.001, 0.01, and 0.1 w/v%. After incubation, the relative amount of biofilm was assayed using a biofilm formation assay kit according to the manufacturer's instructions, and the absorbance was measured at 595 nm using a microplate reader. In addition, the metabolic activity of the bacteria in the biofilm was assayed using a biofilm viability assay kit (DOJINDO Laboratories) according to the manufacturer's instructions by measuring the absorbance at 450 nm using the microplate reader.

2.7. Statistical Analysis

For the antibacterial and antibiofilm assays, six wells were used for each condition to determine average and SD values. One-way analysis of variance (ANOVA) and Tukey's post hoc multiple-comparison test were used to determine the differences between the average values of the groups. Statistical significance was set at $p < 0.05$.

3. Results

3.1. Morphological Analysis

The two products, CF-CaP2h and CF-CaP24h, were particles with different morphologies. As shown in the FESEM and TEM images (Figure 3a,c), CF-CaP2h consisted of nearly spherical particles with a primary particle diameter of ~30 nm. In contrast, CF-CaP24h consisted of irregularly shaped particles with indistinct boundaries (Figure 3b,d).

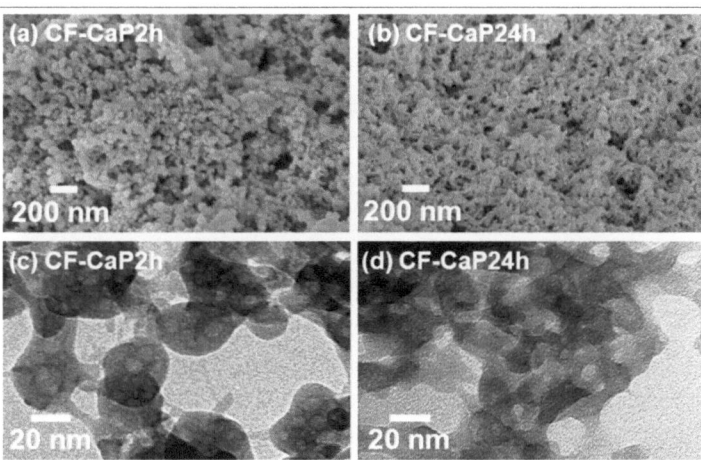

Figure 3. (a,b) FESEM and (c,d) TEM images of (a,c) CF-CaP2h and (b,d) CF-CaP24h.

3.2. Chemical Analysis

Both particles, CF-CaP2h and CF-CaP24h, were composed of CaP and CF. In the SEM-EDX spectra (Figure 4a), strong peaks of Ca and P were detected in both CF-CaP2h and CF-CaP24h, indicating that these particles mainly consisted of CaP. Peaks of nitrogen or fluoride, which are component elements specific to CF, were not detected in the SEM-EDX spectra. On the other hand, in the FTIR spectra (Figure 4b), peaks of O-C-O asymmetric vibration (1585 cm^{-1}) [32] and N-H bending vibration (1615 cm^{-1}) [33], ascribed to CF, were detected in both CF-CaP2h and CF-CaP24h in addition to the distinctive peaks ascribed to CaP: P-OH stretching vibration (872 cm^{-1}) [34], PO$_4^{3-}$ stretching vibration (1029–1051 cm^{-1}) [35], and CO$_3^{2-}$ asymmetric stretching (1483 and 1413 cm^{-1}) [36]. This suggested the presence of CF in both CaP particles.

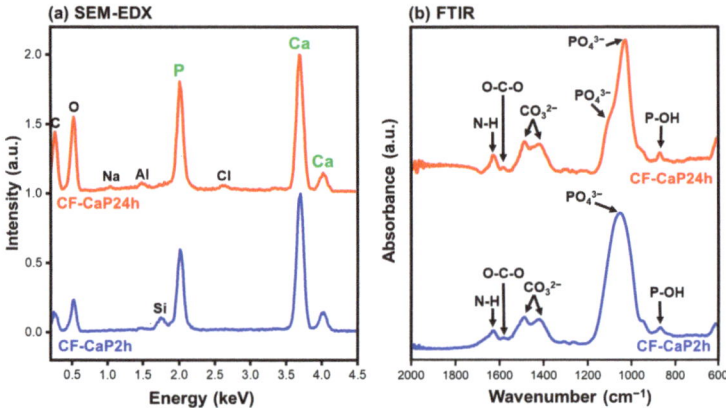

Figure 4. (a) SEM-EDX and (b) FTIR spectra of CF-CaP2h and CF-CaP24h. The peaks of Al and Si in (a) are from the sample holders.

The CF-immobilization efficiency, amount (mg/tube) and content (w/w%) of the immobilized CF, and yield of the particles were greater for CF-CaP24h than that for CF-CaP2h. The amount of CF immobilized in the CaP particles was 2.5-fold greater for CF-CaP24h (1.35 ± 0.02 mg) than that for CF-CaP2h (0.54 ± 0.01 mg), as shown in Figure 5a. Since the yields of particles obtained from the supersaturated CaP solution (per one tube) were 12.9 mg and 15.8 mg for CF-CaP2h and CF-CaP24h, respectively, the CF content in the particles was 4.22 ± 0.09 and 8.48 ± 0.14 w/w% for CF-CaP2h and CF-CaP24h, respectively. From the amount of immobilized CF, the immobilization efficiencies of CF were calculated as 27.3 ± 0.5 and 67.8 ± 1.0% for CF-CaP2h and CF-CaP24h, respectively (Figure 5b).

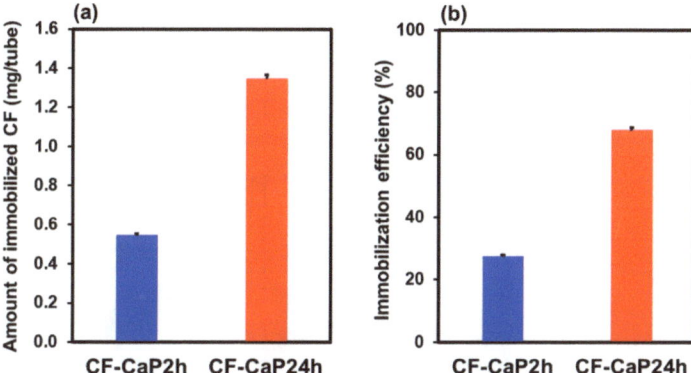

Figure 5. (**a**) Amount of immobilized CF and (**b**) immobilization efficiency of CF in CF-CaP2h and CF-CaP24h (n = 6, average + SD).

3.3. Crystalline Structural Analysis

The CaP phase in CF-CaP2h was amorphous, whereas that in CF-CaP24h was Ca-deficient, low-crystalline hydroxyapatite. In the XRD pattern of CF-CaP2h (Figure 6a), a broad peak was observed at approximately 30°, which was attributed to CaP in the amorphous phase [37]. No other peaks ascribed to crystalline CaP phases were detected. In contrast, CF-CaP24h exhibited peaks ascribed to low-crystalline hydroxyapatite (Figure 6a). Based on the ICP-OES result (Figure 6b), the Ca/P elemental ratio of CF-CaP2h was 1.43 ± 0.02, which increased to 1.53 ± 0.01 for CF-CaP24h, most likely due to the amorphous-to-crystalline transformation in the CaP phase by prolonged aging [37]. The Ca/P elemental ratio of CF-CaP24h was lower than that of stoichiometric hydroxyapatite (1.67), indicating that the CaP phase in CF-CaP24h was Ca-deficient hydroxyapatite. As shown in Figure 4b, a single broad peak of PO_4^{3-} stretching vibration (1051 cm^{-1}) in CF-CaP2h was split into a sharp, strong peak (1029 cm^{-1}) and a shoulder peak (1109 cm^{-1}) in CF-CaP24h, which is a phenomenon observed for the phase transformation from amorphous CaP to hydroxyapatite [38,39]. These results revealed that the amorphous CaP phase in CF-CaP2h was converted to a crystalline hydroxyapatite phase in CF-CaP24h during prolonged aging (from 2 to 24 h). The Ca/P elemental ratio of hydroxyapatite precipitated from aqueous solutions increases up to nearly 1.67 through maturation with increasing aging time. Considering the relatively low Ca/P elemental ratio of CF-CaP24h, it most probably still contained residual amorphous phase and would have therefore undergone further maturation if aged for more than 24 h.

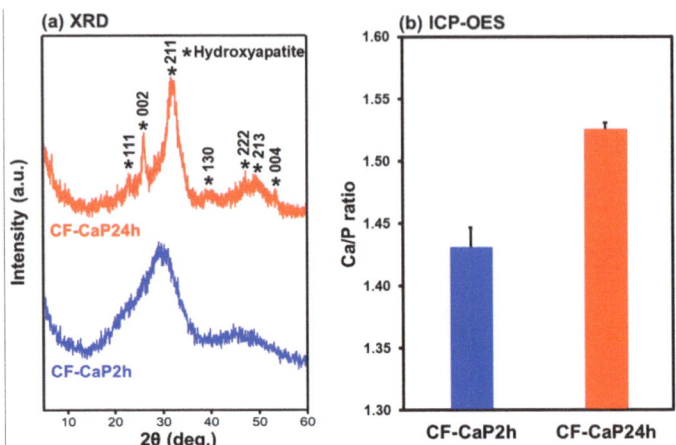

Figure 6. (a) XRD patterns and (b) Ca/P elemental ratios of CF-CaP2h and CF-CaP24h (n = 3, average + SD).

3.4. CF-Release Assay

CF-CaP24h allowed slower CF release than CF-CaP2h in the physiological salt solution. Figure 7 shows the release profiles of CF (percentage and concentration) from CF-CaP2h and CF-CaP24h during 72 h incubation. In this assay, the suspension of particles (net CF concentration, 0.40 mg/mL) stored in the dialysis tube was kept in the physiological salt solution to separate the particles from the test solution (physiological salt solution). For both CF-CaP2h and CF-CaP24h, the concentration of CF in the physiological salt solution increased over time. Because particles (larger than 30 nm) cannot pass through the dialysis tube (pore size of ~2.5 nm), the CF detected in the physiological salt solution was derived from the CF released from CF-CaP2h and CF-CaP24h. Free CF showed a faster increase in the CF concentration in the physiological salt solution (Figure 7). This indicates that the diffusion of CF through the dialysis tube was not the rate-determining step in the CF-release assay for CF-CaP2h and CF-CaP24h. Thus, the rate of increase in the CF concentration of the physiological salt solution reflects the CF-release rate from these particles. In other words, the CF release was faster for CF-CaP2h than for CF-CaP24h. This difference between CF-CaP2h and CF-CaP24h was likely caused by the different crystalline structures of their CaP matrices.

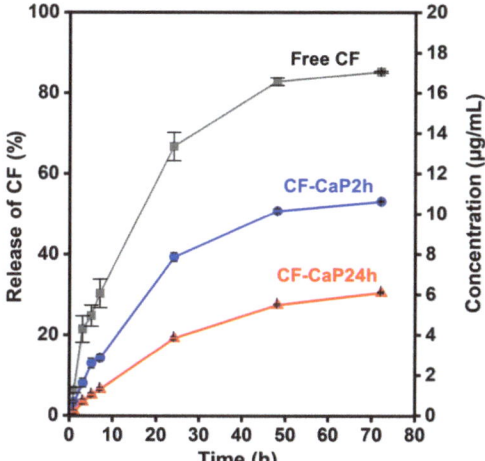

Figure 7. Changes in the percentage of CF detected in the physiological salt solution among the net CF dose added to the dialysis tube (left axis) and CF concentration (right axis) of the physiological salt solution during incubation of CF-CaP2h (blue circle), CF-CaP24h (red triangle), and free CF (grey square) in the dialysis tube for up to 72 h (n = 3, average ± SD).

3.5. Antibacterial Assay

Both CF-CaP2h and CF-CaP24h showed dose-dependent antibacterial activity against all the tested bacteria. At a lower dose (0.001 w/v%), neither CF-CaP2h nor CF-CaP24h exhibited antibacterial activity against any tested bacteria, as shown in Figure 8. At a medium dose (0.01 w/v%), both particles showed antibacterial activity against all tested bacteria except for *A. naeslundii* (only CF-CaP24h was effective). At a higher dose (0.1 w/v%), both particles showed antibacterial activity against all tested bacteria. CF-CaP24h exhibited stronger antibacterial activity than CF-CaP2h against *S. mutans* (Figure 8a) and *A. naeslundii* (Figure 8b) at a medium dose (0.01 w/v%). Against *P. gingivalis*, the opposite trend (stronger for CF-CaP2h) was observed at medium and higher doses (0.01 and 0.1 w/v%), although the difference between the two particles was not statistically significant (Figure 8c).

In the assay with *S. mutans* and *A. naeslundii*, the pH of the bacterial suspension decreased, which was alleviated by higher doses of CF-CaP2h and CF-CaP24h. Figure 9 shows the changes in the pH of the bacterial suspensions after 24 h incubation in the presence of various doses of CF-CaP2h and CF-CaP24h. The pH value of the *S. mutans* suspension decreased by 3.1 after incubation in the absence of the particles (Ctrl), whereas the decrease in pH was less than 0.8 in the presence of higher doses (0.01 and 0.1 w/v%) of CF-CaP2h and CF-CaP24h (Figure 9a). This indicated that these particles had an acid-neutralizing effect [40]. A similar effect was observed for *A. naeslundii*; the decrease in pH (1.7) of the *A. naeslundii* suspension during incubation was reduced to 0.5 in the presence of a higher dose (0.1 w/v%) of CF-CaP2h and CF-CaP24h (Figure 9b). At a medium dose (0.01 w/v%), only CF-CaP24h exerted an acid-neutralizing effect, and CF-CaP2h had no apparent effect on the pH of the bacterial suspension (*A. naeslundii*). For *P. gingivalis*, only a slight decrease in the pH of the bacterial suspension was observed, irrespective of the presence (at any concentration) or absence of the particles (Figure 9c).

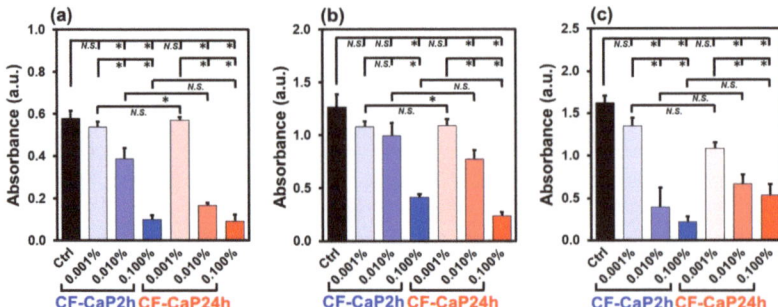

Figure 8. Relative number of living bacteria (absorbance at 450 nm) after the incubation of (**a**) *S. mutans*, (**b**) *A. naeslundii*, and (**c**) *P. gingivalis* in the presence of CF-CaP2h and CF-CaP24h at various concentrations: 0 (Ctrl), 0.001, 0.01, and 0.1 w/v% (n = 6, average + SD, * p < 0.05, N.S.: not significant).

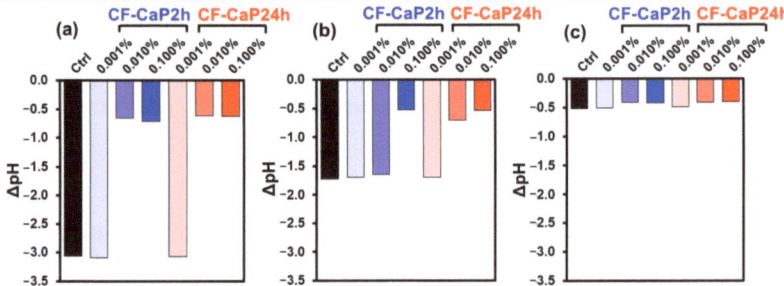

Figure 9. pH changes in suspensions of (**a**) *S. mutans*, (**b**) *A. naeslundii*, and (**c**) *P. gingivalis* after incubation for 24 h in the presence of CF-CaP2h and CF-CaP24h at various doses: 0 (Ctrl), 0.001, 0.01, and 0.1 w/v%.

3.6. Biofilm Formation Assay

Both CF-CaP2h and CF-CaP24h inhibited the biofilm formation at higher doses. In this study, we performed two assays using biofilms formed by *S. mutans*. Both biofilm formation (Figure 10a) and the metabolic activity of the bacterial biofilm (Figure 10b) were inhibited in the presence of CF-CaP2h and CF-CaP24h at higher doses of 0.01 and 0.1 w/v%.

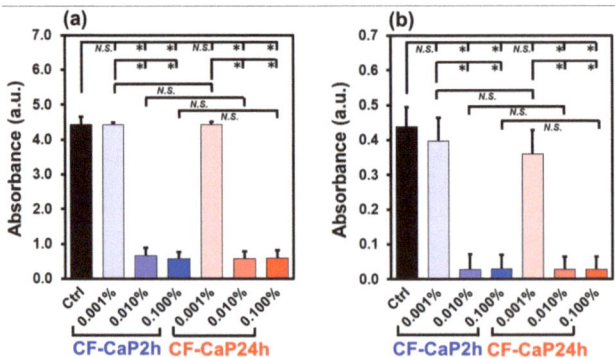

Figure 10. (**a**) Relative amounts of biofilms (absorbance at 595 nm) and (**b**) relative metabolic activity of the bacterial (*S. mutans*) biofilm (absorbance at 450 nm), after incubation of *S. mutans* in the presence of CF-CaP2h and CF-CaP24h at various doses: 0 (Ctrl), 0.001, 0.01, and 0.1 w/v% (n = 6, average + SD, * p < 0.05, N.S.: not significant).

4. Discussion

CF-immobilized CaP particles with different crystalline phases were successfully prepared by the coprecipitation process in the highly supersaturated CaP solution supplemented with CF by varying the aging time (2 and 24 h). The probable mechanism for the formation of the CF-immobilized CaP particles is as follows (Figure 11): First, homogeneous nucleation of CaP (amorphous phase nucleation) occurred in the supersaturated CaP solution, and the nuclei grew into nearly spherical CaP particles with a primary particle size of ~30 nm after aging for 2 h (Figure 3a,c), while retaining their amorphous state (Figure 6a). Meanwhile, the CaP particles immobilized CF, probably due to the electrostatic interactions between the ionized carboxyl groups in CF and the calcium ions in CaP [18,41]. Electrostatic interactions between the protonated piperazinyl groups in CF and the phosphate ions in CaP might also be involved in the CF immobilization in the CaP particles [42]. At this stage (2 h), approximately 27% of CF in the solution was immobilized in the CaP particles (Figure 5b). In the subsequent aging stage (from 2 to 24 h), the nearly spherical CaP particles grew further, immobilizing the residual CF in the solution and converting into irregularly shaped particles (Figure 3d). This morphological change was caused by the transformation of the CaP phase; the isotropic amorphous CaP phase was converted into anisotropic crystalline hydroxyapatite (Figure 6a). This phase transformation occurs spontaneously because hydroxyapatite is the most stable phase in a supersaturated environment with a nearly neutral pH [29,37] and accounts for the increased Ca/P elemental ratio in the long-aged particles (Figure 6b). In the final stage of aging (24 h), approximately 68% of CF in the solution was immobilized in the CaP particles (Figure 5b), resulting in an increased amount (~2.5 times in mg/tube) and content (~2 times in w/w%) of CF in the particles aged for 24 h (CF-CaP24h) compared with those aged for 2 h (CF-CaP2h).

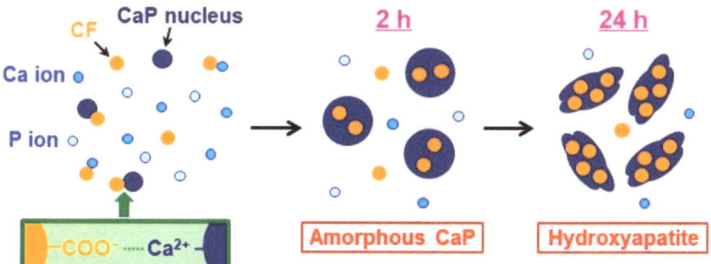

Figure 11. Schematic showing the formation of CF-immobilized CaP particles in the supersaturated CaP solution.

Despite the higher CF content, CF-CaP24h released CF in the physiological salt solution more slowly than CF-CaP2h. A major cause of this difference was the lower solubility of crystalline hydroxyapatite in CF-CaP24h than that of amorphous CaP in CF-CaP2h under the tested conditions, as reported previously [30]. This suggests that the CF release from these particles is associated with the partial dissolution of their CaP matrix. The difference in the specific surface areas of CF-CaP2h and CF-CaP24h, as observed by TEM (Figure 3c,d), might also be involved in their different CF-release profiles.

Both CF-CaP2h and CF-CaP24h exhibited antibacterial activities against *S. mutans*, *A. naeslundii*, and *P. gingivalis* at higher doses (Figure 8). The dose–response relationship differed depending on the type of particles and bacteria. In the three doses tested in this study, the minimum effective dose of CF-CaP24h was 0.01 w/v% (net CF dose of 8.5 µg/mL) for all the tested bacteria, whereas that of CF-CaP2h was 0.1 w/v% (net CF dose of 42 µg/mL) for *A. naeslundii* and 0.01 w/v% (net CF dose of 4.2 µg/mL) for the other two bacteria. These results are reasonable considering the minimal inhibitory concentration (MIC) of CF (1 µg/mL [22] and 4 µg/mL [21] for *S. mutans*, 3.9 µg/mL [25] and 0.063-4 µg/mL [26] for *A. naeslundii*, and 0.064-0.25 µg/mL [24] and 0.019 µg/mL [23] for

P. gingivalis). At lower doses, the concentration of CF released from the particles in the bacterial suspension was likely to be below the MIC.

Despite the slower CF release in the physiological salt solution, CF-CaP24h exhibited a higher antibacterial activity against *S. mutans* and *A. naeslundii* than CF-CaP2h at the medium dose of 0.01 w/v% (Figure 8a,b). This might be due to the acidification of the bacterial suspension caused by these acid-producing bacteria (Figure 9a,b), which accelerates the dissolution of the CaP matrix, not only of amorphous CaP but also of hydroxyapatite [43]. The net CF dose in the bacterial suspension provided by CF-CaP24h was approximately double than that provided by CF-CaP2h, reflecting the higher CF content in the former. Therefore, CF-CaP24h can release a higher CF concentration than CF-CaP2h in an acidified bacterial suspension via accelerated CaP matrix dissolution. The dissolution of the CaP matrix may be responsible for the acid-neutralizing effect of these particles, as reported in our previous study [12]. At a medium dose (0.01 w/v%), CF-CaP24h exhibited an acid-neutralizing effect on *A. naeslundii*, whereas CF-CaP2h did not. This can be attributed to the difference in the CaP phase between the two particles, hydroxyapatite (with hydroxide) in CF-CaP24h and amorphous CaP (without hydroxide) in CF-CaP2h.

The degree of acidification of the bacterial suspension by *P. gingivalis* was much lower than that by *S. mutans* and *A. naeslundii* (Figure 9). The pH values of the suspension of *P. gingivalis* decreased from 7.1–7.2 to 6.6–6.8 after incubation for 24 h, irrespective of the type of particles and their doses. Under this pH range, the release profile of CF from the particles should be similar to that in the physiological salt solution (pH 7.4 at 37 °C). Therefore, CF-CaP2h would likely release more CF than CF-CaP24h in the *P. gingivalis* suspensions. This may account for the relatively stronger (in average value) antibacterial activity of CF-CaP2h than that of CF-CaP24h at medium (0.01 w/v%) and higher (0.1 w/v%) doses (Figure 8c).

Both CF-CaP2h and CF-CaP24h showed antibiofilm activity against *S. mutans* at higher doses (Figure 10). In the three doses tested in this study, the minimum effective dose was 0.01 w/v% for both CF-CaP2h (net CF dose of 4.2 µg/mL) and CF-CaP24h (net CF dose of 8.5 µg/mL) in the two assays. According to a previous report, the half-maximal inhibitory concentration of CF against biofilm formation by *S. mutans* is 3.9 µM (~1.3 µg/mL) [44], which is consistent with our results.

Overall, our data suggest that the CF-immobilized CaP particles have the potential to be used as dental disinfectants against oral bacteria. The prepared particles are small; hence, they may be delivered to narrow spaces, such as dental fissures, pits, and periodontal pockets, which are regions of predilection for caries and periodontal diseases. When these particles are delivered to these regions, they are expected to release CF and exhibit antibacterial and antibiofilm activities against oral bacteria, along with an acid-neutralizing effect. These particles would therefore be effective in the prevention and treatment of oral diseases including dental caries and periodontal disease. The release of CF from the particles is mediated by the dissolution of the CaP matrix into calcium and phosphate ions. Thus, these particles have a favorable secondary effect on tooth remineralization.

Despite presenting some credible findings, there are several limitations to this study. First, the release of CF was assayed using a neutralized physiological salt solution, which differs from the actual intraoral conditions. Hence, the effects of oral components and changes in the conditions (temperature, pH, etc.) on the properties and efficacy of the particles should be investigated in future research. Second, neither the storage stability nor the intraoral stability of the particles has yet been examined, and the intraoral kinetics of the particles remains unknown. Further modifications to the particles might be required to improve their functionalities, such as water-dispersibility, stability, and retention at the target sites. More detailed in vitro and in vivo studies are also required to confirm the potential of the CF-immobilized CaP particles.

5. Conclusions

CF-immobilized CaP particles were fabricated via a coprecipitation process using a supersaturated CaP solution. As the aging time in the coprecipitation process increased from 2 to 24 h, the CaP phase in the resulting particles transformed from amorphous to low-crystalline hydroxyapatite, and their Ca/P elemental ratio, yield, and CF content increased. The particles aged for 24 h released CF in the physiological salt solution more slowly than those aged for 2 h. Both particles exhibited antibacterial and antibiofilm activities, along with an acid-neutralizing effect against *S. mutans*, *P. gingivalis*, and *A. naeslundii*, whose dose–response relationship was slightly different. Aging time in the coprecipitation process was identified as a controlling factor affecting the physiochemical properties of the resulting CF-immobilized CaP particles and their functionality as a dental disinfectant against oral bacteria.

Author Contributions: Conceptualization, A.P., A.O. and H.M.; methodology, A.P., A.O., M.N., T.I. and E.N.; validation, A.P., M.N. and T.I.; formal analysis, A.P. and T.I.; investigation, A.P., T.I. and E.N.; resources, A.O., M.N., E.N. and H.M.; data curation, A.P., T.I. and M.N.; writing—original draft preparation, A.P. and M.N.; writing—review and editing, A.O., T.I., E.N. and H.M.; visualization, A.P., M.N., T.I. and A.O.; supervision, A.O. and H.M.; project administration, A.O.; funding acquisition, A.P., A.O., M.N., E.N. and H.M. All authors have read and agreed to the published version of the manuscript.

Funding: This study was supported by JSPS KAKENHI Grant Numbers JP22KF0412, JP22F21044, JP22H05148, and JP22K10012, and the Amada Foundation, Japan.

Institutional Review Board Statement: Not applicable.

Informed Consent Statement: Not applicable.

Data Availability Statement: Data are contained within the article.

Acknowledgments: We thank M. Zhang from AIST for the ICP-OES measurements, and W. Ding from AIST for the FTIR measurements. The TEM observation was supported by "Advanced Research Infrastructure for Materials and Nanotechnology in Japan (ARIM)" of the Ministry of Education, Culture, Sports, Science and Technology (MEXT).

Conflicts of Interest: The authors declare no conflicts of interest.

References

1. Li, X.; Liu, Y.; Yang, X.; Li, C.; Song, Z. The oral microbiota: Community composition, influencing factors, pathogenesis, and interventions. *Front. Microbiol.* **2022**, *13*, 895537. [CrossRef] [PubMed]
2. Matsumoto-Nakano, M. Role of *Streptococcus mutans* surface proteins for biofilm formation. *Jpn. Dent. Sci. Rev.* **2018**, *54*, 22–29. [CrossRef] [PubMed]
3. Hussain, M.; Stover, C.M.; Dupont, A. *P. gingivalis* in periodontal disease and atherosclerosis–Scenes of action for antimicrobial peptides and complement. *Front. Immunol.* **2015**, *6*, 45. [CrossRef] [PubMed]
4. Dige, I.; Raarup, M.K.; Nyengaard, J.R.; Kilian, M.; Nyvad, B. *Actinomyces naeslundii* in initial dental biofilm formation. *Microbiology* **2009**, *155*, 2116–2126. [CrossRef] [PubMed]
5. Rajeshwari, H.R.; Dhamecha, D.; Jagwani, S.; Rao, M.; Jadhav, K.; Shaikh, S.; Puzhankara, L.; Jalalpure, S. Local drug delivery systems in the management of periodontitis: A scientific review. *J. Control. Release* **2019**, *307*, 393–409.
6. Bapat, R.A.; Joshi, C.P.; Bapat, P.; Chaubal, T.V.; Pandurangappa, R.; Jnanendrappa, N.; Gorain, B.; Khurana, S.; Kesharwani, P. The use of nanoparticles as biomaterials in dentistry. *Drug Discov. Today* **2019**, *24*, 85–98. [CrossRef]
7. Sokolova, V.; Epple, M. Biological and medical applications of calcium phosphate nanoparticles. *Chem. Eur. J.* **2021**, *27*, 7471–7488. [CrossRef]
8. Dorozhkin, S.V. Nanosized and nanocrystalline calcium orthophosphates. *Acta Biomater.* **2010**, *6*, 715–734. [CrossRef] [PubMed]
9. Zalite, V.; Lungevics, J.; Vecstaudza, J.; Stipniece, L.; Locs, J. Nanosized calcium deficient hydroxyapatites for tooth enamel protection. *J. Biomed. Mater. Res.* **2022**, *110*, 1354–1367. [CrossRef]
10. Xu, J.; Shi, H.; Luo, J.; Yao, H.; Wang, P.; Li, Z.; Wei, J. Advanced materials for enamel remineralization. *Front. Bioeng. Biotechnol.* **2022**, *10*, 985881. [CrossRef]
11. Xie, C.; Lu, H.; Li, W.; Chen, F.M.; Zhao, Y.M. The use of calcium phosphate-based biomaterials in implant dentistry. *J. Mater. Sci. Mater. Med.* **2012**, *23*, 853–862. [CrossRef] [PubMed]

12. Nakamura, M.; Oyane, A.; Shimizu, Y.; Miyata, S.; Saeki, A.; Miyaji, H. Physicochemical fabrication of antibacterial calcium phosphate submicrospheres with dispersed silver nanoparticles via coprecipitation and photoreduction under laser irradiation. *Acta Biomater.* **2016**, *46*, 299–307. [CrossRef] [PubMed]
13. Cao, G.; Jiang, Y.; Chen, F.; Lu, B.; Tan, S.; Feng, V.; Qi, S.; He, S.; Xu, Y.; Chen, X. Antibacterial silver-doped calcium phosphate synthesized by an enzymatic strategy for initial caries treatment. *Ceram. Int.* **2020**, *46*, 22466–22473. [CrossRef]
14. Yang, M.; Ren, J.; Zhang, R. Novel gallium-doped amorphous calcium phosphate nanoparticles: Preparation, application and structure study. *J. Non-Cryst. Solids* **2017**, *466–467*, 15–20. [CrossRef]
15. Chen, X.; Tang, Q.L.; Zhu, Y.J.; Zhu, C.L.; Feng, X.P. Synthesis and antibacterial property of zinc loaded hydroxyapatite nanorods. *Mater. Lett.* **2012**, *89*, 233–235. [CrossRef]
16. Kovtun, A.; Kozlova, D.; Ganesan, K.; Biewald, C.; Seipold, N.; Gaengler, P.; Arnold, W.H.; Epple, M. Chlorhexidine-loaded calcium phosphate nanoparticles for dental maintenance treatment: Combination of mineralising and antibacterial effects. *RSC Adv.* **2012**, *2*, 870–875. [CrossRef]
17. Ghosh, S.; Wu, V.; Pernal, S.; Uskoković, V. Self-setting calcium phosphate cements with tunable antibiotic release rates for advanced antimicrobial applications. *ACS Appl. Mater. Interfaces* **2016**, *8*, 7691–7708. [CrossRef] [PubMed]
18. Kumar, G.S.; Govindan, R.; Girija, E.K. In situ synthesis, characterization and *in vitro* studies of ciprofloxacin loaded hydroxyapatite nanoparticles for the treatment of osteomyelitis. *J. Mater. Chem. B* **2014**, *2*, 5052–5060. [CrossRef]
19. Sangeetha, K.; Ashok, M.; Girija, E.K.; Vidhya, G.; Vasugi, G. Strontium and ciprofloxacin modified hydroxyapatites as functional grafts for bone prostheses. *Ceram. Int.* **2018**, *44*, 13782–13789. [CrossRef]
20. Sharma, D.; Patel, R.P.; Zaidi, S.T.R.; Sarker, M.M.R.; Lean, Q.Y.; Ming, L.C. Interplay of the quality of ciprofloxacin and antibiotic resistance in developing countries. *Front. Pharmacol.* **2017**, *21*, 546. [CrossRef]
21. Carreira, C.d.M.; dos Santos, S.S.F.; Jorge, A.O.C.; Lage-Marques, J.L. Antimicrobial effect of intracanal substances. *J. Appl. Oral Sci.* **2007**, *15*, 453–458. [CrossRef] [PubMed]
22. Chotitumnavee, J.; Parakaw, T.; Srisatjaluk, R.L.; Pruksaniyom, C.; Pisitpipattana, S.; Thanathipanont, C.; Amarasingh, T.; Tiankhum, N.; Chimchawee, N.; Ruangsawasdi, N. In vitro evaluation of local antibiotic delivery via fibrin hydrogel. *J. Dent. Sci.* **2019**, *14*, 7–14. [CrossRef]
23. Nalawade, T.M.; Bhat, K.G.; Sogi, S. Antimicrobial activity of endodontic medicaments and vehicles using agar well diffusion method on facultative and obligate anaerobes. *Int. J. Clin. Pediatr. Dent.* **2016**, *9*, 335–341. [PubMed]
24. Eick, S.; Schmitt, A.; Sachse, S.; Schmidt, K.H.; Pfister, W. In vitro antibacterial activity of fluoroquinolones against *Porphyromonas gingivalis* strains. *J. Antimicrob. Chemother.* **2004**, *54*, 553–556. [CrossRef]
25. Elshikh, M.; Moya-Ramiırez, I.; Moens, H.; Roelants, S.; Soetaert, W.; Marchant, R.; Banat, I.M. Rhamnolipids and lactonic sophorolipids: Natural antimicrobial surfactants for oral hygiene. *J. Appl. Microbiol.* **2017**, *123*, 1111–1123. [CrossRef]
26. Barberis, C.; Budia, M.; Palombarani, S.; Rodriguez, C.H.; Ramírez, M.S.; Arias, B.; Bonofiglio, L.; Famiglietti, A.; Mollerach, M.; Almuzara, M.; et al. Antimicrobial susceptibility of clinical isolates of *Actinomyces* and related genera reveals an unusual clindamycin resistance among *Actinomyces urogenitalis* strains. *J. Glob. Antimicrob. Resist.* **2017**, *8*, 115–120. [CrossRef] [PubMed]
27. Shubhra, Q.T.H.; Oyane, A.; Nakamura, M.; Puentes, S.; Marushima, A.; Tsurushima, H. Rapid one-pot fabrication of magnetic calcium phosphate nanoparticles immobilizing DNA and iron oxide nanocrystals using injection solutions for magnetofection and magnetic targeting. *Mater. Today Chem.* **2017**, *6*, 51–61. [CrossRef]
28. Bigi, A.; Boanini, E. Calcium phosphates as delivery systems for bisphosphonates. *J. Funct. Biomater.* **2018**, *9*, 6. [CrossRef]
29. Nakamura, M.; Bunryo, W.; Narazaki, A.; Oyane, A. High immobilization efficiency of basic protein within heparin-immobilized calcium phosphate nanoparticles. *Int. J. Mol. Sci.* **2022**, *23*, 11530. [CrossRef]
30. Kadkhodaie-Elyaderani, A.; de Lama-Odría, M.d.C.; Rivas, M.; Martínez-Rovira, I.; Yousef, I.; Puiggalí, J.; del Valle, L.J. Medicated scaffolds prepared with hydroxyapatite/streptomycin nanoparticles encapsulated into polylactide microfibers. *Int. J. Mol. Sci.* **2022**, *23*, 1282. [CrossRef]
31. Pal, A.; Oyane, A.; Nakamura, M.; Koga, K.; Nishida, E.; Miyaji, H. Fluoride-incorporated apatite coating on collagen sponge as a carrier for basic fibroblast growth factor. *Int. J. Mol. Sci.* **2024**, *25*, 1495. [CrossRef] [PubMed]
32. Nugrahani, I.; Tjengal, B.; Gusdinar, T.; Horikawa, A.; Uekusa, H. A comprehensive study of a new 1.75 hydrate of ciprofloxacin salicylate: SCXRD structure determination, solid characterization, water stability, solubility, and dissolution study. *Crystals* **2020**, *10*, 349. [CrossRef]
33. Sahoo, S.; Chakraborti, C.K.; Mishra, S.C. Qualitative analysis of controlled release ciprofloxacin/carbopol 934 mucoadhesive suspension. *J. Adv. Pharm. Technol. Res.* **2011**, *2*, 195–204. [CrossRef] [PubMed]
34. Jin, B.; Liu, Z.; Shao, C.; Chen, J.; Liu, L.; Tang, R.; De Yoreo, J.J. Phase transformation mechanism of amorphous calcium phosphate to hydroxyapatite investigated by liquid-cell transmission electron microscopy. *Cryst. Growth Des.* **2021**, *21*, 5126–5134. [CrossRef]
35. Manoj, M.; Mangalaraj, D.; Ponpandian, N.; Viswanatan, C. Core–shell hydroxyapatite/Mg nanostructures: Surfactant free facile synthesis, characterization and their in vitro cell viability studies against leukaemia cancer cells (K562). *RSC Adv.* **2015**, *5*, 48705–48711. [CrossRef]
36. Kumar, K.C.V.; Subha, T.J.; Ahila, K.G.; Ravindran, B.; Chang, S.W.; Mahmoud, A.H.; Mohammed, O.B.; Rathi, M.A. Spectral characterization of hydroxyapatite extracted from black sumatra and fighting cock bone samples: A comparative analysis. *Saudi J. Biol. Sci.* **2021**, *28*, 840–846. [CrossRef] [PubMed]

37. Dorozhkin, S.V. Synthetic amorphous calcium phosphates (ACPs): Preparation, structure, properties, and biomedical applications. *Biomater. Sci.* **2021**, *9*, 7748–7798. [CrossRef]
38. Pleshko, N.; Boskey, A.; Mendelsohn, R. Novel infrared spectroscopic method for the determination of crystallinity of hydroxyapatite minerals. *Biophys. J.* **1991**, *60*, 786–793. [CrossRef]
39. Tao, J. FTIR and raman studies of structure and bonding in mineral and organic–mineral composites. In *Methods in Enzymology*; De Yoreo, J.J., Ed.; Academic Press: Cambridge, MA, USA, 2013; Volume 532, pp. 533–556.
40. Moreau, J.L.; Sun, L.; Chow, L.C.; Xu, H.H.K. Mechanical and acid neutralizing properties and bacteria inhibition of amorphous calcium phosphate dental nanocomposite. *J. Biomed Mater. Res. Part B Appl. Biomater.* **2011**, *98B*, 80–88. [CrossRef]
41. Nardecchia, S.; Gutierrez, M.C.; Serrano, M.C.; Dentini, M.; Barbetta, A.; Ferrer, M.L.; del Monte, F. In situ precipitation of amorphous calcium phosphate and ciprofloxacin crystals during the formation of chitosan hydrogels and its application for drug delivery purposes. *Langmuir* **2012**, *28*, 15937–15946. [CrossRef]
42. Ikawa, N.; Kimura, T.; Oumi, Y.; Sano, T. Amino acid containing amorphous calcium phosphates and the rapid transformation into apatite. *J. Mater. Chem.* **2009**, *19*, 4906–4913. [CrossRef]
43. Astasov-Frauenhoffer, M.; Varenganayil, M.M.; Decho, A.W.; Waltimo, T.; Braissant, O. Exopolysaccharides regulate calcium flow in cariogenic biofilms. *PLoS ONE* **2017**, *12*, e0186256. [CrossRef] [PubMed]
44. Mekky, A.E.M.; Sanad, S.M.H. Novel bis(pyrazole-benzofuran) hybrids possessing piperazine linker: Synthesis of potent bacterial biofilm and MurB inhibitors. *Bioorg. Chem.* **2020**, *102*, 104094. [CrossRef] [PubMed]

Disclaimer/Publisher's Note: The statements, opinions and data contained in all publications are solely those of the individual author(s) and contributor(s) and not of MDPI and/or the editor(s). MDPI and/or the editor(s) disclaim responsibility for any injury to people or property resulting from any ideas, methods, instructions or products referred to in the content.

materials

Article

Pushout Bond Strength in Coronal Dentin: A Standardization Approach in Comparison to Shear Bond Strength

Franz-Josef Schröter and Nicoleta Ilie *

Department of Conservative Dentistry and Periodontology, University Hospital, Ludwig-Maximilians-Universität München, Goethestr. 70, D-80336 Munich, Germany; josi.schroeter@web.de
* Correspondence: nilie@dent.med.uni-muenchen.de

Abstract: To find an alternative that is closer to clinical reality in terms of cavity geometry and configuration factor, this study investigated the pushout test on in vitro adhesive testing to coronal dentin when compared to the established shear test, both in a standardized approach. For a feasible comparison between both tests, the pushout specimen was adjusted in thickness (1.03 ± 0.05 mm) and cavity diameter (1.42 ± 0.03 mm) to receive a bonding area (4.63 ± 0.26 mm^2) that matches that of the shear test (4.57 ± 0.13 mm^2). Though, the configuration factor between both tests differs largely (pushout 1.5 ± 0.08; shear bond 0.20 ± 0.01). The bond strength of five different adhesives (n = 20) was investigated for both tests. The pushout test registered a high number of invalid measurements (30%) due to concomitant dentin fracture during testing. In contrast to the shear test, the pushout test failed to discriminate between different adhesives ($p = 0.367$). Both tests differed largely from each other when comparing adhesive groups. When solely looking at the valid specimens, Weibull modulus reached higher values in the pushout approach. Conclusively, the pushout test in this specific setup does not distinguish as precisely as the shear bond test between different adhesives and needs adaption to be routinely applied in adhesive dentistry.

Keywords: bond strength; shear test; pushout test; Weibull; dental adhesives; c-factor

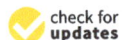

Citation: Schröter, F.-J.; Ilie, N. Pushout Bond Strength in Coronal Dentin: A Standardization Approach in Comparison to Shear Bond Strength. *Materials* **2023**, *16*, 5667. https://doi.org/10.3390/ma16165667

Academic Editors: Josip Kranjčić and Tina Poklepovic Pericic

Received: 24 July 2023
Revised: 9 August 2023
Accepted: 12 August 2023
Published: 17 August 2023

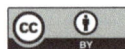

Copyright: © 2023 by the authors. Licensee MDPI, Basel, Switzerland. This article is an open access article distributed under the terms and conditions of the Creative Commons Attribution (CC BY) license (https://creativecommons.org/licenses/by/4.0/).

1. Introduction

The factors influencing in vitro bond strength results of dental adhesives involve the used substrate (bovine or human; dentin or enamel), storage condition, specimen's geometry, film thickness as well as loading condition and modulus of elasticity [1,2]. Since sound human teeth are rarely extracted, in vitro testing focuses on the usage of third molars. They are among the only teeth that are extracted in advance of eruption due to prophylactic reasons. Even though unerupted teeth appear moister when compared to erupted teeth [1], they are at least neither carious nor filled. While morphological changes with increasing tooth age do take place [3], bond strength performance appears to be unaffected by these changes [4].

Aside from the influence of the used substrate, the testing methods vary in the given results. Throughout the development of in vitro bond strength testing on tooth structure, two test methods have been established as the main setups for bond strength testing of dental adhesives, representing 83% of the reported studies in the given review: the micro-tensile and macro-shear test [5]. Depending on the bonding area, a distinction can be made between micro (<3 mm^2) and macro (>3 mm^2) tests [6].

Both of those two established methods come with advantages and disadvantages. Among the advantages of the micro-tensile test is obtaining numerous specimens out of one tooth, since sticks usually have a bonding area of 1 mm^2, instead of the >3 mm^2 required for macro-shear testing. Further, more adhesive failures are supposed to occur when compared to the shear test, where cohesive failures represent a mentionable problem [1].

On the other hand, fabrication of specimens for micro-tensile bond strength testing is labor intensive and technically demanding, because challenging factors in handling, such as quick dehydration of specimens, further come into place [1]. Cutting the sticks induces stress at the bonding interface, which leads to pre-testing failures during sample preparation, as indicated by the 35.4% pre-testing failures reported when bonding to enamel and 18.2% when bonding to dentin during preparation with a diamond saw [7]. Large criticism arises, as the reporting of pre-testing failures often is sparse [8], with only 30% of papers overall even mentioning pre-testing failures [2]. Further, it is important to accurately report and discern between pre-testing failures and manipulation errors, as pre-testing failures contain failures that occur before tensile testing that are not attributed to human handling, and manipulation errors occur during testing that are attributed to human manipulation [9].

When looking at the shear test, its widespread use can be explained by the plain test protocol, simple specimen preparation and efficient use of substrate, as up to eight specimens can be received out of one tooth. In comparison to the preparation of micro-tensile specimens, tooth cutting takes place prior to adhesive bonding, lowering the irritation of the bonding interface. Also, tooth pieces can be embedded in methacrylate resin in order to improve handling, while micro-tensile sticks remain free of a surrounding substance [10,11]. Meanwhile, both—shear and micro-tensile test—are criticized for the occurrence of cohesive failures, which do not allow exact calculation of bond strength values [12] and are recommended to be excluded from statistical analysis [2]. Amongst others, cohesive failures lead to the scattering of test results, which complicates the comparison between studies [13]. This scattering can be associated with alignment errors [14] and microcracks during cutting [7] in the case of the micro-tensile test, and stress concentration near the loading site due to test configuration and specimen geometry in the case of the shear test [15].

Since these two tests both have varying setups, a detailed description of the used approach or the reference to the applied ISO (International Organization for Standardization) standard needs to be provided in order to establish one generally accepted and conducted testing method for adhesive bond strength testing [2,6,8]. As an alternative testing method, an extrusion (pushout) test for dental purposes was first described in 1970, where a cylinder was pushed out of a disk of dental material in varying plunger diameters to simulate the masticatory cycle, reflecting qualities of clinical relevance [16]. An important factor of clinical relevance in such tests is represented by the configuration factor (c-factor) that describes the ratio of bonded to unbonded surface, as an approximate c-factor of 1.7 represented by the pushout approach is closer to the clinical situation than the 0.2 simulated in shear and tensile tests [17,18]. As polymerization shrinkage stress increases simultaneously with c-factor [17], a pushout approach compared to shear or tensile tests might be better suited for clinical prediction, as in vitro specimens should be subjected to polymerization shrinkage stress prior to bond strength testing [19].

Nowadays, the pushout test is not employed as a universal bond strength test and is commonly used to measure retention of fiber posts to root canal dentin [6]. In the few studies in which the test was not only used to determine the bond strength to human root dentin, it displays significantly higher bond strength values in crown dentin when compared to root dentin [20,21]. Endodontically treated roots are cut into slices of up to 2 mm thickness, exposing a small portion of filled root canal in a slightly conical form [22]. A crucial step is the central positioning of the steel plunger on the filling [23], which is used to push out the tested substrate. Critique on the pushout test arises, because of the great variability of the test setup. Variables like plunger size, testing speed, slice thickness and preparation method in terms of borehole size and taper influence results. Further, when testing root canal fillings, the calculation of the true diameter is hardly feasible as root canals are not perfectly round in shape [24]. First attempts to standardize the pushout test as a method to test adhesion to coronal dentin have been made to bovine teeth [25], yet remain to be established. On a positive note, and in contrast to the micro-tensile test, almost no stress at the bonding interface takes place during specimen production, as slices are cut in advance of dentin bonding. Also, there is no need to demount them in any specific matrices' holder, as in shear tests.

Thus, the present work investigated the applicability of a standardized pushout test setup for adhesive dentistry in comparison to the macro-shear test and shines light on the question of whether the pushout test is equally suited to attain reliable bond strength values of dental adhesives to coronal dentin. The null hypothesis was therefore that with similar bonding surface areas, bonding procedure and test conditions, the outcome of both tests is similar.

2. Materials and Methods

Four experimental and one gold-standard self-etch adhesives (Table 1) are used to compare bond strength results of the pushout and shear test. The synthesis and exact compositions of the four experimental adhesives, namely Exp. 1.1–2.2, are addressed elsewhere (submitted paper), as this paper focuses on the comparison of both tests, rather than the influence of the adhesives' components.

Table 1. Chemical composition of used materials as provided by the manufacturer.

Name	Composition	LOT
Exp. 1.1	bis-GMA, TEGDMA, HEMA, polyacrylic acid, initiators, green tea-extract	-
Exp. 1.2	bis-GMA, TEGDMA, HEMA, polyacrylic acid, initiators	-
Exp. 2.1	bis-GMA, TEGDMA, HEMA, polyacrylic acid, initiators, tricalcium-phosphate, chitosan, green tea-extract	-
Exp. 2.2	bis-GMA, TEGDMA, HEMA, polyacrylic acid, initiators, tricalcium-phosphate, chitosan	-
CSE	Primer: 10-MDP, HEMA, DM, initiators Bond: 10-MDP, bis-GMA, HEMA, DM, initiators	2P0372 420696
AF	ormocer, 84 wt.% Ba-Al-Si-glass	2111693

Abbreviations: Exp. = experimental adhesive; CSE = Clearfil SE Bond; AF = Admira Fusion x-tra; bis-GMA = bisphenol-A-diglycidyl-methacrylate; TEGDMA = triethylene-glycol-dimethacrylate; HEMA = 2-hydroxyethyldimethylacrylate; 10-MDP = 10-methacryloyloxydecyl-dihydrogenphosphate; DM = dimethylacrylate; ormocer = organically modified ceramic; Ba-Al-Si-glass = barium-aluminum-silicate-glass.

Clearfil SE Bond (CSE; Kuraray Noritake Dental Inc., Kurashiki, Japan) worked as the gold-standard reference and its primer was used for all groups. Primer and adhesive were applied with a microbrush for 20 s each, followed by gentle air drying. Any excess bonding agent was removed with a disposable paper fabric. Light curing was performed for 10 s with a light-curing unit (Bluephase®Style, Ivoclar Vivadent, Schaan, Liechtenstein) with a light-emitting window of 10 mm diameter and an irradiance of 1544 ± 207 mW/cm^2. A low shrinkage resin-based composite (RBC; Admira Fusion x-tra, AF, VOCO GmbH, Cuxhaven, Germany; LOT 2111693) was applied with gentle pressure through a ball-end plunger to ensure good alignment to dentin. Any excess material was removed, followed by light curing for 20 s.

2.1. Pushout Test Specimen Preparation

In total, 47 sound human third molars, stored in 0.2% sodium azide solution at room temperature for no more than three months, were used to produce five groups (n = 20) of test specimens. Teeth were cut with a low-speed diamond saw (IsoMet, Buehler, Lake Bluff, IL, USA) in a vertical direction to produce 1 ($\pm$0.1) mm thick slices. Slices were measured with a digital caliper. Tooth slices were continuously stored in distilled water to prevent dehydration of exposed dentin. Specimens were then mounted in a vertical drilling machine (Degussa Dental GmbH, Hanau, Germany) to ensure consistent, perpendicular drilling in the dentin surface. The borehole was positioned in coronal dentin, above the pulp chamber to cut dentinal tubules crosswise and with >1 mm distance to pulp chamber and enamel. The holes were drilled with a parallel chamfer dental diamond burr (Komet Dental, Lemgo, Germany) with a diameter of 1.4 mm and a medium grain size of 107 µm under constant water cooling. Calculation of the bonding area followed the formula for lateral surfaces of cylinders: $A = 2 \times \pi \times r \times h$, where A is the lateral area, r the radius and h the height of the cavity. The dimensions were chosen to match the bonding area of the shear test setup. After drilling, specimens underwent bonding procedure and cavity filling. In addition to the regular specimens, seven test specimens of the adhesive Exp. 1.2 without the use of primer were produced. Specimens were then stored in artificial saliva in a thermal oven at 37 °C for 24 h.

2.2. Shear Test Specimen Preparation

A total of 20 sound human third molars were used to equally produce five groups (n = 20) of test specimens for the shear test setup. Teeth were cut horizontally to expose coronal dentin, followed by size-dependent sectioning which resulted in a maximum specimen count of eight per tooth. Pieces were embedded in methacrylate resin (Technovit 4004, Kulzer, Hanau, Germany; Powder LOT K010164; Liquid LOT K010108) in a stainless-steel cylinder of 16 mm in diameter. Specimens were randomly allocated to each group; a standardized smear layer was produced with P1200 silicon carbide paper, and they were bonded within 24 h after cutting. Following bonding procedure, specimens were mounted in a matrix holder (Ultradent Products, South Jordan, UT, USA) with a cylindrical split mold (Ultradent Products, South Jordan, UT, USA) for RBC buildups of 2.5 mm in height and 2.4 mm in diameter of the same restorative material following ISO 29022 [26]. Calculation of the bonding area took place by measuring the buildups' diameters twice followed by calculation of a mean radius r for each specimen. Bonding area calculation then followed the formula of circle areas: $A = \pi \times r^2$. Also, seven specimens using adhesive Exp. 1.2 were produced without the usage of primer. Storing condition was equal to the pushout specimens.

2.3. Mechanical Testing Methods

The universal testing machine (Z2.5, Zwick/Roell, Ulm, Germany) operated at a crosshead speed of 0.5 mm/min until failure and was used for both test setups.

The pushout test was carried out with a round metal plunger (1.2 mm diameter) on a stainless-steel ring to enable free dislodgement of the filling. The plunger was positioned centrally on the filling and placement was controlled by 2.4× magnifying glasses. The specimen was loaded until failure, i.e., dislodgement of the filling or disruption of the specimen, and the pushout force at failure was measured. Because the test setup resulted in a frequent fracture of tooth slices as it will be shown later, additional specimens were manufactured in order to receive n = 20 specimens eligible for statistical evaluation, which resulted in a total of 142 pushout test specimens.

Shear bond strength testing followed an adaption of ISO 29022 [26] from a notched-edge to a straight-edge chisel. The maximum load at fracture was measured.

Bond strength (BS) was calculated by dividing the maximum load at failure through the individual bonding area of each specimen with the following formula:

$$BS = F/A$$

where BS represents the calculated bond strength, F the maximum load at failure and A the individual bonding area.

2.4. Microscopic Analysis

Microscopic analysis was performed with a light microscope (Stemi 508, Carl Zeiss Microscopy GmbH, Göttingen, Germany), photographed with a camera extension (Axiocam color 305, Carl Zeiss Microscopy GmbH, Göttingen, Germany) and pictured with AxioVision 4.8.2 computer software. The plunger position was assessed based on the margins of the plunger indentation within the restorative material. Whenever plunger margins were entirely in the restorative material and more than 50 μm distant from dentin, they were classified as central (Figure 1A); when margins were <50 μm away, they were classified as margin (Figure 1B) and lastly, whenever margins intersected dentin for >50 μm (Figure 1C), they were classified as overlapping. Further, light microscopy was used to determine whether a fracture within dentin was visible. If a fracture line was visible in dentin (Figure 1C) on top and on bottom of the specimen, it was classified as invalid and therefore excluded from statistical analysis.

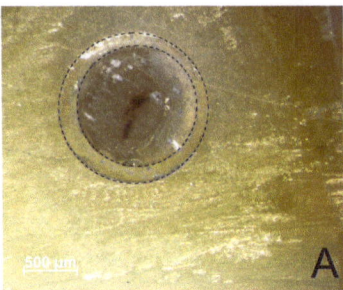 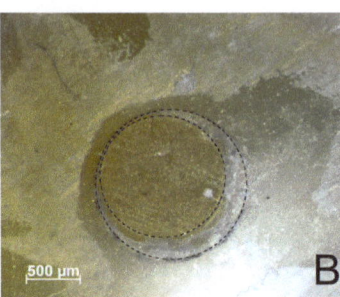 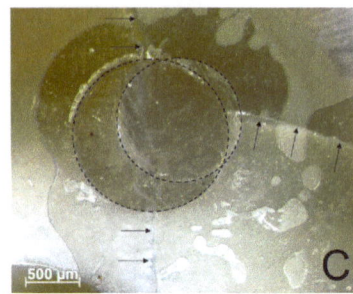

Figure 1. Showcase pictures of the plunger positions central (**A**), margin (**B**) and overlapping (**C**). Cavity circumference is marked by the large, dotted circle, plunger indentation by the smaller, dotted circle. Arrows indicate the visible fracture line within dentin.

2.5. Statistical Analysis

SPSS (IBM SPSS Statistics, Version 28, International Business Machines Cooperation, NY, USA) was used to analyze data. The Shapiro–Wilk test was used to check for normal distribution, and Levene's test to assess equality of variances. One-way analysis of variances (ANOVA) with Dunnett's post hoc test compared groups within one test setup. Students t-test for independent variables compared each group with its corresponding group of the other test setup as well as both tests without the use of the adhesives' primer. A three-way ANOVA was used to evaluate the influence of the parameters' adhesive, plunger position and dentin fracture causing invalid measurement. Results were considered significant for $p < 0.05$.

Lastly, the reliability of all groups was assessed by Weibull analysis. The model describes the probability of failure for brittle materials at uniform stress with the following formula:

$$P_f = 1 - \exp(-(\frac{\sigma}{\sigma_0})^m)$$

where σ is the measured bond strength, σ_0 the characteristic strength at probability of failure $P_f(\sigma_0) = 0.63$ and m the Weibull modulus. The doubled logarithm of this expression $\ln[\ln(\frac{1}{1-P_f})] = m\ln(\sigma) - m\ln(\sigma_0)$ results in a straight line. The upward gradient of that line represents m. R^2 expresses the fit of variances of the observed data towards the projected ideal linear function.

2.6. Ethical Approval

No consultation obligation by the institutional ethics committee is needed for this research project. The study was approved under the project number KB 20/032.

3. Results

A total of 42 specimens were excluded from the pushout test due to observed dentin fracture after measurement. The number of valid measurements has been upgraded to 100. The mean slice thickness was 1.03 (±0.05) mm, and the mean cavity diameter 1.42 (±0.03) mm. The mean bonding area of the 100 valid specimens was 4.63 (±0.26) mm^2, while the unbonded area was 3.18 (±0.14) mm^2. Meanwhile, the mean bonding area of the shear test specimens was 4.57 (±0.13) mm² and 23.51 (±1.55) mm² for the unbonded surface, respectively. Division of the bonded by the unbonded area resulted in a c-factor of 1.5 (±0.08) for the pushout and 0.20 (±0.01) for the shear test specimens. Table 2 displays the mean bond strength, Weibull modulus and R^2 values for both test setups.

Table 2. Bond strength values in MPa and Weibull modulus with 95% confidence interval in brackets, and R^2 values for both test setups. Superscript letters indicate significant difference within the test setup itself. Asterisk (*) indicates significant differences between the corresponding groups of each test.

	Pushout			Shear		
	BS	m	R^2	BS	m	R^2
Exp. 1.1	16.5 (15.0; 18.1) *	5.9 (4.61; 7.25)	0.82	12.6 (9.5; 15.6) [a,c]	2.1 (1.92; 2.25)	0.97
Exp. 1.2	14.2 (12.2; 16.2) *	3.8 (3.14; 4.45)	0.88	7.0 (5.1; 8.9) [b]	1.9 (1.80; 2.01)	0.99
Exp. 2.1	16.3 (14.4; 18.1) *	5.0 (4.26; 5.79)	0.91	12.5 (11.0; 14.1) [a]	4.0 (3.48; 4.48)	0.93
Exp. 2.2	16.5 (14.1; 18.4) *	3.5 (3.29; 3.78)	0.98	9.3 (8.1; 10.5) [b,c]	4.3 (3.81; 4.79)	0.94
CSE	16.5 (14.3; 18.7)	4.1 (3.62; 4.49)	0.95	15.9 (12.8; 18.9) [a]	2.9 (2.44; 3.32)	0.91

Abbreviations: BS = bond strength; m = Weibull modulus; R^2 = fit of variances to the projected ideal linear function within Weibull statistics; Exp. = experimental adhesive; CSE = Clearfil SE Bond.

The Shapiro–Wilk test confirmed normal distribution for all groups except for Exp. 1.1 ($p = 0.033$) within the pushout test. Data were therefore considered normally distributed. Levene's test approved equality of variances for the pushout test ($p = 0.386$), but not for the shear test ($p < 0.001$). Thus, ANOVA with Dunnett's post hoc test was used to check for significant differences within each test setup. While no differences were found in the pushout test (n = 100; $p = 0.367$), differences in the shear test were found ($p < 0.001$). When comparing the two test setups, students t-test showed significant differences between the groups Exp. 1.1 ($p = 0.02$), Exp. 1.2 ($p < 0.001$), Exp. 2.1 ($p = 0.002$) and Exp. 2.2 ($p < 0.001$), but not for CSE ($p = 0.724$). To visualize the differences in bond strength, the boxplot of both tests is provided (Figure 2).

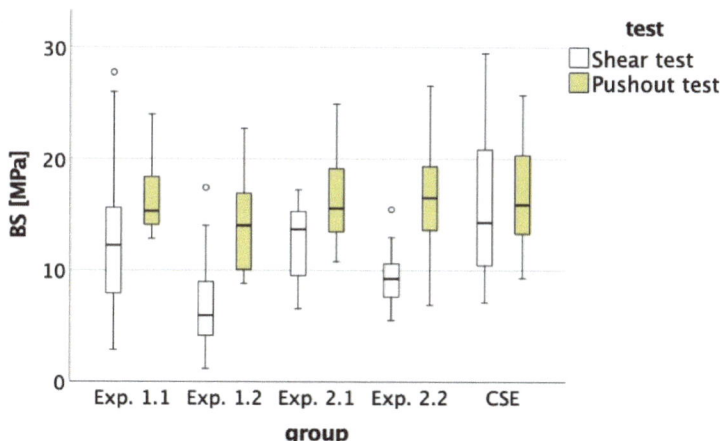

Figure 2. Boxplot for the pushout test and the shear test of the bond strengths (BS) of each group.

The valid measurements (n = 100) were neither influenced by adhesive group ($p = 0.858$) nor plunger position ($p = 0.339$). Regarding the Weibull modulus, a general trend to higher values was observed in the pushout test. While Exp. 2.2 was inferior to the shear test values, all other groups surpassed the shear test values with CSE, Exp. 1.1 and Exp. 1.2 differing significantly. For the Weibull distribution, see Figure 3.

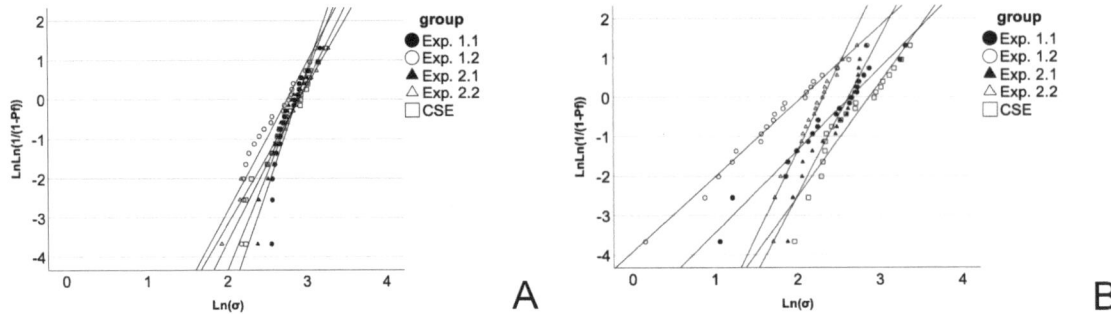

Figure 3. Weibull distribution for the pushout test (**A**) and the shear test (**B**) strength data.

The results of the Exp. 1.2 specimens without the primer are shown in Table 3. One of the seven pushout specimens was invalid during evaluation, which led to its exclusion. T-test for independent variables showed a significant difference between both tests ($p < 0.001$).

Table 3. Comparison of bond strength (BS) values (MPa ± standard deviation) of Exp. 1.2 without primer. Asterisk (*) indicates significant differences between both test setups.

	n	BS
Pushout test	6	14.9 (2.3) *
Shear test	7	2.1 (1.2)

In total, 42 of 142 specimens were declared invalid due to dentin fracture during evaluation. Table 4 shows the error frequency for each group. Of all measurements (n = 142), the used adhesive ($p = 0.263$) and the occurrence of dentin fractures and therefore invalid declaration ($p = 0.655$) had no influence on bond strength, while the plunger position influenced bond strength slightly ($\eta_p^2 = 0.057$) but significantly ($p = 0.03$).

Table 4. Produced specimens in total and count of errors for each test group.

	Total	Invalid
Exp. 1.1	26	6
Exp. 1.2	28	8
Exp. 2.1	33	13
Exp. 2.2	33	13
CSE	22	2
total	142	42

The plunger position of the valid specimens (n = 100) is displayed in Figure 4A. An ANOVA with only the centered plungers also showed no significant differences within the pushout test ($p = 0.399$). In comparison, Figure 4B shows the plunger position for the 42 invalid specimens, where an overlap was found in 6 cases, marginal position 17 and central position 19 times. The plunger position had no influence on bond strength values of invalid specimens (n = 42; $p = 0.088$).

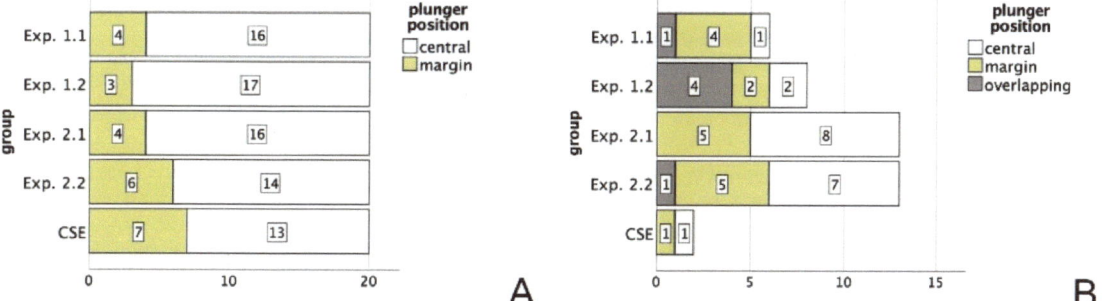

Figure 4. Plunger positions of the valid (**A**) and invalid (**B**) specimens.

4. Discussion

The aim to draw a scientifically correct comparison between a shear bond and a pushout test needed multiple requirements: Firstly, all specimens were manufactured with equal materials, inside the same laboratory and by the same operator. This renders a comparison between the two tests possible, as a comparison between different laboratories was shown to be difficult [27], since even small differences in local geometry of adhesive interface influence the bond strength results significantly [28]. Secondly, a standardized, reproducible specimen production as stipulated by the literature was conducted [2,6,8] and compared to the already standardized and recognized ISO 29022 method of the shear bond test while ultimately, similar bonded surface areas for both tests were manufactured in order to adequately compare bond strength values as well as their reliability. This resulted in cutting the teeth in vertical slices with a mean thickness of 1.03 (±0.05) mm and by drilling with a chamfer of 1.4 mm diameter in a mean cavity of 1.42 (±0.03) mm diameter, leading to a mean dentin bonding area of 4.63 (±0.26) mm^2, comparable to the 4.57 (±0.13) mm^2 area of the shear test.

As polymerization shrinkage of RBCs takes place during light curing, resulting in shrinkage stress [29], specimens for both test methods were produced using the same restorative material and curing conditions. While the used RBC was chosen, because of the low 1.24% polymerization shrinkage [30], shrinkage stress further correlates with the c-factor. The lower the c-factor, the smaller the shrinkage stress. Calculation of the c-factor resulted in a 7.5 times higher value in the pushout test setup compared to the shear test setup, which is in accordance with the results found in other studies [17]. Conclusively, one would assume that shrinkage stresses are higher in the pushout test specimen, which results in imperfect alignment of RBC to the cavity walls ultimately causing quicker failure and thus inferior bond strength values. Though, this can be rejected with the present results as it might be explained by the perfectly parallel cavity walls causing friction during dislodgement that were high enough to overshadow the disadvantages of the higher c-factor.

When addressing bonding areas, Weibull statistics cannot be overlooked, as it is used to determine the reliability of brittle materials by assigning the likelihood of failure to a numeric value, namely the Weibull modulus m. For larger areas, the probability for a critical flaw, such as pores, inclusions or microcracks, to be on the bonding interface is much higher than for smaller areas, resulting in higher bond strengths for smaller areas [31]. In order to minimize the influence of area, bonding areas of both tests closely matched each other. Though, the pushout test found mostly higher m values when compared to the shear test (Table 2), represented by the steeper upward gradient in Figure 3. Four out of five groups exceeded the shear tests' values, which means that the pushout setting is less susceptible to critical flaws, such as cracks and pores, than the shear test. As non-uniform stress distribution leads to quicker failures of test specimens [2], because the crack propagates from a critical flaw on the bonding interface [31], the higher m in the pushout test might be associated with a more evenly distributed stress, as it was already shown that a homogenous stress distribution when testing glass fiber posts is attainable, revealed by finite element analysis [32]. This leads to a higher m and consequently a higher reliability of measured values in the pushout test, which might be attributed to a less technique-sensitive test protocol compared to the shear test.

As the bonding area was predetermined by the shear bond strength standard ISO 29022, geometry of the pushout test specimen was adapted in slice thickness and cavity diameter. The 1 mm dentin slice thickness was chosen for more than just the reason of matching areas: when comparing literature, slices of usually 1–2 mm thickness are used [24] and 1 mm thickness further allows for a uniform stress distribution [33]. Though, it might be too thin to withstand dentin fracture outside the bonding interface (Figure 1C), which was considered as invalid. Whilst not being considered a pre-testing failure, it can be classified as a manipulation error and is therefore excluded from statistical analysis analogous to the ADM guidelines for micro-tensile testing [9]. As 42 specimens were invalid (30%), an improvement of this test setup's reliability might be achieved by embedding the specimens in methacrylate resin, as in the shear test, to increase specimen stability. Also, conducting the test under water might help by hindering dehydration of test specimens. Still, testing of aged specimens is challenging, when an identical specimen count per group is desired in order to adequately compare results. As it is criticized in the literature that the reporting of pre-testing failures in micro-tensile testing is often missing [8], this also applies to the pushout test, as fractures outside the adhesive interface as found in the present study (Table 4) are not addressed in any reviews on the study design of pushout tests [24,34,35].

In addition to the thickness of the dentin slices, which determines the height of the cavity, the diameter of the borehole was adjusted to 1.4 mm. This led to an adjustment of the plunger diameter to 1.2 mm for two reasons: when comparing our study design with other protocols, a plunger that is 0.2 mm smaller than the diameter of posts can be used [36] and it furthermore represents 85% of the boreholes' mean diameter, which in turn should not affect bond strength values [37]. Though, as a plunger size of 70–90% of the canal diameter does not affect bond strength values and smaller strengths are found when the diameter is below 55% [37], the plunger diameter of a smaller size should be chosen to ensure perfect positioning and prevent manipulation errors, while still keeping a standardized diameter, as varying diameters can additionally alter bond strength values [38]. Regarding manipulation errors, the plunger was ideally placed centrally on the filling in order to support uniform stress distribution, which was controlled with magnifying glasses prior to testing. Afterwards, the positioning was controlled microscopically, showing that 136 of the 142 tested specimens had either a central or margin position, while a poor (overlapping) position accounted for only 4% of all measurements. Each one of them resulted in an invalid measurement due to dentin fracture (Figure 4B). Therefore, even though the applied plunger diameter is in the proper range given by the literature [37], a slightly smaller plunger might ease the positioning. The importance of good plunger alignment is also displayed in the small ($\eta_p^2 = 0.057$), though significant, influence on bond strength values, when considering all measurements, but is usually not addressed in the literature, retrospectively [22,35].

Apart from specimen geometries, another similarity between the two tests was the orientation of the dentinal tubules. Dentinal tubules run radially from the pulp chamber to the dentin surface [39]. During shear test specimen preparation, the horizontal cut above the pulp chamber intersects the tubules nearly perpendicular to their course, which results in the crosswise bonding of tubules. By cutting the tooth vertically and drilling a perpendicular hole in the slice for the pushout test, the dentinal tubules are intersected in the same manner as in the shear test. Although shear bond strength seems to be independent of dentin tubule orientation [40], equal penetration of the tubules during bonding procedure allows for a better comparison of both test methods.

Since the five adhesives did not differ from each other within the pushout setup, a difference when compared to the shear test results seems obvious. All pushout groups but CSE had significantly higher bond strength values than their corresponding shear test groups (Table 2, Figure 2), which leads to the rejection of the null hypothesis. The fact that the differences seen in the shear test do not appear in the pushout test suggests that the adhesive agent is not the decisive factor for bond strength or fracture resistance in this specific setup. Therefore, a few specimens without priming were produced to investigate the influence of flawed application of the adhesive system on bond strength (Table 3). The difference is strikingly obvious, which supports the theory of the measured values' independency from the adhesives' performance. Reasonable explanations could be that—as mentioned above—the parallel cavity wall configuration causes friction between RBC and dentin. Usually, the pushout test finds application in endodontological, laboratory trials to test the adhesion of root canal fillings and fiber posts to tooth substrate [34]. Due to the root canal treatment, the canal diameter goes from large to small, resulting in a conical shape of the cavity. Even the conical shape yields friction [37], parallel walls presumably even more. But an exact standard as to which taper needs to be applied has not yet been established, as taper varies largely due to the root canal treatment method, including a taper of 0% [24]. Furthermore, the softer gutta-percha shows lower bond strength (5.86 ± 1.22 MPa) when compared to epoxy resin cones (17.23 ± 4.53 MPa; 16.16 ± 4.73 MPa) and deforms due to compressive stress. Contrarily, stiffer core materials are more resistant to deformation and allow a more linear load profile until dislodgement, resulting in higher bond strength values for stiffer materials that lay in the same range of the bond strengths we found for our materials (Table 2) [37]. This linear load profile might also result in a higher susceptibility to friction, explained by the similar results of all evaluated groups throughout the pushout test.

Summarized, even though the pushout test is closer to reality in terms of c-factor and cavity configuration, it is inferior to the shear test in discerning bond strengths of different adhesives in this specific, standardized setup in vitro. Aside from the perfectly parallel cavity walls, the predetermined bonding area by the shear test as well as the high occurrence of invalid measurements and the slightly too large plunger can be considered as limitations within this study and might influence results, when being changed. Thus, conical cavity walls, alteration in specimen geometry (e.g., thickness, drilling diameter), embedding of specimens in methacrylate resin and testing under water might change the pushout test's outcome. Also, the testing of aged specimens might be helpful to its long-term applicability. Though, materials are not as susceptible to inherent flaws as in the shear test, shown by the mainly higher Weibull modulus, leading to a higher reliability of measured values in this setup. While more conical cavity walls might help with the problem of friction, the question remains whether it could be better to discern between adhesive groups than the established methods. Lastly, as demanded for the micro-tensile test, pre-testing and manipulation errors within the pushout test must also be accurately reported.

5. Conclusions

Within the limitations of the present study, it suggests that the standardized pushout test in this specific setup is inferior to the shear test in measuring adhesives' bond strength values but is less prone to inherent flaws explained by higher Weibull moduli. Further adjustments are necessary in order to routinely apply the pushout test to adhesive dentistry, including the need to accurately report pre-testing failures and manipulation errors.

Author Contributions: F.-J.S.: Investigation, writing—original draft preparation, formal analysis, visualization; N.I.: Conceptualization, methodology, resources, data curation, writing—review and editing, visualization, supervision, project administration. All authors have read and agreed to the published version of the manuscript.

Funding: This research received no external funding.

Informed Consent Statement: Not applicable.

Data Availability Statement: The raw data required to reproduce these findings are available upon request.

Acknowledgments: The authors appreciate VOCO, Germany, for the donation of the used ormocer.

Conflicts of Interest: The authors declare no conflict of interest.

References

1. Pashley, D.H.; Sano, H.; Ciucchi, B.; Yoshiyama, M.; Carvalho, R.M. Adhesion testing of dentin bonding agents: A review. *Dent. Mater.* **1995**, *11*, 117–125. [CrossRef] [PubMed]
2. Scherrer, S.S.; Cesar, P.F.; Swain, M.V. Direct comparison of the bond strength results of the different test methods: A critical literature review. *Dent. Mater.* **2010**, *26*, e78–e93. [CrossRef] [PubMed]
3. Murray, P.E.; Stanley, H.R.; Matthews, J.B.; Sloan, A.J.; Smith, A.J. Age-related odontometric changes of human teeth. *Oral Surg. Oral Med. Oral Pathol. Oral Radiol. Endod.* **2002**, *93*, 474–482. [CrossRef] [PubMed]
4. Oliveira, G.C.; Oliveira, G.M.; Ritter, A.V.; Heymann, H.O.; Swift, E.J.; Yamauchi, M. Influence of tooth age and etching time on the microtensile bond strengths of adhesive systems to dentin. *J. Adhes. Dent.* **2012**, *14*, 229–234. [CrossRef] [PubMed]
5. De Munck, J.; Mine, A.; Poitevin, A.; Van Ende, A.; Cardoso, M.V.; Van Landuyt, K.L.; Peumans, M.; Van Meerbeek, B. Meta-analytical review of parameters involved in dentin bonding. *J. Dent. Res.* **2012**, *91*, 351–357. [CrossRef]
6. Salz, U.; Bock, T. Testing adhesion of direct restoratives to dental hard tissue—A review. *J. Adhes. Dent.* **2010**, *12*, 343–371. [CrossRef]
7. Sadek, F.T.; Monticelli, F.; Muench, A.; Ferrari, M.; Cardoso, P.E.C. A novel method to obtain microtensile specimens minimizing cut flaws. *J. Biomed. Mater. Res. Part. B Appl. Biomater.* **2006**, *78B*, 7–14. [CrossRef]
8. Armstrong, S.; Geraldeli, S.; Maia, R.; Raposo, L.H.; Soares, C.J.; Yamagawa, J. Adhesion to tooth structure: A critical review of "micro" bond strength test methods. *Dent. Mater.* **2010**, *26*, e50–e62. [CrossRef]
9. Armstrong, S.; Breschi, L.; Özcan, M.; Pfefferkorn, F.; Ferrari, M.; Van Meerbeek, B. Academy of Dental Materials guidance on in vitro testing of dental composite bonding effectiveness to dentin/enamel using micro-tensile bond strength (μTBS) approach. *Dent. Mater.* **2017**, *33*, 133–143. [CrossRef]
10. McDonough, W.G.; Antonucci, J.M.; He, J.; Shimada, Y.; Chiang, M.Y.M.; Schumacher, G.E.; Schultheisz, C.R. A microshear test to measure bond strengths of dentin–polymer interfaces. *Biomaterials* **2002**, *23*, 3603–3608. [CrossRef]
11. Beck, F.; Ilie, N. Antioxidants and Collagen-Crosslinking: Benefit on Bond Strength and Clinical Applicability. *Materials* **2020**, *13*, 5483. [CrossRef]
12. Versluis, A.; Tantbirojn, D.; Douglas, W.H. Why do Shear Bond Tests Pull Out Dentin? *J. Dent. Res.* **1997**, *76*, 1298–1307. [CrossRef] [PubMed]
13. Van Noort, R.; Noroozi, S.; Howard, I.C.; Cardew, G. A critique of bond strength measurements. *J. Dent.* **1989**, *17*, 61–67. [CrossRef] [PubMed]
14. Cho, B.H.; Dickens, S.H. Effects of the acetone content of single solution dentin bonding agents on the adhesive layer thickness and the microtensile bond strength. *Dent. Mater.* **2004**, *20*, 107–115. [CrossRef] [PubMed]
15. DeHoff, P.H.; Anusavice, K.J.; Wang, Z. Three-dimensional finite element analysis of the shear bond test. *Dent. Mater.* **1995**, *11*, 126–131. [CrossRef]
16. Roydhouse, R.H. Punch-Shear Test for Dental Purposes. *J. Dent. Res.* **1970**, *49*, 131–136. [CrossRef]
17. Feilzer, A.J.; De Gee, A.J.; Davidson, C.L. Setting Stress in Composite Resin in Relation to Configuration of the Restoration. *J. Dent. Res.* **1987**, *66*, 1636–1639. [CrossRef]
18. Frankenberger, R.; Krämer, N.; Oberschachtsiek, H.; Petschelt, A. Dentin bond strength and marginal adaption after NaOCl pre-treatment. *Oper. Dent.* **2000**, *25*, 40–45.
19. da cunha Mello, F.S.; Feilzer, A.J.; de Gee, A.J.; Davidson, C.L. Sealing ability of eight resin bonding systems in a Class II restoration after mechanical fatiguing. *Dent. Mater.* **1997**, *13*, 372–376. [CrossRef]
20. Kurtz, J.S.; Perdigão, J.; Geraldeli, S.; Hodges, J.S.; Bowles, W.R. Bond strengths of tooth-colored posts, effect of sealer, dentin adhesive, and root region. *Am. J. Dent.* **2003**, *16*, 31a–36a.
21. Marques de Melo, R.; Galhano, G.; Barbosa, S.H.; Valandro, L.F.; Pavanelli, C.A.; Bottino, M.A. Effect of adhesive system type and tooth region on the bond strength to dentin. *J. Adhes. Dent.* **2008**, *10*, 127–133. [PubMed]
22. Zicari, F.; Couthino, E.; De Munck, J.; Poitevin, A.; Scotti, R.; Naert, I.; Van Meerbeek, B. Bonding effectiveness and sealing ability of fiber-post bonding. *Dent. Mater.* **2008**, *24*, 967–977. [CrossRef] [PubMed]
23. Castellan, C.S.; Santos-Filho, P.C.; Soares, P.V.; Soares, C.J.; Cardoso, P.E. Measuring bond strength between fiber post and root dentin: A comparison of different tests. *J. Adhes. Dent.* **2010**, *12*, 477–485. [CrossRef] [PubMed]
24. Brichko, J.; Burrow, M.F.; Parashos, P. Design Variability of the Push-out Bond Test in Endodontic Research: A Systematic Review. *J. Endod.* **2018**, *44*, 1237–1245. [CrossRef]
25. Borges, B.C.; Souza-Junior, E.J.; da Costa Gde, F.; Pinheiro, I.V.; Sinhoreti, M.A.; Braz, R.; Montes, M.A. Effect of dentin pre-treatment with a casein phosphopeptide-amorphous calcium phosphate (CPP-ACP) paste on dentin bond strength in tridimensional cavities. *Acta Odontol. Scand.* **2013**, *71*, 271–277. [CrossRef]

26. *ISO 29022*; Dentistry—Adhesion—Notched-Edge Shear Bond Strength Test. International Organization for Standardization: Geneva, Switzerland, 2013.
27. Sudsangiam, S.; van Noort, R. Do dentin bond strength tests serve a useful purpose? *J. Adhes. Dent.* **1999**, *1*, 57–67.
28. Van Noort, R.; Cardew, G.E.; Howard, I.C.; Noroozi, S. The effect of local interfacial geometry on the measurement of the tensile bond strength to dentin. *J. Dent. Res.* **1991**, *70*, 889–893. [CrossRef]
29. Ilie, N.; Kunzelmann, K.H.; Hickel, R. Evaluation of micro-tensile bond strengths of composite materials in comparison to their polymerization shrinkage. *Dent. Mater.* **2006**, *22*, 593–601. [CrossRef]
30. Rizzante, F.A.P.; Duque, J.A.; Duarte, M.A.H.; Mondelli, R.F.L.; Mendonça, G.; Ishikiriama, S.K. Polymerization shrinkage, microhardness and depth of cure of bulk fill resin composites. *Dent. Mater. J.* **2019**, *38*, 403–410. [CrossRef]
31. Quinn, J.B.; Quinn, G.D. A practical and systematic review of Weibull statistics for reporting strengths of dental materials. *Dent. Mater.* **2010**, *26*, 135–147. [CrossRef]
32. Soares, C.J.; Santana, F.R.; Castro, C.G.; Santos-Filho, P.C.; Soares, P.V.; Qian, F.; Armstrong, S.R. Finite element analysis and bond strength of a glass post to intraradicular dentin: Comparison between microtensile and push-out tests. *Dent. Mater.* **2008**, *24*, 1405–1411. [CrossRef]
33. Goracci, C.; Tavares, A.U.; Fabianelli, A.; Monticelli, F.; Raffaelli, O.; Cardoso, P.C.; Tay, F.; Ferrari, M. The adhesion between fiber posts and root canal walls: Comparison between microtensile and push-out bond strength measurements. *Eur. J. Oral Sci.* **2004**, *112*, 353–361. [CrossRef]
34. Collares, F.M.; Portella, F.F.; Rodrigues, S.B.; Celeste, R.K.; Leitune, V.C.B.; Samuel, S.M.W. The influence of methodological variables on the push-out resistance to dislodgement of root filling materials: A meta-regression analysis. *Int. Endod. J.* **2016**, *49*, 836–849. [CrossRef] [PubMed]
35. Goracci, C.; Grandini, S.; Bossù, M.; Bertelli, E.; Ferrari, M. Laboratory assessment of the retentive potential of adhesive posts: A review. *J. Dent.* **2007**, *35*, 827–835. [CrossRef]
36. Rathke, A.; Frehse, H.; Muche, R.; Haller, B. Durability of fiber post-to-composite bonds achieved by physical vapor deposition and tribochemical silica coating. *J. Adhes. Dent.* **2014**, *16*, 559–565. [CrossRef]
37. Pane, E.S.; Palamara, J.E.; Messer, H.H. Critical evaluation of the push-out test for root canal filling materials. *J. Endod.* **2013**, *39*, 669–673. [CrossRef] [PubMed]
38. Nagas, E.; Uyanik, O.; Durmaz, V.; Cehreli, Z.C. Effect of plunger diameter on the push-out bond values of different root filling materials. *Int. Endod. J.* **2011**, *44*, 950–955. [CrossRef]
39. Linde, A.; Goldberg, M. Dentinogenesis. *Crit. Rev. Oral Biol. Med.* **1993**, *4*, 679–728. [CrossRef] [PubMed]
40. Asande Adebayo, O.; Francis Burrow, M.; John Tyas, M. Bonding of one-step and two-step self-etching primer adhesives to dentin with different tubule orientations. *Acta Odontol. Scand.* **2008**, *66*, 159–168. [CrossRef]

Disclaimer/Publisher's Note: The statements, opinions and data contained in all publications are solely those of the individual author(s) and contributor(s) and not of MDPI and/or the editor(s). MDPI and/or the editor(s) disclaim responsibility for any injury to people or property resulting from any ideas, methods, instructions or products referred to in the content.

MDPI AG
Grosspeteranlage 5
4052 Basel
Switzerland
Tel.: +41 61 683 77 34

Materials Editorial Office
E-mail: materials@mdpi.com
www.mdpi.com/journal/materials

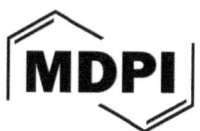

Disclaimer/Publisher's Note: The title and front matter of this reprint are at the discretion of the Guest Editors. The publisher is not responsible for their content or any associated concerns. The statements, opinions and data contained in all individual articles are solely those of the individual Editors and contributors and not of MDPI. MDPI disclaims responsibility for any injury to people or property resulting from any ideas, methods, instructions or products referred to in the content.

www.ingramcontent.com/pod-product-compliance
Lightning Source LLC
LaVergne TN
LVHW072345090526
838202LV00019B/2481